PHOSPHOLIPIDS IN THE NERVOUS SYSTEM

VOLUME 1: METABOLISM

Phospholipids in the Nervous System

Volume 1: Metabolism

Editors

Lloyd A. Horrocks, Ph.D.
Department of Physiological Chemistry
College of Medicine
The Ohio State University
Columbus, Ohio 43210

G. Brian Ansell, Ph.D., D.Sc.
Department of Pharmacology
University of Birmingham Medical School
Birmingham B15 2TJ, United Kingdom

Giuseppe Porcellati, M.D., Ph.D
Istituto di Biochimica
Universitá di Perugia Policlinico
06100 Perugia, Italy

Raven Press ■ New York

Raven Press, 1140 Avenue of the Americas, New York, New York 10036

Made in the United States of America

International Standard Book Number 0-89004-805-3
Library of Congress Catalog Number 81-40731

Preface

"Phospholipids are the centre, life, and chemical soul of all bioplasm whatsoever, that of plants as well as animals," according to Thudichum in the preface of his book published in 1884. Today we know that they account for about one-fourth of the dry weight of the human brain. They are important as the backbone of all cellular membranes. During the last several years it has become apparent that the metabolism of phospholipids is important in the functional activity of the nervous system. Many of these new developments are described in this book.

The products of methylation of ethanolamine glycerophospholipids include choline plasmalogens and phosphatidylcholine. Lipid methylation has biological roles in membrane fluidity and Ca^{2+} influx. Different enzymes for the exchange of ethanolamine, choline, and serine are distributed asymmetrically and in different membranes. The ethanolamine and choline phosphotransferases also have different locations in membranes, which may contribute to asymmetry of phospholipids in the membranes.

Turnover of polyunsaturated fatty acids in phospholipids involves deacylation–reacylation and *de novo* biosynthesis. The acyl-CoA synthetase and reacylation are localized in endoplasmic reticulum. Reacylation with arachidonate is greatest for phosphatidylcholine and phosphatidylinositol. The rate-limiting step, deacylation, is more active in neuronal perikarya than in astroglia. New HPLC methods are available for the separation of the molecular species of phospholipids. Ischemia and hypoxia cause a rapid release of fatty acids from phospholipids and an inhibition of reincorporation. Administration of cytidine nucleotides stimulates reincorporation and prevents the accumulation of free fatty acids.

Choline metabolism in phospholipids and acetylcholine, recycling, and outflow from brain is described. Carbamylcholine stimulates the synthesis of phosphatidylcholine, which may be involved in the regulation of GABAergic neurons. Phosphatidylserine affects cholinergic fibers by antagonizing some effects of scopolamine and increasing levels of acetylcholine in the caudate. A direct uptake of double-labeled phosphatidylserine into brain is reported.

New assay methods for sphingomyelinase are described. Plasmalogenase is localized in the plasma membrane of oligodendroglia, but is absent from myelin. Enzymes for synthesis of acidic phospholipids are transported in axons. Phospholipids are transported to nerve endings by axonal flow of smooth endoplasmic reticulum. Polar groups are turned over in nerve endings.

Phosphatidylinositol is hydrolyzed by a cytosolic calcium-dependent phospholipase C which is activated by phosphatidate and phosphatidylglycerol and inhibited by phosphatidylcholine. The distribution of this enzyme and the turnover of phosphatidylinositol in all membrane fractions in adrenal medulla suggest that Ca^{2+} gating is not regulated by phosphatidylinositol turnover. The effects of some pharmacological agents on the metabolism of inositol glycerophospholipids in iris muscle are described. An increased synthesis of phosphatidylinositol bisphosphate may be associated with reduced conduction velocity in sciatic nerve of diabetic rats. Cationic amphiphilic drugs such as propanolol inhibit phosphatidate phosphohydrolase and cause membranous cytoplasmic inclusions.

v

Michell has summed up with his reactions to several of the new concepts. Also included are abstracts of posters presented at a satellite symposium of the International Society for Neurochemistry that was held in Birmingham, England in September, 1981.

This volume is for all those interested in how the nervous system functions at a molecular level including reactions to injury and drugs. It will also appeal to all biochemists working with membranes and lipid metabolism.

Lloyd A. Horrocks
G. Brian Ansell
Giuseppe Porcellati

Acknowledgments

We offer our special appreciation to Francesco Della Valle and Cristina Schirato of Fidia Research Labs, Abano Terme, Italy for their support of the symposium. Members of the local organizing committee, J. N. Hawthorne, R. H. Michell, C. E. Rowe, and S. Spanner, and staff of the University of Birmingham, also contributed a great deal to the success of the symposium.

Contents

Abstracts

Contributors

A. A. Abdel-Latif
Department of Cell and Molecular Biology
Medical College of Georgia
Augusta, Georgia 30912

C.-D. Agardh
Laboratory of Experimental Brain Research
University Hospital
S-221 85 Lund, Sweden

B. W. Agranoff
Neuroscience Laboratory
Mental Health Research Institute;
and Department of Biological Chemistry
The University of Michigan
Ann Arbor, Michigan 48109

R. A. Akhtar
Department of Cell and Molecular Biology
Medical College of Georgia
Augusta, Georgia 30912

S. G. A. Alivisatos
Department of Physiology
University of Athens Medical School
Athens (609), Greece

C. Alling
Department of Psychiatry and Neurochemistry
University of Goteborg
Goteborg, Sweden

V. Andreoli
Biochemistry Department
The Medical School
University of Perugia
06100 Perugia, Italy

G. B. Ansell
Department of Pharmacology
University of Birmingham Medical School
Birmingham B15 2TJ, United Kingdom

F. Aporti
Department of Biochemistry
Fidia Research Laboratories
35031 Abano Terme, Italy

D. Aravantinos
Department of Physiology
University of Athens Medical School
Athens (609), Greece

J. Axelrod
Laboratory of Clinical Science
National Institutes of Health
Bethesda, Maryland 20205

M. I. Aveldaño de Caldironi
Department of Physiological Chemistry
Ohio State University
Columbus, Ohio 43210

N. Azila
Department of Biochemistry
University Hospital and Medical School
Nottingham NG7 2UH, United Kingdom

P. R. Bar
Institute of Molecular Biology
University of Utrecht
Utrecht, The Netherlands

A. Battistella
Department of Biochemistry
Fidia Research Laboratories
35031 Abano Terme, Italy

N. G. Bazán
LSU Eye Center
Louisiana State University Medical Center
School of Medicine
New Orleans, Louisiana 70112

M. E. Bell
Department of Biochemical and Biophysical
Sciences
University of Houston
Houston, Texas 77004

A. Benenson
Centre de Neurochimie du CNRS
67084 Strasbourg Cedex, France

L. Binaglia
Institute of Biological Chemistry
University of Perugia
06100 Perugia, Italy

W. D. Blaker
Biological Sciences Research Center and
Department of Biochemistry and Nutrition
University of North Carolina at Chapel Hill
Chapel Hill, North Carolina 27514

A. L. Bleyaert
Department of Anesthesiology and Critical Care
Medicine
University of Pittsburgh
Pittsburgh, Pennsylvania 15261

J. K. Blusztajn
Laboratory of Neuroendocrine Regulation
Department of Nutrition and Food Science
Massachusetts Institute of Technology
Cambridge, Massachusetts 02139

A. C. Bonetti
Department of Pharmacology
University of Florence
50134 Florence, Italy

R. Borsato
Department of Biochemistry
Fidia Research Laboratories
Abano Terme, Italy

K. Bradbury
Department of Pathology
University of Leeds
Leeds LS2 9JT, United Kingdom

P. Broom
School of Pharmacy
Portsmouth Polytechnic
Portsmouth, England

P. J. Brophy
Department of Biochemistry
University of Stirling
Stirling FK9 4LA, Scotland

M. Brunetti
Istituto di Chimica Biologica
Università di Perugia
06100 Perugia, Italy

G. Calderini
Fidia Research Laboratories
Department of Biochemistry
Abano Terme, Italy

J. W. Callahan
Departments of Pediatrics and Biochemistry
University of Toronto
Toronto, Ontario, Canada

A. Camacho
Department of Physiology
University of Florida School of Medicine
Gainesville, Florida 32610

B. Canguilhem
Institut de Physiologic
Faculté de Medecine de Strasbourg
Strasbourg, France

E. M. Carey
Department of Biochemistry
University of Sheffield
Sheffield S10 2TN, United Kingdom

A. Carruthers
Department of Biochemistry
University of Sheffield
Sheffield S10 2TN, United Kingdom

L. Corazzi
Institute of Biological Chemistry
The Medical School
University of Perugia
Perugia, Italy

F. T. Crews
Department of Pharmacology
University of Florida School of Medicine
Gainesville, Florida 32610

Z. Dabrowiecki
Department of Physiological Chemistry
Ohio State University
Columbus, Ohio 43210

F. Dainou
Centre de Neurochimie du CNRS
U44 de l'INSERM
67084 Strasbourg Cedex, France

D. J. Davidson
Departments of Pediatrics and Biochemistry
University of Toronto
Toronto, Ontario, Canada

R. M. C. Dawson
Biochemistry Department
ARC Institute of Animal Physiology
Babraham, Cambridge CB2 4AT, United
*   Kindgom*

H. Debuch
Institut für Physiologische Chemie
Lehrstuhl II
Universität zu Köln
D-5000 Köln 41 (Lindenthal)
Federal Republic of Germany

G. Deliconstantinos
Department of Physiology
University of Athens Medical School
Athens (609), Greece

G. E. DeMedio
Istituto di Chimica Biologica
University di Perugia
06100 Perugia, Italy

L. Di Giamberardino
Département de Biologie
CEN Saclay
91191 Gif-sur-Yvette Cedex, France

F. J. Doherty
Department of Biochemistry
University of Birmingham
Birmingham B15 2TT, United Kingdom

R. V. Dorman
Department of Physiological Chemistry
Ohio State University
Columbus, Ohio 43210

H. Dreyfus
Centre de Neurochimie du CNRS
U44 de l'INSERM
67084 Strasbourg Cedex, France

B. Droz
Département de Biologie
CEN Saclay
91191 Gif-sur-Yvette Cedex, France

L. Dubourg
Laboratoire de Biochimie Medicale A
Université de Bordeaux II
Bordeaux, France

A. D. Edgar
Centre de Neurochimie du CNRS
67084 Strasbourg Cedex, France

J. Eichberg
Department of Biochemical and Biophysical
  Sciences
University of Houston
Houston, Texas 77004

J. Engel
Department of Pharmacology
University of Goteborg
Goteborg, Sweden

S. K. Fisher
Neuroscience Laboratory
Mental Health Research Institute;
and Department of Biological Chemistry
The University of Michigan
Ann Arbor, Michigan 48109

C. Font
Medical Physiology Department A
The Panum Institute
Copenhagen University
Copenhagen, Denmark 2200

K. A. Foster
Department of Biochemistry
University of Nottingham Medical School
Queen's Medical Centre
Nottingham NG7 2UH, United Kingdom

E. Francescangeli
Biochemistry Department
The Medical School
University of Perugia
06100 Perugia, Italy

N. Freeman
Department of Biochemistry
University of Sheffield
Sheffield S10 2TN, United Kingdom

K. A. Frey
Neuroscience Laboratory
The University of Michigan
Ann Arbor, Michigan 48109

L. Freysz
Centre de Neurochimie du CNRS
67084 Strasbourg Cedex, France

H. Gainer
National Institute of Child Health and Human
  Development
National Institutes of Health
Bethesda, Maryland 20205

A. Gaiti
Department of Biochemistry
University of Perugia
Perugia, Italy

S. Gatt
Laboratory of Neurochemistry
Hebrew University—Hadassah Medical School
Jerusalem, Israel

U. Gerken
Laboratory for Nerve Tissue Culture
Institute for Physiological Chemistry
5300 Bonn, Federal Republic of Germany

M. Giesing
Laboratory for Nerve Tissue Culture
Institute for Physiological Chemistry
5300 Bonn, Federal Republic of Germany

C. Giordano
Università Cattolica del Sacro Cuore
Centro Radioisotopi
00135 Rome, Italy

W. H. Gispen
Institute of Molecular Biology
University of Utrecht
Utrecht, The Netherlands

N. M. Giusto
Istituto de Investigaciones Bioquimicas
UNS-CONICET
Bahia Blanca, Argentina

A. Gjedde
Medical Physiology Department A
The Panum Institute
Copenhagen University
Copenhagen, Denmark 2200

G. Goracci
Biochemistry Department
The Medical School
University of Perugia
06100 Perugia, Italy

R. M. Gould
Institute for Basic Research in Developmental
  Disabilities
Staten Island, New York 10314

N. C. C. Gray
Department of Biochemistry
Health Sciences Centre
University of Western Ontario
London, Ontario N6A 5C1, Canada

J. Gunawan
Institut für Physiologische Chemie
Lehrstuhl II
Universität zu Köln
D-5000 Köln 41 (Lindenthal)
Federal Republic of Germany

A. J. Hansen
Medical Physiology Department A
The Panum Institute
Copenhagen University
Copenhagen, Denmark 2200

H. W. Harder
Department of Physiological Chemistry
Ohio State University
Columbus, Ohio 43210

G. Hauser
Ralph Lowell Laboratories
Mailman Research Center
McLean Hospital
Belmont, Massachusetts 02178

J. N. Hawthorne
Department of Biochemistry
University Hospital and Medical School
Nottingham NG7 2UH, United Kingdom

K. Hirasawa
Biochemistry Department
ARC Institute of Animal Physiology
Babraham, Cambridge CB2 4AT, United
  Kingdom

F. Hirata
Laboratory of Clinical Science
National Institutes of Health
Bethesda, Maryland 20205

R. W. Holz
Department of Pharmacology
Medical School
University of Michigan
Ann Arbor, Michigan 48109

L. A. Horrocks
Department of Physiological Chemistry
Ohio State University
Columbus, Ohio 43210

M. G. Ilincheta de Boschero
Istituto de Investigaciones Bioquimicas
UNS-CONICET
Bahia Blanca, Argentina

H. K. Illig
Institut für Physiologische Chemie
Lehrstuhl II
Universität zu Köln
D-5000 Köln 41 (Lindenthal)
Federal Republic of Germany

R. F. Irvine
Biochemistry Department
ARC Institute of Animal Physiology
Barbraham, Cambridge CB2 4AT, United
  Kingdom

Y. Ishima
Laboratory of Neurophysiology
Tomobe Hospital Medical Centre
Tomobe, Nishiibaragigun
Ibaragi, Japan

J. Jolles
Institute of Molecular Biology
University of Utrecht
Utrecht, The Netherlands

C. S. Jones
Departments of Pediatrics and Biochemistry
University of Toronto
Toronto, Ontario, Canada

F. B. Jungalwala
Department of Biochemistry
E. K. Shriver Center
Waltham, Massachusetts 02254

K. Kaibuchi
Department of Biochemistry
Kobe University School of Medicine
Kobe 650, Japan

J. N. Kanfer
Department of Biochemistry
Faculty of Medicine, University of Manitoba
Winnipeg, Manitoba, Canada R3E OW3

U. Kikkawa
Department of Biochemistry
Kobe University School of Medicine
Kobe 650, Japan

H. L. Koenig
Département de Biologie
CEN Saclay
91191 Gif-sur-Yvette Cedex, France

F. LeBaron
Department of Biochemistry
University of New Mexico
Albuquerque, New Mexico 87131

S. Liljequist
Department of Pharmacology
University of Goteborg
Goteborg, Sweden

J. C. Louis
Centre de Neurochimie du CNRS
U44 de l'INSERM
67084 Strasbourg Cedex, France

N. Louros
Department of Physiology
University of Athens Medical School
Athens (609), Greece

P. Mandel
Centre de Neurochimie du CNRS
67084 Strasbourg Cedex, France

P. Mantovani
Department of Biochemistry
Fidia Research Laboratories
35031 Abano Terme, Italy

R. Massarelli
Centre de Neurochimie du CNRS
U44 de l'INSERM
67084 Strasbourg Cedex, France

P. Massari
Università Cattolica del Sacro Cuore
Centro Radioisotopi
00135 Rome, Italy

Y. Masuzawa
Teikyo University
Sagamiko
Tsukuigun, Kanagawa

T. Matsubara
Department of Biochemistry
Kobe University School of Medicine
Kobe 650, Japan

S. Mazzari
Department of Biochemistry
Fidia Research Laboratories
35031 Abano Terme, Italy

A. McGivney
Laboratory of Microbiology and Immunology
National Institutes of Health
Bethesda, Maryland 20205

R. C. McKenzie
Department of Biochemistry
University of Stirling
Stirling FK9 4LA, Scotland

M. Mersel
Centre de Neurochimie du CNRS
67084 Strasbourg Cedex, France

D. M. Michaelson
Department of Biochemistry
Tel-Aviv University
Ramat Aviv, Israel

R. H. Michell
Department of Biochemistry
University of Birmingham
Birmingham B15 2TT, United Kingdom

R. Minakuchi
Department of Biochemistry
Kobe University School of Medicine
Kobe 650, Japan

D. Montaudon
Laboratoire de Biochimie Medicale A
University de Bordeaux II
Bordeaux, France

P. Morell
Biological Sciences Research Center and
Department of Biochemistry and Nutrition
University of North Carolina at Chapel Hill
Chapel Hill, North Carolina 27514

R. Mozzi
Centre de Neurochimie du CNRS
U44 de l'INSERM
67084 Strasbourg Cedex, France

R. Mozzi
Biochemistry Department
The Medical School
University of Perugia
06100 Perugia, Italy

P. P. N. Murthy
Neuroscience Laboratory
University of Michigan
Ann Arbor, Michigan 48109

J. P. Nemmer
Department of Anesthesiology and Critical Care
Medicine
University of Pittsburgh
Pittsburgh, Pennsylvania 15261

E. M. Nemoto
Department of Anesthesiology and Critical Care
Medicine
University of Pittsburgh
Pittsburgh, Pennsylvania 15261

Y. Nishizuka
Department of Biochemistry
Kobe University School of Medicine
Kobe 650, Japan

P. Orlando
Università Cattolica del Sacro Cuore
Centro Radioisotopi
00135 Rome, Italy

H. Pant
National Institute on Alcohol Abuse and
Alcoholism
Rockville, Maryland 20852

A. S. Pappu
Veterans Administration Hospital
La Jolla, California 92161

P. Van Paridon
Biochemical Laboratory
Rijksuniversiteit Utrecht
Padualaan 8
Utrecht 25606, Netherlands

M. F. Pediconi
INIBIBB
UNS-CONICET
8000 Bahia Blanca, Argentina

R. Pellkofer
Institut für Organische Chemie und Biochemie
de Universitat Bonn
Gerhard-Domagk-Str. 1
D-5300 Bonn 1, Federal Republic of Germany

G. Pepeu
Department of Pharmacology
Florence University
50134 Florence, Italy

R. G. Peterson
Department of Anatomy
Indiana University School of Medicine
Indianapolis, Indiana 46223

I. Phillips
Department of Physiology
University of Florida School of Medicine
Gainesville, Florida 32610

I. Pinchasi
Department of Biochemistry
Tel-Aviv University
Ramat Aviv, Israel

G. Porcellati
Institute of Biological Chemistry
University of Perugia
06100 Perugia, Italy

A. Raz
Department of Biochemistry
Tel-Aviv University
Ramat Aviv, Israel

S. Rehncrona
Laboratory of Experimental Brain Research
E-Blocket
University Hospital
S-221 85 Lund, Sweden

J. Robert
Laboratoire de Biochimie Medicale A
Université de Bordeaux II
Bordeaux, France

E. B. Rodriguez de Turco
INIBIBB
UNS-CONICET
8000 Bahia Blanca, Argentina

R. Roberti
Institute of Biological Chemistry
University of Perugia
06100 Perugia, Italy

A. D. Roses
Duke University Medical Center
Durham, North Carolina 27710

C. E. Rowe
Department of Biochemistry
University of Birmingham
Birmingham B15 2TT, United Kingdom

K. Sandhoff
Institut für Organische Chemis und Biochemie
der Universitat Bonn
Gerhard-Domagk-Str. 1
D-5300 Bonn 1, Federal Republic of Germany

K. Sano
Department of Biochemistry
Kobe University School of Medicine
Kobe 650, Japan

S. Sanyal
Department of Biochemistry
E. K. Shriver Center
Waltham, Massachusetts 02254

L. H. Schrama
Institute of Molecular Biology
State University of Utrecht
Utrecht, The Netherlands

M. Schwartzman
Department of Biochemistry
Tel-Aviv University
Ramat Aviv, Israel

P. Shankaran
Departments of Pediatrics and Biochemistry
University of Toronto
Toronto, Ontario, Canada

G. K. Shiu
Department of Anesthesiology and Critical Care
   Medicine
University of Pittsburgh
Pittsburgh, Pennsylvania 15261

D. Siepi
Biochemistry Department
The Medical School
University of Perugia
06100 Perugia, Italy

B. K. Siesjo
Laboratory of Experimental Brain Research
E-Blocket
University Hospital
S-221 85 Lund, Sweden

H. Singh
Experimental and Clinical Medical Research
   Centre
Polish Academy of Sciences
Dworkowa 3
00-784 Warsaw, Poland

E. Siemkowicz
Medical Physiology Department A
The Panum Institute
Copenhagen University
Copenhagen, Denmark 2200

R. Siraganian
Laboratory of Microbiology and Immunology
National Institutes of Health
Bethesda, Maryland 20205

P. J. Somerharju
Biochemical Laboratory
Rijksuniversiteit Utrecht
Padualaan 8
Utrecht 2506, Netherlands

S. Spanner
Department of Pharmacology
University of Birmingham Medical School
Birmingham B15 2TJ, United Kingdom

K. P. Strickland
Department of Biochemistry
Health Sciences Centre
University of Western Ontario
London, Ontario N6A 5C1, Canada

J. Strosznajder
Experimental and Clinical Medical Research
   Centre
Polish Academy of Sciences
Dworkowa 3
00-784 Warsaw, Poland

G. Y. Sun
Sinclair Comparative Medicine Research Farm
   and Biochemistry Department
University of Missouri
Columbia, Missouri 65201

Y. Takai
Department of Biochemistry
Kobe University School of Medicine
Kobe 650, Japan

A. D. Toews
Biological Sciences Research Center and
   Department of Biochemistry and Nutrition
University of North Carolina at Chapel Hill
Chapel Hill, North Carolina 27514

G. Theodosiadis
Department of Physiology
University of Athens Medical School
Athens (609), Greece

E. C. Tjeenk Willink
Department of Pharmacology
University of Florida School of Medicine
Gainesville, Florida 32610

G. Toffano
Department of Biochemistry
Fidia Research Laboratories
35031 Abano Terme, Italy

G. Trovarelli
Istituto di Chimica Biologica
Universita di Perugia
06100 Perugia, Italy

M. Tytell
Department of Anatomy
Bowman Gray School of Medicine
Wake Forest University
Winston-Salem, North Carolina 27103

J. M. Vance
Duke University Medical Center
Durham, North Carolina 27710

M. Vanrollins
Department of Physiological Chemistry
Ohio State University
Columbus, Ohio 43210

A. Vecchini
Institute of Biological Chemistry
The Medical School
University of Perugia
Perugia, Italy

G. C. Velley
Psychophysiological Laboratory
French University
75006 Paris, France

G. Vincendon
Centre de Neurochimie du CNRS
67084 Strasbourg Cedex, France

K. Waku
Teikyo University
Sagamiko
Tsukuigun, Kanagawa

A. Weir
School of Pharmacy
Portsmouth Polytechnic
Portsmouth, England

E. Westerberg
Laboratory of Experimental Brain Research
E-Blocket
University Hospital
S-221 85 Lund, Sweden

G. L. White
School of Pharmacy
Portsmouth Polytechnic
Portsmouth, England

T. Wieloch
Laboratory of Experimental Brain Research
E-Blocket
University Hospital
S-221 85 Lund, Sweden

K. W. A. Wirtz
Biochemical Laboratory
Rijksuniversiteit Utrecht
Padualaan 8
Utrecht 2506, Netherlands

B. Witter
Institut für Physiologische Chemie
Lehrstuhl II
Universität zu Köln
D-5000 Köln 41 (Lindenthal)
Federal Republic of Germany

H. Woelk
Department of Psychiatry
Neurochemistry Unit
University of Giessen
Giessen, Federal Republic of Germany

R. J. Wurtman
Laboratory of Neuroendocrine Regulation
Department of Nutrition and Food Science
Massachusetts Institute of Technology
Cambridge, Massachusetts 02139

L. H. Yamaoka
Duke University Medical Center
Durham, North Carolina 27710

B. Yu
Department of Biochemistry
Kobe University School of Medicine
Kobe 650, Japan

A. Zanotti
Department of Biochemistry
Fidia Research Laboratories
Abano Terme, Italy

S. H. Zeisel
Laboratory of Neuroendocrine Regulation
Department of Nutrition and Food Science
Massachusetts Institute of Technology
Cambridge, Massachusetts 02139

Phospholipids in the Nervous System, Vol. 1: Metabolism, edited by L. Horrocks, et al. Raven Press, New York © 1982.

Phospholipid Synthesis by Interconversion Reactions in Brain Tissue

R. Mozzi, G. Goracci, D. Siepi, E. Francescangeli, V. Andreoli, *L. A. Horrocks, and G. Porcellati

*Biochemistry Department, The Medical School, University of Perugia, 06100 Perugia, Italy; *Department of Physiological Chemistry, The Ohio State University, Columbus, Ohio 43210*

Phospholipids are continuously renewed in brain and, concurrently with their de novo synthesis, several reactions which change only some components of the molecule take place in the cell, leading to the interconversion of a molecule into another, generally with a lower requirement of energy. These reactions are connected with the turnover and rearrangement of membrane phospholipids and contribute to the compositional maintenance of the membrane and consequently to its functional integrity.

There is no doubt, in fact, that different tissues and subcellular components possess a typical phospholipid composition and that most membrane functions require a certain physical state of the membrane itself. For instance, enzymic reactions and transport are influenced by the fluidity of the membrane, which in turn depends on several factors, including fatty acid composition.

The interconversion reactions are responsible for the turnover of different portions of the phospholipid molecule, and, at least in some cases, this conversion occurs where the new molecule is required.

Base-exchange and methylation of phosphatidylethanolamine to phosphatidylcholine produce changes at the level of the polar head groups leading to the interconversion of phospholipid classes. Another possibility of interconversion is represented by the reversibility of choline and ethanolamine phosphotransferase activities, which has been recently demonstrated in brain (13). Diglycerides, formed by the reversal of these enzymic activities from membrane-bound phospholipid and CMP can be reutilized, together with the CDP-bases, for the synthesis of new phospholipid molecules. This chapter will first deal with methylation reactions and then with reversal of phosphotransferases.

INTERCONVERSION BY N-METHYLATION

Phosphatidyl choline can be formed by the methylation of phosphatidylethanolamine. Phosphatidyl-N-monomethylethanolamine and phosphatidyl-N,N-dimethylethanolamine represent the intermediates of the pathway and

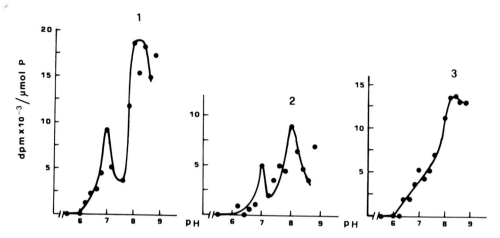

Fig. 1. The effect of pH on the incorporation of methyl groups into brain microsomal phosphatidylcholine (1), phosphatidyl-N,N-dimethylethanolamine (2) and phosphatidyl-N-monomethylethanolamine (3). Brain microsomes (0.2-0.3 mg protein) were incubated for 20 min at 37°C in a medium (final volume of 80 μl) containing 2.66 μM S-adenosyl-L-[methyl-^{3}H]methionine (15 Ci/mmol) and 60 mM succinate-NaOH (pH 5.0-5.5) or cacodylate (5.0-7.0) or phosphate (6.0-7.8) or Tris-HCl (7.2-8.8) buffers. Samples were treated with 80 μl cold TCA and the precipitates, washed three times, were extracted with chloroform-methanol (2:1, v/v) and filtered and washed. Extracts, dried under nitrogen, were resuspended in chloroform-methanol (2:1, v/v) and chromatographed (21). Authentic phosphatidyl-N-monomethylethanolamine and phosphatidyl-N,N-dimethylethanolamine standards were chromatographed with the samples. Synthesized compounds were identified by cochromatography with standards. Data taken from reference 23.

S-adenosylmethionine (SAM) is the methyl donor. The mechanism is an example of a direct conversion. Although three successive methylations are required, phosphatidyl-N-monomethylethanolamine and phosphatidyl-N,N-dimethylethanolamine are in fact still phospholipid molecules.

This methylation was first demonstrated in liver by Bremer and Greenberg (4). In 1979, Mozzi and Porcellati (22) and Blusztajn and Wurtman (2) have independently reported its occurrence in brain, and a similar finding was also made by Crews et al. (5).

By incubating rat brain cortex homogenate with labelled SAM, Mozzi and Porcellati have demonstrated an incorporation of methyl groups into phosphatidylcholine (22). The incorporation is greatly enhanced by the addition of phosphatidyl-N,N-dimethylethanolamine to the incubation medium (22). In 1980, Mozzi et al. (23) have further reported that brain cortex microsomes are responsible for synthesizing phosphatidylcholine by the same pathway. The pH dependence for methyl group incorporation into phosphatidyl-N-monomethylethanolamine, phosphatidyl-N,N-dimethylethanolamine and phosphatidylcholine is shown in Fig. 1.

The first methyl group transfer possesses an optimum pH value around 8.2, whereas the incorporation of the successive methyl groups presents another peak around pH 7.0.

These results, together with others (2,22,23), indicate that two enzymes are involved for methyl group incorporation in brain, as reported for adrenal medulla by Hirata et al. (17). Incubation of microsomes at pH values higher than 8.8 indicates the presence of another peak of maximal incorporation, although the instability of the SAM molecule at these pH values affects the reproducibility of the results.

The data here reported refer to cerebral microsomes from 28-30 day-old-rats. The age affects noticeably the activity of the methylation pathway (23).

The heterogeneity of brain and the different distribution of SAM in rat brain areas (31) may indicate a specific localization of this pathway related to particular cell functions. To verify this hypothesis, Mozzi et al. (25) have examined the methylation pathway in different brain areas as shown in Fig. 2.

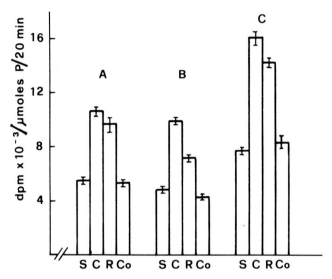

Fig. 2. The incorporation of methyl groups into phosphatidyl-N-monomethylethanolamine (A), phosphatidyl-N,N-dimethylethanolamine (B), and phosphatidylcholine (C) of homogenates from different brain areas of the rat. Brain areas from 5 to 6 rats (28-30 days old) were prepared as described in the text. Homogenates (0.4-0.6 mg protein) were incubated in a medium (final volume of 80 µl) containing 60 mM Tris-HCl buffer (pH 8.2) and 1.4 µM S-adenosyl-L-[methyl-^{3}H]methionine (specific activity of 62 Ci/mmol). The incubation was carried out for 20 min at 37°C and the reaction was stopped as reported in Fig. 1. Results are the mean with S.E.M. from three experiments. S=striatum; C=cerebellum; R=the rest; Co=cortex.

More precisely, rat brains from 28-30 day-old-animals have been divided into three well-defined parts: the cortex, the cerebellum and the striatum. The remainder, taken as a fourth portion, was called "the rest". The homogenates were incubated at pH 8.2 with labelled SAM and the incorporation into phosphatidyl-N-monomethylethanolamine, phosphatidyl-N,N-dimethylethanolamine and phosphatidylcholine was measured. Fig. 2 shows that brain cortex and striatum possess a lower methyltransferase activity than cerebellum and the rest of brain, either into phosphatidylcholine or into partially methylated forms. These results may indicate an involvement of the enzymic mechanisms in particular physiological processes. In this connection, Crews et al. (5) have reported that brain synaptosomes can synthesize phosphatidylcholine by the methylation pathway and it is possible that its activity in particular brain areas is due to a different distribution into cell types.

Recently, Mozzi et al. (26) have confirmed some preliminary results about the synthesis of choline plasmalogen by the methylation pathway (23,24). Fig. 3 shows the incorporation of methyl groups into phosphatidylcholine and into choline plasmalogen in the rat brain homogenate. Choline plasmalogen incorporates methyl groups from SAM with a linear time-activity relationship, although the degree of incorporation is lower than into phosphatidylcholine. The addition of ethanolamine plasmalogen increases the rate of incorporation of methyl groups into choline plasmalogen (Table 1), depending on the amount of ethanolamine plasmalogen added to the incubation mixture. A small decrease is observed for the incorporation into phosphatidylcholine.

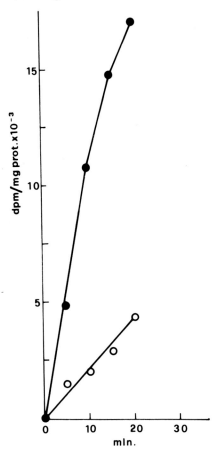

Fig. 3. Incorporation of methyl groups from SAM into phosphatidylcholine (black circles) and choline plasmalogen (white circles). Whole homogenates from brain were incubated in a final volume of 80 μl containing 1.8 μM S-adenosyl-L-[methyl-^{3}H]methionine (specific activity of 68 Ci/mmol) and 60 mM Tris-HCl buffer (pH 8.2). After incubation for various time intervals, lipids were extracted (15) and chromatographed according to Horrocks and Sun (18) to separate choline plasmalogen from phosphatidylcholine. Identity of compounds synthesized was carried out by co-chromatography with authentic standards (11).

Table 1.   The effect of the addition of beef heart ethanolamine
           plasmalogen on the incorporation of labelled
           methyl groups into choline lipids[d]

Ethanolamine plasmalogen added (μmol)	Incorporation ratios	
	A	B
0.054	1.15	0.88
0.100	1.30	0.86
0.143	1.58	0.82
0.160	1.67	0.82

[a]Incubation was carried out as described in Fig. 3. Different amounts of ethanolamine plasmalogen were added to the incubation medium by sonicating for 15 min at 37°C under a continuous nitrogen stream using a 100 W MK-2 ultrasonic disintegrator (MSE, England). Ethanolamine plasmalogen was prepared and purified, as described elsewhere (26). Data represent the ratios between the incorporation in brain homogenate obtained in the presence of added ethanolamine plasmalogen and in its absence. A= incorporation into plasmalogen; B=incorporation into phosphatidylcholine.

Table 2.   The incorporation of methyl groups into phosphatidylcholine,
           "methylated" ethanolamine plasmalogens and choline plasmalogen
           of rat brain homogenates[d]

Phosphatidylcholine	"Methylated"ethanolamine plasmalogens	Choline plasmalogen
11,407	10,543	7,744
10,021	8,206	8,543
8,726*	6,176*	1,414*
10,089*	6,834*	1,082*
13,000	10,010	3,313
17,020	7,045	4,358

[a]Whole rat brain homogenates were incubated as described in Fig. 3. The data, expressed as dpm/mg of protein/20 min, are the results of single experiments. In the experiments indicated with * rats weighing less than normal were used. "Methylated" ethanolamine plasmalogens refer to the mono- and di-methylated forms of plasmalogen.

    Table 2 indicates that the degree of incorporation of methyl groups into choline plasmalogen varies much more than that into phosphatidylcholine and "methylated" ethanolamine plasmalogens. For "methylated" ethanolamine plasmalogens we indicate the mono- and di- methylated forms of plasmalogen itself. The rate of synthesis of choline plasmalogen might depend on the nutritional state and health of the animals, as indicated by the very low incorporation rate observed in two cases when 28 day-old-animals, weighing less than normal, were used (Table 2).
    Experiments with brain microsomes (26) have demonstrated that this fraction also is able to synthesize choline plasmalogen from ethanolamine plasmalogen by the methylation pathway. The degree of incorporation is lower than into phosphatidylcholine (Fig. 4), and the addition of ethanol-

amine plasmalogen increases the rate of methyl group transfer only after 10-20 min of incubation, indicating that the physical state of exogenous substrate is possibly involved in this effect.

The stepwise methylation could be connected in brain with the synthesis of acetylcholine (23,32), since it may provide a mechanism for the formation of choline from ethanolamine. Furthermore, the conversion of phosphatidylethanolamine to phosphatidylcholine is related to changes in membrane fluidity (16) and produces molecular species enriched in polyunsaturated fatty acids (29).

The possibility that the phosphatidylethanolamine pool, synthesized in brain microsomes by the base-exchange reaction (11,12), could be utilized for methylation to phosphatidylcholine has been examined (Mozzi and Porcellati, unpublished results). It is known that the base-exchange reaction produces phosphatidylethanolamine enriched in polyunsaturated fatty acids (6). In this connection, Fig. 5 shows the synthesis of phosphatidylcholine from phosphatidylethanolamine which was synthesized by the base-exchange reaction. More precisely, the particles were first incubated for 20 min at 37°C in the presence of labelled ethanolamine and 2 mM Ca^{2+} to allow a typical base-exchange reaction for phosphatidylethanolamine synthesis to take place (11,12). Cold SAM was then added to the preincubated microsomes, and the methyl group transfer reactions were followed for additional time intervals (Fig. 5). Phosphatidylethanolamine continues to be synthesized, since labelled ethanolamine and Ca^{2+} were not removed.

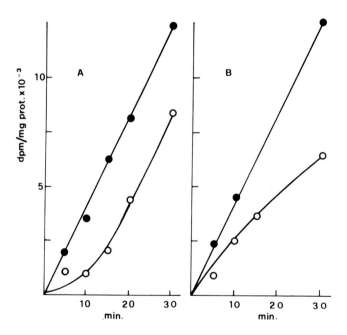

Fig. 4. Incorporation of methyl groups from SAM into phosphatidylcholine (black circles) and choline plasmalogen (white circles). Brain cortex microsomes from 28-30 day-old-rats were prepared in a 0.32 M sucrose-2 mM dithioerythritol (DTE) solution and resuspended in the same medium. Microsomes (1.0-1.5 mg of protein) were incubated and lipids were extracted and analyzed as described in Fig. 3. In A, 74 nmol of ethanolamine plasmalogen were added to the incubation medium, as described in Table 1.

It is very interesting that synthesis of phosphatidyl-N-monomethyl-ethanolamine takes place after SAM addition, indicating that the labelled phosphatidylethanolamine coming from the base-exchange reaction is a substrate for methylation to phosphatidyl-N-monomethyl- ethanolamine. This last lipid is feebly synthesized in the absence of added SAM, utilizing only the small endogenous SAM content of the microsomes. Radioactivity of phosphatidyl-N,N-dimethylethanolamine and phosphatidylcholine, once form-ed, drops to lower values; this indicates a rapid degradation, particular-ly of phosphatidylcholine and phospholipids synthesized by the methylation pathway from this particular phosphatidylethanolamine pool. This degrada-tion might be important for the release of choline (see also ref. 3), and possibly for involvement with acetylcholine production.

More work is needed to clarify the relationships of choline release, acetylcholine production, the stepwise methylation pathway and base-exchange reactions.

INTERCONVERSION BY THE REVERSAL OF CHOLINE AND ETHANOLAMINE PHOSPHOTRANSFERASES

There is no doubt that diacylglycerols play an important role in phospholipid metabolism since they are converted into choline and ethanol-amine phospholipids by cholinephosphotransferase and ethanolaminephospho-transferase, respectively. Despite this fact, noticeable differences in

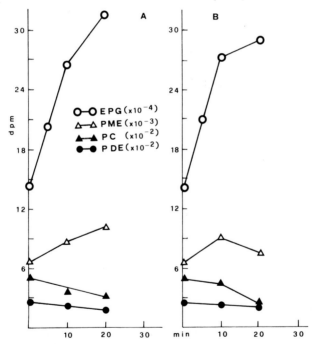

Fig. 5. Methylation of microsomal ethanolamine phosphoglycerides after a base-exchange reaction in brain microsomes. Rat brain microsomes (4.46 mg of protein) were preincubated in a final volume of 805 µl with hepes buffer (60 mM, pH 8.0), 1.98 mM Ca^{2+}, and 1.7 mM [^{14}C]ethanolamine (specific activity 44 mCi/mmol) for 20 min at 37°C. An aliquot of the incubation medium was immediately extracted after pre- incubation (15) to obtain a zero time incubation value. Other aliquots (0.56 mg protein) were incubated for additional time intervals (see figure) with (A) 50 µM cold SAM and with no addition (8). Extraction and analysis of lipids was performed as reported previously (22).

the composition of the molecular species of diacylglycerols and choline and ethanolamine phosphoglycerides have been observed in brain (27), thus indicating that rearrangements of phospholipid molecules occur after de novo synthesis. This is particularly true for choline phosphoglycerides since a rather low specificity of cholinephosphotransferase for different molecular species has been reported (28).

The interconversion of different molecular species of the same phospholipid class can be achieved by the acylation-reacylation cycle (19). On the other hand, it is also possible to utilize diacylglycerols produced from other phosphoglycerides with a different pattern of molecular species. Phosphoinositides can be cleaved by a specific phospholipase C (20) which yields diglycerides.

Recently, the reversibility of the reactions catalyzed by ethanolamine and choline phosphotransferases has been reported to occur in brain (13). The reversal of these reactions utilizes microsomal choline or ethanolamine phosphoglycerides which produce CDP-choline or CDP-ethanolamine, respectively, and diglycerides by reacting with CMP. It is very likely that both nucleotides and diglycerides are reutilized for synthesizing new phospholipid molecules. This mechanism for interconversion of choline phosphoglycerides to ethanolamine phosphoglycerides and vice versa is depicted in Fig. 6. Its importance in the liver has been reported by Sundler et al. (30) who found that 1/4 of diacyl glycerols available for the synthesis of phosphatidylethanolamine originate from phosphatidylcholine by the back reaction.

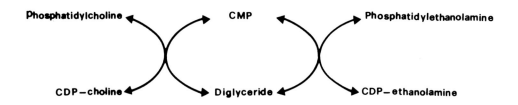

Fig. 6. Interconversion of choline and ethanolamine phosphoglycerides by the back-reaction of phosphotransferases.

In the brain we have carried out experiments to study the utilization of diacylglycerols produced by back-reaction for synthesis of other phospholipid molecules. This study is also connected with the problem of the synthesis of choline plasmalogen. As mentioned above, the biosynthetic pathway of this lipid is largely unknown. The methylation pathway described above or the base-exchange reaction (10) might contribute importantly to their biosynthesis, but do not account for the high rate of turnover of the polar portion of the molecule which was observed after injection of labelled phosphate (8) and choline (7) into the brain. These two studies, in addition, have been performed on cells obtained from cerebral cortex where methyltransferases seem to be less active (25).

The high turnover rate of the polar portion of the choline plasmalogen molecule is consistent with the hypothesis that the lipid acceptor, namely alkenylacylglycerol, is available to the cholinephosphotransferase. Alkenylacylglycerol, however, has not yet been found in brain tissue.

Table 3. The effect of CMP "preincubation" on the synthesis of choline and ethanolamine phosphoglycerides[a]

Lipid subclass	"Preincubated" control microsomes	"Preincubated" microsomes	P
Alkenylacyl-GPE	0.141 ± 0.034 (6)	0.248 ± 0.020 (6)	<0.01
Diacyl-GPE	0.478 ± 0.081 (6)	1.045 ± 0.144 (6)	<0.005
Alkylacyl-GPE	0.122 ± 0.037 (6)	0.405 ± 0.042 (4)	<0.0025
Alkenylacyl-GPC	0.086 ± 0.016 (6)	0.166 ± 0.016 (5)	<0.005
Diacyl-GPC	0.553 ± 0.153 (6)	1.446 ± 0.220 (5)	<0.005
Alkylacyl-GPC	0.024 ± 0.006 (6)	0.083 ± 0.009 (5)	<0.0005

[a]Brain microsomes were prepared as reported previously (14) in the presence of 2 mM EDTA which was subsequently removed. Preincubation conditions were 60 mM Tris-HCl buffer (pH 8.0), 20 mM $MgCl_2$, 0.08 mM DTE, 4 mM CMP (when required), and 2.5 mg microsomal protein/ml. Final volume: 3 ml. Temperature: 37°C. Time: 15 min. Preincubation was stopped by diluting with 0.32 M sucrose. Preincubated microsomes were recovered by centrifugation (105,000 x g for 45 min). Control microsomes were preincubated without CMP addition. Incubation conditions were the same as preincubation, except that 1 mM CDP-[^{14}C-1,2]choline (specific radioactivity of 1.01 nCi/nmol) or 1 mM CDP-[^{14}C-1,2]ethanolamine (specific radioactivity of 1.55 nCi/nmol) was present and 1.5 mg of microsomal protein was used. Final volume: 0.3 ml. Lipid was extracted by the Folch procedure, and analyzed as described by Horrocks and Sun (18). Results are expressed as nmol/mg protein/15 min ± S.E.M. Number of experiments in parentheses.

Our preliminary experiments have been carried out by incubating rat brain microsomes with CMP, thus producing diglycerides which accumulate in the membrane, particularly in the presence of a diglyceride lipase inhibitor such as DFP (diisopropyl fluorophosphate) (14). Diglyceride-enriched microsomes have then been reincubated with labelled CDP-choline or CDP-ethanolamine. The results (Table 3) show that the CMP-treated microsomes react with CDP-ethanolamine and CDP-choline to a greater extent than control microsomes which were preincubated without CMP. An activation of phosphotransferase due to CMP can be ruled out since this nucleotide is known to inhibit the incorporation of CDP-bases into phosphoglycerides as reported by Freysz et al. (9). It is very likely therefore that diglycerides released by back-reaction can be re-utilized for the synthesis of new phospholipid molecules.

Interestingly, CDP-ethanolamine is a better precursor for alkylacyl-GPE and alkenylacyl-GPE than CDP-choline is for the corresponding choline phospholipids. On the contrary, the rate of synthesis of diacyl-GPC is higher than that of diacyl-GPE. This is true both in the control and in the CMP-treated microsomes.

The enhancement of choline plasmalogen synthesis, due to CMP treatment, supports the hypothesis that alkenylacylglycerols may also be formed by the back-reaction. At the moment, we are unable to establish if they really originate from ethanolamine plasmalogen. However, the extent of the increase of the labelling of choline plasmalogen, due to CMP preincubation, is not consistent with an origination of alkenylacylglycerols from choline phosphoglycerides only.

Other experiments have been performed by carrying out the preincubation in a medium containing 3 mM DFP. As shown in Table 4, the presence of DFP greatly enhances the incorporation of CDP-bases into the corresponding glycerophospholipids as compared to CMP-treated microsomes incubated without DFP.

Table 4. The effect of DFP on the synthesis of choline and ethanolamine phosphoglycerides.

Lipid subclass	"Preincubated" control microsomes		"Preincubated" microsomes	
	- DFP	+ DFP	- DFP	+ DFP
Alkenylacyl-GPE	0.110	0.073	0.229	0.299
Diacyl-GPE	0.372	0.260	0.995	1.741
Alkylacyl-GPE	0.064	-	0.335	0.489
Alkenylacyl-GPC	0.101	0.123	0.197	0.494
Diacyl-GPC	0.380	0.301	1.018	2.400
Alkylacyl-GPC	0.013	0.027	0.100	0.210

[a]Preparation, preincubation and incubation conditions are described in Table 3 except 3 mM DFP was added in the preincubation medium when required. Results are expressed as in Table 3. Data represent the mean from two experiments.

The comparison with control microsomes (Table 4) indicates that the observed increase is due to an enlargement of the diglyceride pool since we have observed that DFP alone does not affect the phosphotransferase activities. Furthermore, since alkylacylglycerols and alkenylacylglycerols seem to accumulate better in the presence of DFP, one might assume that the brain microsomal diglyceride lipase, like the platelet enzyme (1), does not possess a specificity for position 1.

In conclusion, diglycerides formed by the back-reaction can be cleaved in the brain by diglyceride lipase but they can also be reutilized for the synthesis of new phospholipid molecules, possibly leading to interconversion. This is particularly important for the synthesis of choline plasmalogen. We have provided evidence with the present contribution that alkenylacylglycerols may originate from ethanolamine plasmalogens and then be converted into choline plasmalogen.

ACKNOWLEDGEMENT

This work was supported by a grant from the Consiglio Nazionale delle Ricerche, Rome (contract No. 80.00543.04/115). The technical assistance of Mr. Antonio Boila is gratefully acknowledged.

REFERENCES

1. Bell, R.L., Kennerly, D.A., Stanford, N., and Majerus, P.W. (1979): Proc. Natl. Acad. Sci. USA, 76:3238-3241.
2. Blusztajn, J.K., Zeisel, S.H., and Wurtman, R.J. (1979): Brain Res., 179:319-327.
3. Blusztajn J.K. and Wurtman, R.J. (1981): Nature, 290:417-418.

4. Bremer, J. and Greenberg, D. (1961): Biochim. Biophys. Acta, 46:205-216.
5. Crews, F.T., Hirata, F., and Axelrod, J. (1980): J. Neurochem., 34: 1491-1498.
6. De Medio, G.E., Woelk, H., Gaiti, A., Porcellati, G., and Fratini, F. (1975) Ital. J. Biochem., 24:335-350.
7. Francescangeli, E., Goracci, G., Piccinin, G.L., Mozzi, R., Woelk, H., and Porcellati, G. (1977): J. Neurochem., 28:171-176.
8. Freysz, L., Bieth, R., and Mandel, P. (1969): J. Neurochem., 16:1417-1424.
9. Freysz, L., Horrocks, L.A., and Mandel, P. (1978): In: Enzymes of Lipid Metabolism, edited by S. Gatt, L. Freysz, and P. Mandel, pp. 253-268, Plenum Press, New York.
10. Gaiti, A., Goracci, G., DeMedio, G.E., and Porcellati, G. (1972): FEBS Letters, 27:116-121.
11. Gaiti, A., Brunetti, M., and Porcellati, G. (1975): FEBS Letters, 49:361-364.
12. Gaiti, A., Brunetti, M., Woelk, H., and Porcellati, G. (1976): Lipids, 11:823-830.
13. Goracci, G., Horrocks, L.A., and Porcellati, G. (1977): FEBS Letters, 80:41-44.
14. Goracci, G., Francescangeli, E., Horrocks, L.A., and Porcellati, G. (1981): Biochim. Biophys. Acta, 664:373-379.
15. Hara, A. and Radin, N.S. (1978): Anal. Biochem., 90:420-426.
16. Hirata, F. and Axelrod, J. (1978): Proc. Natl. Acad. Sci. USA, 75: 2348-2352.
17. Hirata, F., Viveros, O.H., Diliberto, E.J., and Axelrod, J. (1978) Proc. Natl. Acad. Sci. USA, 75:1718-1721.
18. Horrocks, L.A. and Sun, G.Y. (1972): In: Research Methods in Neurochemistry, edited by N. Marks and R. Rodnight, pp. 223-231, Plenum Press, New York.
19. Lands, W.E.M. (1960): J. Biol. Chem., 235:2233-2237.
20. Lapetina, E.G. and Michell, R.M. (1973): Biochem.J., 131:433-442.
21. Katyal, S.L. and Lombardi, B. (1974): Lipids, 9:81-85.
22. Mozzi, R. and Porcellati, G. (1979): FEBS Letters, 100:363-366.
23. Mozzi, R., Andreoli, V., and Porcellati, G. (1980): In: Natural Sulfur Compounds, edited by D. Cavallini, G.E. Gaull, and V. Zappia, pp. 41-54, Plenum Press, New York.
24. Mozzi, R., Siepi, D., Andreoli, V., and Porcellati, G. (1981): Ital. J. Biochem., 30:311-312.
25. Mozzi, R., Siepi, D., Andreoli, V., Piccinin, G.L., and Porcellati, G. (1981): Bull. Mol. Biol. Med., 6:6-15.
26. Mozzi, R., Siepi, D., Andreoli, V., and Porcellati, G. (1981): FEBS Letters, 131:115-118.
27. Porcellati, G. and Binaglia, L. (1976): In: Lipids, edited by R. Paoletti, G. Jacini, and G. Porcellati, Vol. I, pp. 75-88, Raven Press, New York.
28. Roberti, R., Binaglia, L., and Porcellati, G. (1980): J. Lipid Res., 21:449-454.
29. Skurdal D.N. and Cornatzer, W.E. (1975): Intern. J. Biochem., 6: 579-583.
30. Sundler, R., Akesson, B., and Nilsson, A. (1974): Biochim. Biophys. Acta, 337:248-254.
31. Yu, P.H. (1978): Anal. Biochem., 86:498-504.

32. Zeisel, S.H., Blusztajn, J.K., and Wurtman, R.J. (1979): In: Nutrition and the Brain, edited by A. Barbeau and R.J. Wurtman, pp. 47-55, Raven Press, New York.

Phospholipids in the Nervous System, Vol. 1:
Metabolism, edited by L. Horrocks, et al. Raven
Press, New York © 1982.

The Base Exchange Enzymes and Phospholipase D of Rat Brain Microsomes

J. N. Kanfer

Department of Biochemistry, Faculty of Medicine, University of Manitoba, Winnipeg,
Manitoba, Canada R3E 0W3

Early studies on the biosynthesis of phospholipids by liver particulates revealed an active incorporation of radioactive L-serine (7) and choline (5) into phospholipid. In both instances there was no requirement for an energy source, an alkaline pH optimum and a Ca^{+2} requirement. The investigators suggested that a reversal of phospholipase D activity was an attractive explanation for these observations, however this possibility was considered unlikely due to the failure to detect this hydrolytic enzyme in mammalian tissues. This postulate implied that phospholipase D in addition to possessing hydrolytic activity was responsible for catalyzing the incorporation of L-serine, choline and ethanolamine into their corresponding phospholipid. This misconception about the base exchange reactions continued for the next one and a half decades. The reactions being considered are:

Base Exchange

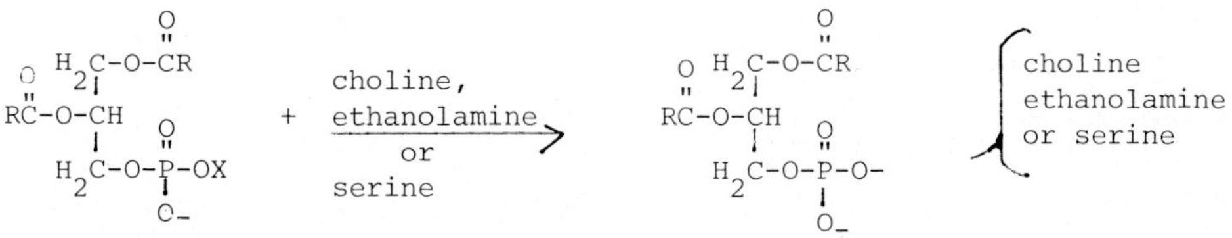

Phospholipase D

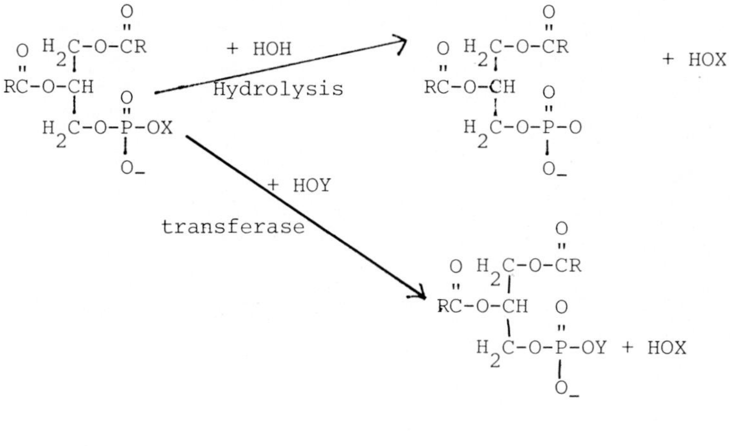

Evidence obtained in this laboratory will be summarized demonstrating that there are at least 3 separate proteins responsible for separately catalyzing these incorporations of each base and a phospholipase D which does not possess base exchange activity. This information has been obtained both with partially purified enzyme preparation and with their membrane-bound forms. A suggestion that more than one enzyme was involved in the base exchange reaction based upon the kinetics and differential Ca^{+2} concentration was made by another active group (6).

SEPARATION OF THE SOLUBILIZED ENZYMES

A major contribution which ultimately led to the separations of these enzymes was the successful solubilization of all 4 activities from rat brain microsomes with the detergent Miranol H2M (12). Early suggestive evidence for the existence of at least 2 separate base exchange enzymes was obtained by differential rates of heat inactivation of the choline incorporatiing enzyme as compared to the serine and ethanolamine activity (11). This indication that separate enzymes were responsible for the 3 base exchange activities prompted an effort at purification.

A protocol utilizing a combination of gel exclusion, ammonium sulfate fractionation and ion exchange chromatography resulted in the physical separation of the 3 activities for the incorporation of ethanolamine, choline and serine without overlap or cross contamination by the other activities as shown in Fig. 1 (9).

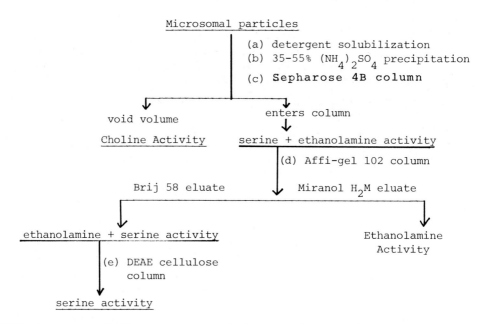

FIG. 1. Protocol for separation of the L-serine, choline and ethanolamine base exchange enzymes.

THE L-SERINE BASE EXCHANGE ENZYME

The L-serine base exchange enzyme is believed to be the sole route for phosphatidylserine biosynthesis in mammals (15) and therefore we embarked upon its further purification. A 37 fold purification was achieved from a starting microsomal suspension. The preparation was devoid of ethanolamine and choline incorporating activity and the presences of these 2 bases did not affect the enzyme's ability to convert serine to phosphatidylserine. Phosphatidylethanolamine was the most effective phospholipid acceptor as shown in Fig. 2.

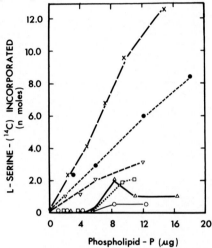

FIG. 2. Effect of varying the acceptor phospholipid using the standard incubation system. X---X, Phosphatidylethanolamine (egg yolk),□--·□, phosphatidic acid;△———△,phosphatidylcholine;▽---▽, phosphatidylserine; 0——-0, phosphatidylinositol; ●---●, asolectin.

The Km values were 0.4 mM for L-serine, 0.25 mM for ethanolamine plasmalogen, and for pig liver phosphatidylethanolamine and for egg yolk phosphatidylethanolamine was 0.67 mM. There was no detectable phospholipase D activity (13). The reaction is simply:

$$\text{Phosphatidylethanolamine} + \text{L-Serine} \xrightarrow{\text{Ca}^{+2}} \text{Phosphatidylserine} + \text{ethanolamine}$$

and not merely a reversal of phospholipase D.

PHOSPHOLIPASE D

The phospholipase D activity solubilized from microsomes by detergent was purified approximately 270 fold and has an apparent molecular weight of 200,000. The purified enzyme cleaved both phosphatidylcholine and phosphatidylethanolamine as substrates with Km values of 0.75 and 0.91 mM respectively. The highly purified enzyme was devoid of any detectable base exchange activity at all pH values from 5 to 8 (Fig.3) (14).

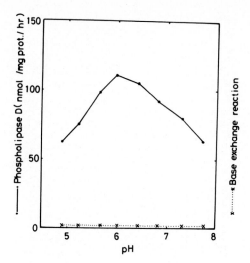

Fig. 3. The effect of varying pH on phospholipase D activity. ββ'-Dimethylglutarate buffer for the pH range of 4.9 to 5.6 and Hepes buffer for the pH range of 6.0 to 7.7 were employed. The assay method was the same as described in Fig. 1 except that various buffers were used.

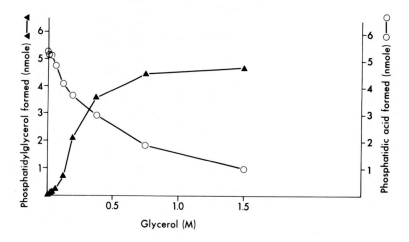

Fig. 4. The effect of glycerol concentration on the formation of phosphatidylglycerol and phosphatidic acid from radioactive lecithin.

Although this phospholipase D does not possess base exchange enzyme activities it does have the capacity to carry out a transphosphatidylation reaction as shown in Fig. 4. Using radioactive lecithin it is apparent that there is a reciprocal relationship between phosphatidylglycerol and phosphatidic acid as glycerol concentration is increased. However, at any given glycerol concentration the total amount of lecithin consumed is constant.

(3). This transphosphatidylation reaction can be form-
ulated as:

Phosphatidylcholine + glycerol $\longrightarrow$ phosphatidylglycerol + choline

The evidence obtained from the solubilized or partially purified
enzymes are consistent with the concept that there are at least 3
separate and specific base exchange enzymes, and at least 1
phospholipase D. It also seems apparent that phospholipase D is
devoid of base exchange activity and that the L-serine base exchange
enzyme is devoid of phospholipase D. Therefore, the original hypothesis
that base exchange activity is merely a reversal of phospholipase D
is invalid and must be discarded.

MICROSOMAL BOUND ACTIVITIES

Early observations on the particulate enzymes revealed that there
were differences in pH optimum, degree of inhibition by structural
analogs and detergents, response to phospholipase treatment, and
differential stability on storage and dialysis (8), as well as heat
stability (11) suggesting that separate enzymes were responsible for
each base exchange activity.

The asymmetric distribution of enzymes (4) and lipid (10) in
biological membranes is a current dogma. An assessment of the topographical distribution of the base exchange enzymes was undertaken.
Trypsin treatment of rat brain microsomes caused a destruction of the
choline base exchange enzyme activity with retention of both the serine
and ethanolamine activities (Table I). In the presence of detergent
all three activities were destroyed (1).

TABLE 1. Base exchange activities in trypsin-treated, intact, and
control rat brain microsomes[a]

Base	Asolectin[c]	Microsomes		
		Intact	Control	Trypsin-treated
Choline	−	4628	2760	440
	+	N.D.[b]	2808	176
Ethanolamine	−	7872	4996	4740
	+	N.D.[b]	3804	4004
Serine	−	15668	6216	5608
	+	21968	13984	14176

[a] cpm incorporated/h by ~150 μg protein in a reaction mixture with
1 μCi per 71 nmol of choline chloride, 0.6 μCi per 150 nmol ethanolamine hydrochloride, and 1 μCi per 20.1 nmol serine.

[b] N.D., not determined.

[c] 30 μg Asolectin microdispersion added where indicated (+).

Since the choline activity is affected preferentially it appears that it is on the cytoplasmic surface and the serine and ethanolamine activities are within the lumen of the microsomal vesicles.

A similar approach was employed to determine the location of phospholipase D of these membranes with both trypsin and pronase. PCMPS is a small molecular weight charged molecule which does not enter the lumen of microsomes and is therefore an adjunct to proteolytic digestion. There is a 20-40% loss of phospholipase D activity with intact particles depending upon the reagent employed. Treatment of detergent disrupted particles results in a 60 to 90% distruction of the activity (Table 2).

TABLE 2.   Effect of proteases and PCMPS on microsomal phospholipase D activity

Microsomes

	Treatment			
	Control	Trypsin	Pronase	PCMPS (600 µM)
Intact	100α	76	61	82
Disrupted	101	48	31	9

α Activities are expressed as a percentage of intact microsomes which had a specific activity of 55 $nmol \cdot mg^{-1} \cdot hr^{-1}$. Microsomes were disrupted by the addition of 0.05% deoxycholate.

These results suggest that phospholipase D is either present on both surfaces of the microsomes or is a transmembrane protein (Chalifour, R. and Kanfer, J.N., unpublished observation).

The effect of varying the temperature of the incubations showed that maximal base exchange activity occurred at 45°C with a transition temperature of 31° calculated from Arrhenius plots (2.). The optimum temperature for phospholipase D activity is 30°C (Fig. 5) with a transition temperature of 16°C (Fig. 6). These values are distinctly different from those obtained for the base exchange enzymes.

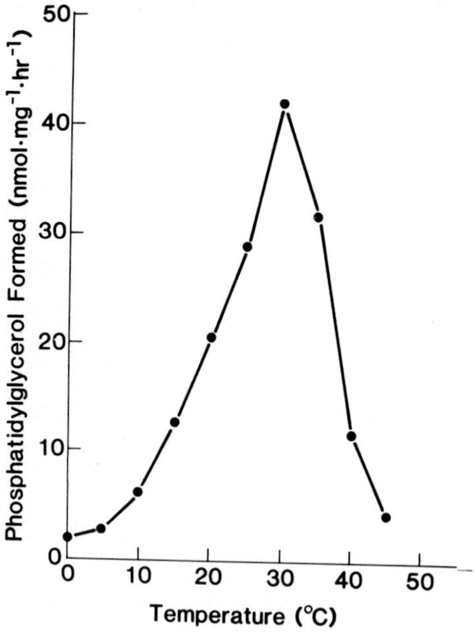

Fig. 5. The effect of incubation temperature on phospholipase D activity of rat brain microsomes.

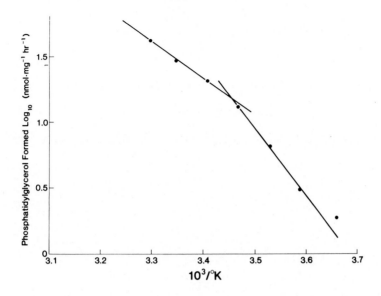

FIG. 6. Arrhenius plot of phospholipase D of rat brain microsomes.

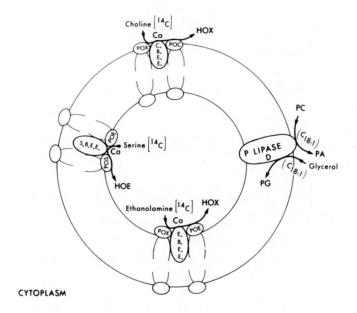

FIG. 7. Topographic localization of the base exchange enzymes and phospholipase D of rat brain microsomes.

The calculated activation energies above and below the transition temperature were different for each of the three base exchange enzymes as were the Kms determined at 27, 37 and 45°C.

These observations suggest that in microsomes, the 3 base exchange enzymes and phospholipase D are in topographically different areas but they also appear to reside in different lipid environments. A model attempting to incorporate these observations is shown in Fig. 7.

ACKNOWLEDGEMENT

This work was supported by grants from the Medical Research Council of Canada and the N.I.H. (NS-16973A)

REFERENCES

1. Buchanan, A.G. and Kanfer, J.N. (1980): <u>J. Neurochem.</u>,34:720.

2. Buchanan, A.G. and Kanfer, J.N. (1980): <u>J. Neurochem.</u>,35:814.

3. Chalifour, R.J., Taki, T. and Kanfer, J.N. (1980): <u>Can. J. Biochem.</u>, 58:1189.

4. De Pierre, J.W. and Ernster (1977): <u>L. Ann. Rev. Biochem.</u>,46:201.

5. Dils, C.R. & Hubscher, G. (1961): <u>Biochim. Biophys. Acta</u>,46:505-513.

6. Gaiti, A., De Medio, G.E., Brunetti, M., Amaducci, L. and Porcellati, G. (1974): <u>J. Neurochem.</u>,23:1153.

7. Hubscher, G., Dils, R.R. and Pover, W.F.R. (1959): <u>Biochim. Biophys. Acta</u>, 36:518-528.

8. Kanfer, J.N. (1972): <u>J. Lipid Res.</u>,13:468.

9. Miura, T. and Kanfer, J.N. (1976):<u>Arch.Biochem. Biophys.</u>,175:654.

10. Op den Kamp, J.A.F. (1979): <u>Ann. Rev. Biochem.</u>,48:47.

11. Saito, M., Bourque, E. And Kanfer, J.N. (1975): <u>Arch. Biochem. Biophys.</u>,169:304.

12. Saito, M. and Kanfer, J.N. (1973): <u>Biochem. Biophys. Res. Commun.</u>, 53:391.

13. Taki, T. and Kanfer, J.N. (1978): <u>Biochim. Biophys. Acta</u>,528:309.

14. Taki, T. and Kanfer, J.N. (1979): <u>J. Biol. Chem.</u>, 254:9761.

15. White A., Handler, P., Smith, E.L., Hill, R.L., and Lehman, I.R. (1978): <u>Principles of Biochemistry</u> p.610. 6th Ed. McGraw Hill.

Phospholipids in the Nervous System, Vol. 1: Metabolism, edited by L. Horrocks, et al. Raven Press, New York © 1982.

Effects of Membrane Fluidity on Mast Cell and Nerve Cell Function

F. T. Crews, *A. Camacho, *Ian Phillips, E. C. Tjeenk Willink, **Gabriella Calderini, †Fusao Hirata, †Julius Axelrod, ‡Anne McGivney, and ‡Reuben Siraganian

*Department of Pharmacology and *Physiology, University of Florida School of Medicine, Gainesville, Florida 32610; **Department of Biochemistry, Fidia Research Laboratories, Abano Terme, Italy; †Laboratory of Clinical Science and ‡Laboratory of Microbiology and Immunology, National Institutes of Health, Bethesda, Maryland 20205*

The secretion of hormones and neurotransmitters as well as receptor mediated signal transduction are processes involving membranes. The initial secretory event involves a stimulus which causes a change in membrane permeability and/or other factors which lead to an increase in the intraneuronal calcium concentration. The increase in intraneuronal calcium concentration activates exocytosis, i.e. a mechanism where the membrane of the transmitter containing granule fuses with the neuronal plasma membrane releasing the granule contents extracellularly. This change in membrane permeability, which is necessary for secretion, is dependent on a change in membrane properties.

Once hormones or neurotransmitters are released they carry out their specific functions by interacting with nerves or other target tissues. The initial event is the recognition of the hormone or transmitter by a receptor macromolecule on the outer surface of the cell membrane. The binding of the transmitter to its receptor then triggers a series of complex chemical and physical reactions in the membrane which permits the cell to carry out its specific function. Each of these reactions, i.e. receptor binding and coupling to ion channels and/or enzymes is dependent on a suitable membrane environment. Thus, the metabolism of lipids as well as the lipid composition of the membrane plays an important role in the transduction of neurotransmitter, hormone and other signals through the cell membrane.

MEMBRANE ASYMMETRY AND STRUCTURE

Phospholipids are the major lipids in plasma membranes and along with cholesterol and glycolipids represent approximately 50% of the total membrane mass with proteins making up the remaining 50%. The major phospholipids in synaptosomal membranes are phosphatidylcholine and phosphatidylethanolamine with phosphatidylserine and phosphatidyl-inositol being present in smaller amounts (83). These phospholipids form a bilayer which provides a fluid matrix for protein organization and movement (70). The arrangement of phospholipids in many plasma membranes have been found to be highly asymmetric. Studies of rat erythrocytes have found that most of the phosphatidylcholine and sphingomyelin are on the outside of the membrane surface and that phosphatidylethanolamine, phosphatidylserine and phosphatidylinositol are confined primarily to the inner surface of the plasma membrane (12,37,84).

Synaptosomal plasma membrane studies have also suggested an asymmetric distribution of phospholipids (35). Membrane asymmetry has also been found in the phospholipids of platelets (18) and influenza virion (79) suggesting that the asymmetric distribution of phospholipids may be a general phenomenon.

In addition to being asymmetrically distributed across the membrane, it is likely that membrane lipids are not uniformly distributed within a given layer. It is well known from experiments in model lipid systems that aqueous dispersions of phospholipids with differing transition temperatures contain both fluid and crystalline domains (55,13). Furthermore, the presence of lipid-protein interactions (48) and cholesterol (30,54) can cause the separation of distinct phases within the bilayer. Although it is difficult to measure changes in the various membrane domains, it is highly probable that changes in the properties and composition of certain membrane regions have marked effects on cell function.

MEMBRANE FLUIDITY

According to the now generally accepted fluid-mosaic model of membrane structure (70), integral membrane proteins have hydrophobic ends embedded in the lipid matrix of the membrane which is at least in some parts fluid. The fluid properties of the lipid matrix has been suggested to play an important role in membrane transport (23), enzyme activity (61), and other cell functions including receptor binding and stimulation (66). Many membrane bound enzymes and receptors have several subunits which interact within the membrane. Changes in the viscosity of the membrane can markedly enhance or depress activity by affecting the rotation, diffusion and association of various subunits. For example, the β-adrenergic-receptor-adenylate cyclase complex includes the β-adrenergic receptor, which binds the transmitter, a guanyl nucleotide regulatory subunit and the catalytic adenylate cyclase subunit (57,17). The β-adrenergic receptor, which is exposed on the outside of the membrane, and the catalytic cyclase, which produces cyclic AMP at the inner surface of the membrane are mobile and float in the membrane (46,77). Activation of adenylate cyclase requires the simultaneous binding of hormone to receptor and intracellular GTP to the guanyl nucleotide subunit (57). By fluidizing turkey erythrocyte membranes using cis-vaccenic acid it has been shown that the rate of β-receptor-cyclase activation is enhanced with increases in membrane fluidity (66). In addition the fluidity of the membrane affects the maximal activity of adenylate cyclase directly. Thus, the rate of subunit diffusion, rotation and collision as well as the maximal activity of enzymes is directly effected by the fluid properties of the lipid matrix in the membrane.

PHOSPHOLIPID METHYLATION AND MEMBRANE FLUIDITY

Recent studies on enzymes altering membrane fluidity have centered on two methyltransferase enzymes that methylate phosphatidylethanolamine to form phosphatidylcholine. Although the methylation pathway is a minor pathway for the synthesis of phosphatidylcholine, evidence suggests that it is involved in both secretion and receptor mediated membrane signal transduction. The two phospholipid methyltransferases have only recently been found to be present in rat brain and have their highest specific activity in the synaptosomal plasma membrane (62) (24). The first enzyme, phospholipid methyltransferase I (PMT I), methylates phosphatidylethanolamine one time to form phosphatidyl-N-monomethylethanolamine. PMT I has an optimum pH of 7.5 and a low apparent K_m for S-adenosyl-L-methionine (SAM) the methyl donor. The second enzyme, phospholipid methyltransferase II (PMT II), catalyzes two successive methylations of phosphatidyl-N-monomethylethanolamine to form phosphatidylcholine. PMT II has an optimum pH of 10.5, a high apparent K_m for S-adenosyl-L-methionine, and can be differentially solubilized by sonication. These observations suggest that the synaptosomal fraction of rat brain contains at least two methyltransferases which catalyze the synthesis of phosphatidylcholine. Blusztajn et al. (9) have demonstrated the formation of phosphatidylcholine by the methylation pathway in calf caudate nucleus. In addition, this group has demonstrated the in vitro formation of free choline from phosphatidylcholine synthesized through the methylation pathway (10). Since these enzymes have been shown to affect transmitter-receptor stimulation in erythrocytes (74), astrocytoma cells (73), and many other cell types (42), it seems likely they are involved in synaptic transmission.

Evidence for the asymmetric localization of phospholipid methyltransferases in synaptosome membranes has been obtained by selective proteolytic digestion using trypsin in intact and lysed synaptosomes (26). Trypsin treatment caused a small reduction, about 13%, in PMT I activity in intact synaptosomes, while in lysed synaptosomes it destroyed 83% of the activity. This suggests PMT I mainly faces the cytoplasmic side of the plasma membrane where trypsin cannot penetrate. Trypsin treatment reduced PMT II activity by 57% in intact synaptosomes, and by 95% in lysed synaptosomes (Fig. 1). The loss of PMT II in intact synaptosomes after trypsin treatment represents the fraction of the enzyme localized on the exterior side of the plasma membrane and indicates that PMT II is mainly present on the outer surface of the membrane. The additional loss of PMT II activity in lysed preparations probably represents PMT II present on vesicles, mitochondria and other intrasynaptosomal particles. These results suggest the asymmetric distribution of the two methyltransferases in the synaptosomal plasma membrane; PMT I, which methylates phosphatidylethanolamine to phosphatidyl-N-monomethylethanolamine, is mainly exposed on the cytoplasmic side, and PMT II, which catalyzes the two successive methylations of phosphatidyl-N-monomethylethanolamine to form phosphatidylcholine, faces the exterior side of the membrane.

Similar experiments using phospholipase C suggested that in intact synaptosomes phosphatidyl-N-monomethylethanolamine is buried within the membrane or located on the cytoplasmic side, whereas phosphatidylcholine and phosphatidyl-N,N-dimethylethanolamine are exposed to the outer surface of the membrane (26). The phospholipid methyltransferase

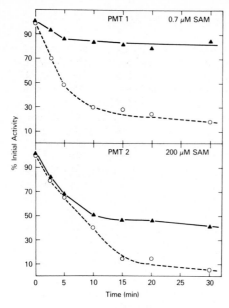

Fig. 1   Effects of trypsin treatment on lysed and intact synaptosomes. Synaptosomes (20 mg of protein) were incubated with trypsin, 1 mg/ml, for various periods of time. At various times, the reaction was stopped with buffer containing 5 mg/ml pancreatic trypsin inhibitor with 2% nonident and assayed for phospholipid methyltransferase I (PMT I) or phospholipid methyltransferase (PMT II) activity as described in Crews et al., (26).
(▲——▲) Intact synaptosomes, (O--O) lysed synaptosomes.

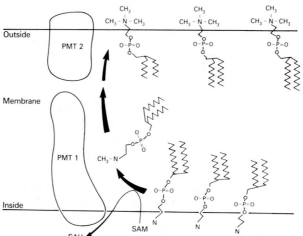

Fig. 2   Schematic diagram of methylation and translocation of phospholipids in synaptosomal membranes. SAM is S-adenosyl-L-
methionine, SAH is S-adenosyl-L-homocysteine.

enzymes have also been found to be asymmetrically distributed in liver microsomal membranes (38) and in rat erythrocyte ghosts (39). These data suggest the stepwise methylation and translocation of a fraction of the methylated phospholipids from the cytoplasmic side to the outside of the membrane (Fig. 2).

The methylation and rapid vectorial rearrangement of phospholipids has been shown to affect membrane fluidity. Using varying concentrations of SAM, it was observed in rat erythrocyte ghosts that the membrane viscosity, as measured by fluorescent polarization, using diphenylhexatriene, decreased in parallel with the synthesis of phosphatidyl-N-monomethylethanolamine (40). Other studies on chicken erythrocytes have found that concanavalin A will increase phospholipid methylation and simultaneously decrease membrane viscosity (64). This study used the electron spin resonance spectra of a stearic acid spin label to estimate membrane viscosity and found that methylation inhibitors could block the concanavalin A induced change in fluidity. These studies suggest that the methylation of phosphatidylethanolamine and the rapid translocation of the methylated phospholipid has an important influence on membrane fluidity.

PHOSPHOLIPID METHYLATION, CA^{2+} FLUX AND EXOCYTOSIS

Mast cells and basophils have been used to study the cellular mechanisms involved in secretion (32,51). The normal stimulus for mast cell secretion is the reaction of a specific antigen with antibodies, i.e. immunoglobulin E (IgE), which are bound to the cell surface. Mast cells exposed to antigen accumulate $^{45}Ca^{2+}$. Furthermore, antigen stimulated $^{45}Ca^{2+}$ accumulation occurs even when the secretory response is inhibited by the cells being deprived of energy (36); thereby supporting the hypothesis that calcium influx is an early event in the secretory response. The mechanism of calcium influx is particularly important since many endogenous regulators of release are thought to act by inhibiting the initial influx of calcium.

The relationship between phospholipid methylation and histamine release was first studied using rat mast cells. Concanavalin A, a lectin which binds membrane glycoproteins (71), was initially used to stimulate the secretion of histamine. Stimulating rat mast cells with concanavalin A resulted in a rapid increase in methylated phospholipids which was followed by the release of histamine (41). After about 3 minutes, there was a fall in the methylated phospholipids suggesting further metabolism of these lipids. More recent studies on phospholipid methylation have used antibodies raised against IgE receptors on rat basophilic leukemia cells (anti-rat basophilic leukemia). It is known that $F(ab')_2$ fragments of anti-rat basophilic leukemia cause an influx of $^{45}Ca^{2+}$ and release histamine by bridging IgE receptors. $F(ab')_2$ fragments of anti-rat basophilic leukemia also induce a rapid increase in phospholipid methylation which precedes $^{45}Ca^{2+}$ influx and histamine release (45). Monovalent Fab' fragments failed to increase phospholipid methylation, induce $^{45}Ca^{2+}$ uptake and release histamine. These findings suggest bridging of IgE receptors is necessary to initiate phospholipid methylation, $^{45}Ca^{2+}$ influx and histamine release.

Changes in phospholipid methylation have also been found during histamine secretion by rat basophilic leukemia cells. Rat basophilic leukemia cells can be readily grown in tissue culture, have IgE receptors and contain histamine, serotonin and other bioactive agents that are found in rat mast cells. There are several rat basophilic leukemia sublines in which the IgE-mediated secretion of histamine is qualitatively similar to secretion from rat mast cells and human basophils (5). Antigen stimulation of rat basophilic leukemia cells results in an initial increase in phospholipid methylation which is followed by a decline in the methylated phospholipids (25), similar to that found in rat mast cells. The increase in phospholipid methylation precedes the release of histamine, and parallels the influx of $^{45}Ca^{2+}$, whereas the decline in the methylated phospholipids closely corresponds in time with the release of histamine and the release of arachidonic acid. The decline in methylated phospholipids has been implicated in the release of arachidonic acid (27).

The relationship between phospholipid methylation, secretion of histamine and arachidonic acid release was further established using the methylation inhibitor 3-deazaadenosine (3-DZA). 3-DZA inhibited phospholipid methylation and histamine release in an almost identical concentration dependent manner whereas other methylations were only slightly affected. 3-DZA also blocked the release of $[^{14}C]$-arachidonic acid from prelabelled cells (25). More recent studies on RBL cells have shown that antigen stimulation of IgE sensitized cells results in an influx of $^{45}Ca^{2+}$ which precedes both histamine and arachidonic acid release. When methylation was inhibited with 3-DZA the influx of $^{45}Ca^{2+}$ was also inhibited (Fig. 3) (27). These findings are consistent with the hypothesis that the initial increase in phospholipid methylation alters membrane viscosity allowing the opening of the Ca^{2+} channel.

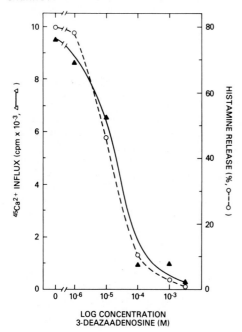

LOG CONCENTRATION
3-DEAZAADENOSINE (M)

Fig. 3   Effects of various concentrations of 3-deazaadenosine and homocysteine thiolac tone on $^{45}Ca^{2+}$ flux and histamine release. Rat basophilic leukemic cells (2 x 10^6 cells/well) sensitized with ovalbumin specific IgE were preincubated with various concentrations of 3-DZA and 2 x 10^{-4} M homocysteine thiolactone for 90 min. Cells were challenged with 10 µg/ml ovalbumin for 30 min as described in Crews et al., (27).

Additional evidence for the critical role of phospholipid methylation in Ca^{2+} influx and histamine release was obtained with mutant rat basophilic leukemic cells (59). Two variant clones of rat basophilic leukemic cells were found which in response to antigen did not release histamine and had no calcium influx (Table 1). However, stimulation with the calcium ionophore did induce calcium flux and histamine release. Both mutant cell lines were found to have IgE receptors suggesting a defect between the receptor and the calcium channel. One cell line was found to have PMT I and almost no PMT II activity. A second variant had PMT II activity and no PMT I activity. Fusion of each cell line at a ratio of 1:1 resulted in the growth of independent hybrids. Hybrids had normal levels of PMT I and PMT II activity and responded to antigen-IgE mediated Ca^{2+} influx and histamine release.

Thus, by fusing two non-secreting cell lines which lacked either PMT I or PMT II, the secretory process was reconstituted. These observations indicate that the cross linking of IgE receptors results in an increase of both phospholipid methytransferases which then allows an influx of Ca^{2+}

TABLE 1. Reconstitution of two phospholipid methyltransferases, Ca^{2+} influx, and histamine release by hybridization of variants defective in one phospholipid methyltransferase.

| Cell Line | Phospholipid Methyltransferase | | IgE Mediated Ca^{2+} Influx | IgE Mediated Histamine Release |
	PMT I	PMT II		
	($pmol$ ^3H-methyl group/mg prot.)		($pmol/10^6$ cells) 30 min	%
2H3	1.71±0.22	21.7±1.9	69.7	58
Variant				
1C1.B1	0.13±0.04	30.2±3.2	0.8	2
2H3.B6	1.04±0.13	4.3±1.3	0.6	2
Hybrid A1	0.82±0.07	20.5±4.7	74.8	28
Hybrid A2	0.70±0.04	17.1±5.0	77.1	33

The two variants were fused and the hybrids grown as described in McGivney et al., (59). The phospholipid methyltransferase enzymes were assayed in membrane fractions by incubations with S-adenosyl-L-[^3H-methyl]-methionine under optimum conditions for each enzyme respectively. $^{45}Ca^{2+}$ (10 µCi/ml) in the presence of 1 mM $CaCl_2$ containing buffer was used to measure $^{45}Ca^{2+}$ influx into cells. The supernatant was sampled for histamine release and the cells were assayed for $^{45}Ca^{2+}$ influx. Histamine release is expressed as percent of the total cellular histamine. Control values for unstimulated Ca^{2+} influx and histamine release were approximately 20 $pmol/10^6$ cells/30 min and 6% respectively.

***

The data suggest the following hypothesis (Fig. 4): antigen stimulation of the cells cross-links and aggregates IgE receptors which increase the methylation of phospholipids resulting in a decrease in membrane viscosity. This decrease in viscosity probably occurs primarily in a specific domain where receptors, the phospholipid methyltransferases, the calcium ion channel and other enzymes are localized. The change in viscosity could allow the opening of the Ca^{2+} channel. Thus, rapid changes in lipid metabolism may alter the membrane fluidity in a highly localized domain within the membrane and thereby cause changes in the activity and coupling of proteins within this domain.

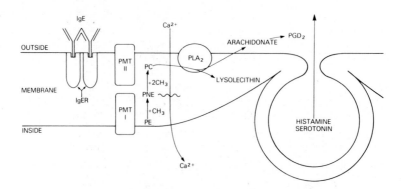

Fig. 4   Schematic diagram of events during antigen IgE mediated
stimulation of histamine and arachidonic acid release. IgE is
immunoglobin E and IgER is immunoglobin E receptor. PE is
phosphatidylethalnolamine which is methylated to phosphatidyl-
N-monomethalethanolamine (PNE), which would alter local
membrane microviscosity allowing calcium influx. PC is
phosphatidylcholine which can be hydrolyzed by phospholipase
A_2 (PLA_2) to lysolecithin, and arachidonate which is
metabolized to PGD2, prostaglandin D2.

CHOLESTEROL/PHOSPHOLIPID MOLAR RATIO AND MEMBRANE FLUIDITY

Although receptor stimulation may rapidly alter membrane fluid properties, the viscosity of the membrane is also affected by relatively
slow changes in composition. One change in composition that is known
to alter membrane viscosity is a change in the cholesterol phospholipid
molar ratio (C/P ratio). The interaction of the rigid backbone of cholesterol with phospholipid acyl chains increases the degree of order
and restricts movement in the membrane interior (16). This increased
order tends to increase viscosity (i.e. decrease fluidity), to abolish
any phase transitions in membrane phospholipids and to alter the rota-
tional freedom and position of proteins within the membrane lipid
matrix (68).
   To determine if increases in the C/P ratio altered receptor cross-
linking and/or the other processes necessary for histamine release we
incorporated cholesterol into rat peritoneal mast cells. Since cholesterol is known to equilibrate between membranes and proteins we were
able to incorporate cholesterol by incubating mast cells in buffer containing 1% bovine serum albumin which had been saturated with cholesterol. Several hours of incubation were required to reach equilibrium
between the cells and protein bound cholesterol. During this time
there was a progressive decrease in the concanavalin A stimulated release of histamine (Fig. 5). After four hours of incubation with
cholesterol the stimulated release of histamine was decreased by
approximately 60%. At this time point approximately 6 μmoles of cholesterol were incorporated into 10^5 mast cells. It is likely that
the increased cholesterol content restricts the movement of membrane
proteins which are necessary for the release process.

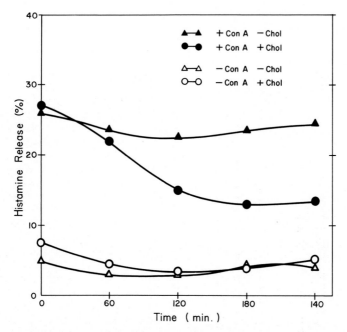

Fig. 5   Effects of cholesterol incorporation on concanavalin A
stimulated histamine release from rat paritoneal mast cells.
Cells were incubated with buffer containing cholesterol for
the various time periods shown. Aliquots were taken and the
cells were washed free of the cholesterol containing media and
then cells were stimulated with concanavalin A (10 µg/ml) and
the release of histamine determined after a 45 min
incubation.

   Although the addition of cholesterol to mast cells was in vitro,
there are physiological and pharmacological conditions which change the
C/P ratio in vivo. We examined the C/P ratio in the synaptosomal
plasma membrane (SPM). This membrane can be purified from brain tissue
(47) and is a critical membrane for normal nerve cell communication.
   One drug studied for changes in the C/P ratio of SPM was ethanol.
Ethanol and other anesthetics are thought to affect the nervous system
by disrupting excitable membranes (67). This suggested that tolerance
and physical dependence upon ethanol could be the result of an alteration in neuronal membranes during chronic exposure. The SPM from control rats, rats acutely treated with ethanol, rats dependent and intoxicated with ethanol, i.e. prodromal dependent rats, and rats undergoing
ethanol withdrawal were prepared and the C/P ratio determined (28).
There was a significant increase in the C/P ratio of SPM from rats
dependent and intoxicated with ethanol as compared to the SPM of control rats and acutely treated with ethanol (Fig. 6). Cholesterol
incorporation into membranes has been shown to increase membrane organization (69). An increased C/P ratio has also been found in the membranes of ethanol tolerant mice (20). Synaptic membranes prepared from
tolerant mice are resistant to ethanol induced fluidization in vitro,
i.e. they have become tolerant to the disruptive effects of ethanol
(19). The disruptive effects of ethanol on membranes are to some
extent opposite to those of cholesterol. Cells may respond to the disruptive effects of ethanol by increasing the C/P ratio in their
membranes. It is possible that under certain conditions cells can
regulate their membrane fluidity by altering the C/P ratio. Certainly

the evidence suggests that tolerance and dependence to ethanol are related to alterations in nerve cell membrane organization and composition.

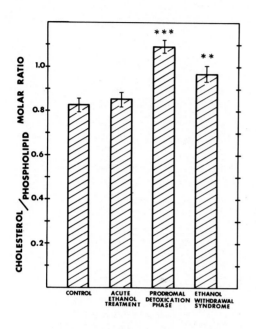

Fig. 6   The cholesterol/ phospholipid molar ratio of SPM prepared from rats after various alcohol treatments. Controls were treated with water. Acute ethanol treatment involves a group of non-fasted animals which were given a single dose of ethanol (5 g/kg) 4 hrs prior to sacrifice. Prodromal detoxication phase group consisted of animals which were rendered physically dependent upon ethanol but were sacrificed while still intoxicated. The animals undergoing ethanol withdrawal syndrome were treated with ethanol as the prodromal group and were decapitated at least 6 hrs after the onset of overt signs and symptoms of the ethanol withdrawal syndrome as described by Majchrowicz (1975).

In addition to the ethanol induced changes in the C/P ratio of SPM, we have found that during aging there are changes in membrane C/P ratio. The SPM from rats of various ages was prepared and its lipid composition compared to that of whole brain. In whole brain the C/P ratio increased in young rats between two and five months of age and then remained relatively constant. In contrast the C/P ratio of SPM changed very little in rats two to twenty months of age. However, the C/P ratio in SPM of rats twenty-four months of age was increased almost two-fold over the C/P ratio of SPM in 20 month old rats (Fig. 7). This alteration in the SPM composition would be expected to alter synaptic transmission and may be related to changes in brain function which occur during aging.

To investigate the effects of changes in the C/P ratio on synaptic transmission we studied carbachol stimulation of pyramidal neurons in the CA1 region of rat hippocampal brain slices. Since cholesterol transfer occurs between proteins rich in cholesterol to membranes containing smaller amounts we incorporated cholesterol into hippocampal slices by perfusing them with buffered Yamamoto's solution containing 1% bovine serum albumin saturated with cholesterol (Fig. 8). Recordings were made through a glass micro-pipette filled with 3 M NaCl saturated with fast green dye as described previously (15). The cholinergic agonist carbachol consistently excited cells in the hippocampus. Atropine blocked the carbachol effect suggesting muscarinic receptor mediated stimulation of firing. Incorporation of cholesterol markedly reduced carbachol induced firing of the hippocampal purkinje cells (Fig. 8). When the response to carbachol was almost completely

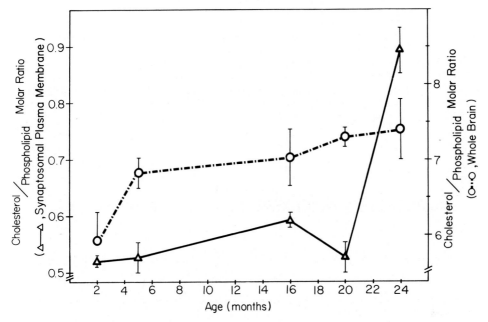

Fig. 7   Cholesterol/phospholipid molar ratio in whole rat brain and in purified synaptosomal plasma membrane. Rats of various ages were decapitated and their brains rapidly frozen. On the day of analysis, brains were thawed and homogenized in 0.32 M sucrose. An aliquot was taken to determine total cholesterol and phospholipid content. Synaptosomal plasma membranes were prepared as described by Jones and Matus (47) and the content of cholesterol and phospholipid determined.

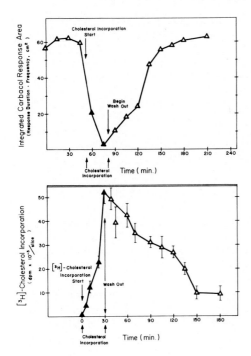

Fig. 8   Cholesterol incorporation and carbachol stimulation of hippocampal cells. Slices of rat hippocampus were perfused. Upper graph shows the integrated area of the carbachol stimulated response from a typical experiment. Lower graph: The incorporation of cholesterol into hippocampal slices was determined by perfusing the slices with media containing [^{3}H]cholesterol (1 μCi/ml) bound to bovine serum albumin. Wash out of cholesterol involved perfusion with the same buffer containing albumin but no cholesterol.

inhibited, perfusion buffers were changed and the cholesterol was
washed out of the slice by perfusion with buffer containing albumin
alone (Fig. 9). Removal of cholesterol restored the carbachol response
to near control levels. Characteristic action potentials were used to
establish the identity of the cell, i.e. that the return of firing
occured in the same cell. It is possible that cholesterol incorporation disrupts the binding and/or stimulus transduction of acetylcholine
like agents in neuronal membranes.

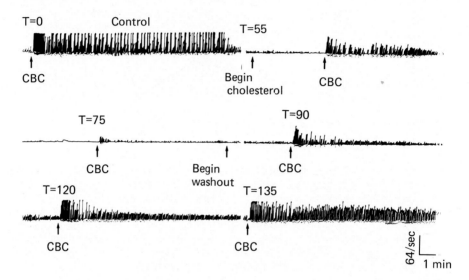

Fig. 9   Effects of cholesterol incorporation on carbachol (CBC) stimu-
          lation of hippocampal pyramidal cells. Slices of rat hippo-
          campus were sandwiched between nylon netting. Recordings were
          made through a glass micropipette from hippocampal pyramidal
          cells in CA1. Carbachol (CBC) was added at the times indica-
          ted. Slices were constantly perfused at a rate of 5 ml/min
          with Yamamoto's buffer containing 1% bovine serum albumin. A
          typical control response is shown at time 0 (T=0). Typical
          responses could be obtained for 4 to 6 hours. Arrows show
          beginning of perfusion with buffer saturated with cholesterol
          and the beginning of cholesterol wash out, i.e. buffer with
          no cholesterol.

CONCLUSIONS

The role of membrane organization in cell function is just beginning
to be understood.
The fluid properties of the membrane lipid matrix have major effects
on membrane function. The phospholipid methyltransferase enzymes can
rapidly increase membrane fluidity and thereby alter certain cellular
processes. This rapid change in viscosity is thought to occur in a
localized domain containing receptors, ion channels, and various other
proteins important for membrane signal transduction. It is possible

that many transmitters and hormones transmit their signals by rapidly changing membrane fluidity.

The physiological and pharmacological factors that alter membrane fluidity by changing the C/P ratio are much slower than the rapid changes with phospholipid methylation. In addition, it is not clear whether changes in bulk fluidity, the formation of distinct lipid domains or some other effect of cholesterol on membrane structure is responsible for the physiological changes that occur in cholesterol enriched membranes. However, it is clear that the regulation of cholesterol and phospholipid content provides the cell with many potential ways to alter cell membrane function. Further studies on the regulation as well as the localization of the various membrane fluid domains are likely to be exciting and physiologically important.

REFERENCES

1. Anderson,P.,Slorach,S.A.,and Uvnas,B.(1973):Acta Physiol.Scand., 88:359-372.
2. Axelrod,J.(1974):Science,184:1341-1348.
3. Balint,J.A.,Beeler,D.A.,Teble,D.H.,and Spritzer,H.L.(1967):J.Lipid Res.,8:486-493.
4. Barnett,R.(1977):pp.427-445,Academic Press Inc.NY.
5. Barsumian,E.,Siraganina,R.P.,and Petrino,M.G.(1981):European J. Immunol.,11:317-323
6. Bhattacharya,A.and Vonderhaar,B.K.(1979):Proc.Natl.Acad.Sci.USA, 76:4489-4493.
7. Bilezikian,J.P.,Spiegel,A.M.,Gammon,D.E.and Aurback,G.D.(1977): Mol.Pharmacol.,13:786-791.
8. Bloj,B.and Zilversmit,D.B.(1976):Biochemistry,15:1277-1283.
9. Blusztajn,J.K.,Zeisel,S.H.and Wurtman,R.J.(1979):Brain Res., 179:319-327.
10. Blusztajn,J.K.and Wurtman,R.J.(1981):Nature,290:417-418.
11. Bremer,J.and Greenberg,D.M.(1961):Biochim.Biophys.Acta,46:205-218.
12. Bretscher,M.S.(1972):J.Mol.Biol.,71:523-528.
13. Brulet,P.,and McConnell,H.M.(1976):J.Am.Chem.Soc.,98:1514-1518.
14. Burwen,S.J.and Satir,B.H.(1977):J.Cell Biol.,73:660-671.
15. Camacho,A.,and Phillips,I.(1981):in preparation.
16. Cantor,C.R.and Schimmmel.(1980):In"Biophysical Chemistry Part III", pp.1350-1351,W. H.Freeman and Co.,San Francisco.
17. Cassel,D.and Salinger,Z.(1976):Biochim.Biophys.Acta,452:538-551.
18. Chap,H.J.,Zwaal,R.F.,and Van Deenen,L.L.M.(1977): Biochim.Biophys.Acta,467:146-164.
19. Chin,J.H.and Goldstein,D.B.(1977):Science,196:684-685.
20. Chin,J.H.,Parsons,L.M.and Goldstein,D.B.(1978): Biochim.Biophys.Acta, 513:358-363.
21. Chiu,T.C.,and Babitch,J.A.(1977):J.Biol.Chem.,252:3862-3869.
22. Cockcroft,S.,and Gomperts,B.D.(1979):Biochem.J.,178:681-687.
23. Coleman,R.(1973):Biochim.Biophys.Acta,300:1-30.
24. Crews,F.T.,Hirata,F.,and Axelrod,J.(1980):J.Neurochem., 34:1491-1498.
25. Crews,F.T.,Hirata,F.,Axelrod,J.,and Siraganian,R.P.(1980): Biochem.Biophys.Res.Commun.,93:42-49.
26. Crews,F.T.,Hirata,F.,and Axelrod,J.(1980):Neurochem.Res., 5:983-991.

27. Crews,F.T.,Morita,Y.,McGivney,A.,Hirata,F.,Siraganian,R.P.,and Axelrod,J. (1981a):Arch.Biochem.Biophys.,(in press).
28. Crews,F.T.,Majchrowicz,E.,and Meeks,R.(1981):Molecular Pharmacol., (in press).
29. Dawson,R.M.C.(1959):J.Biol.Chem.,247:7218-7223.
30. DeKruff,B.,Van Dijck,P.W.,Demel,R.A.,Schuiff,A.,Brants,F.,and Van Deenen,L.L.M.(1974):Biochim.Biophys.Acta,356:1-7.
31. DeRobertis,E.,and VazFerreira,A.(1957):Exp.Cell Res.,12:568-574.
32. Douglas,W.W.(1978):Ciba Foundation Symposium,54:61-87.
33. Fewtrell,C.,Kessler,A.,and Metzger,H.(1979):Adv.Inflam.Res., 1:205-221.
34. Fisher,K.A.(1976):Proc.Natl.Acad.Sci.USA,73:173-177.
35. Fontaine,R.N.,Harris,R.A.,and Schroeder,F.(1980): J.Neurochem., 34:269-277.
36. Foreman,J.C.,Hallett,M.B.,and Mongar,J.L.(1977): J.Physiol., 271:193-205.
37. Gordesky,S.E.,and Marinetti,G.V.(1973):Biochem.Biophys.Res.Commun., 50:1027-1031.
38. Higgins,J.A.(1981):Biochim.Biophys.Acta,640:1-5.
39. Hirata,F.,and Axelrod,J.(1978):Proc.Natl.Acad.Sci.,75:2348-2352.
40. Hirata,F.,and Axelrod,J.(1978):Nature,275:219-220.
41. Hirata,F.,Axelrod,J.,and Crews,F.T.(1979):Proc.Natl.Acad.Sci.USA, 76:4813-4816.
42. Hirata,F.,and Axelrod,J.(1980):Science,209:1082-1090.
43. Hokin,L.E.,and Hokin,M.R.(1954):J.Biol.Chem.,209:549-558.
44. Irvine,R.F.,Hemington,N.,and Dawson,R.M.(1979):Eur.J. Biochem., 99:525-530.
45. Ishizaka,T.,Hirata,F.,Ishizaka,K.,and Axelrod,J.(1980):Proc.Natl. Acad.Sci.USA,77:862-865.
46. Jacobs,S.,and Cuatrecasas,P.(1976):Biochim.Biophys.Acta, 433:482-495.
47. Jones,D.H.,and Matus,A.I.(1974):Biochim.Biophys.Acta,356:276-287.
48. Jost,P.C.,Griffith,O.H.,Capaldi,R.A.and Vanderkooi,G.(1973):Proc. Natl.Acad.Sci.USA,70:480-492.
49. Kahlenberg,A.,Walker,C.,and Rothrlick,R.(1974):Can.J.Biochem., 52:803-808.
50. Kannagi,R.,Koizumi,K.,Hata-Tanoue,S.,and Masuda,T.(1980):Biochem. Biophys.Res.Commun.,96:711-718.
51. Kazimierczak,W.,and Diamant,B.(1978):Prog.Allergy,24:295-365.
52. Kental,S.L.,and Lombardi,B.(1976):Lipids,11:513-516.
53. Kishimoto,A.,Takai,Y.,Mori,T.,Kikkawa,W.,and Nishizuka,Y.(1980): J.Biol.Chem.,255:2273-2276.
54. Klausner,R.D.,Kleinfeld,A.,Hoover,R.L.,and Karnovsky,M.(1980): J.Biol.Chem.,255:1286-1295.
55. Lee,A.G.,Birdsall,N.J.,Metcalf,J.C.,Toon,P.A.and Warren,G.B.(1974): Biochemistry,13:3699-3705.
56. Leonard,J.and Rothman,J.E.(1976):Proc.Natl.Acad.Sci.USA,73:391-395.
57. Levitski,A.(1977):Biochem.Biophys.Res.Commun.,74:1154-1159.
58. Low,M.G.,and Finean,J.B.(1977):Biochem.J.,162:235-240.
59. McGivney,A.,Crews,F.T.,Hirata,F.,Axelrod,J.,and Siraganian,R. Proc.Natl.Acad.Sci.USA,(in press,1981).
60. Majchrowicz,E.(1975):Psychopharmacologia,43:245-254.
61. Melchoir,D.L.and Stein,J.M.(1976):Ann.Rev.Biophys.Bioeng.,5:205-238.
62. Mozzi,R.,and Porcellati,G.(1979):FEBS Letters,100:363-366.

63. Mukherjee,C.,and Lefkowitz,R.J.(1976):<u>Proc.Natl.Acad.Sci.USA</u>, 73:1494-1499.
64. Nakajima,M.,Tamura,E.,Irimura,T.,Toyoskima,S.,Hirano,H.,and Osawa,T.(1981):<u>J.Biochem.</u>,89:665-675.
65. Poznansky,M.and Lange,Y.(1976):<u>Nature</u>,London,259:420-421.
66. Rimon,G.,Hanski,E.,Brown,S.,and Levitzki,A.(1978):<u>Nature</u>, 276:394-396.
67. Seeman,P.(1972):<u>Pharmacol.Rev.</u>,24:583-655.
68. Shinitzky,M.and Inbor,M.(1976):<u>Biochim.Biophys.Acta</u>, 433:133-149.
69. Shinitzky,M.and Barenholz,Y.(1978):<u>Biochimi.Biophys.Acta</u>, 515:367-394.
70. Singer,S.J.,and Nicolson,G.L.(1972):<u>Science</u>,175:720-731.
71. Siraganian,R.P.(1976):<u>In</u>"Mitogens in Immunology" edited by J.J. Oppenheim and D.L. Rosenstreich,pp.69-84,Academic Press,New York.
72. Strickland,K.P.(1973):<u>In</u>"Form and Function of Phospholipids" edited by G.B. Ansell,R.M.C. Dawson and J.N. Hawthorne,pp.9-42, Elsevier,Amsterdam.
73. Strittmatter,W.J.,Hirata,F.,Axelrod,J.,Mallorga,P.,Tallman,J.F.,and Henenberry,R.C.(1979):<u>Nature</u>,282:857-859.
74. Strittmatter,W.J.,Hirata,F.and Axelrod,J.(1979):<u>Science</u>, 204:1205-1207.
75. Sydbom,A.,and Uvnas,B.(1976):<u>Acta Physiol.Scand.</u>,97:222-232.
76. Taurog,J.D.,Mendoza,G.R.,Hook,W.A.,Siraganian,R.P.,and Metzger,H.(1977): <u>J.Immunol.</u>,119:1757-1761.
77. Tolkovsky,A.M.,and Levitzki,A.(1978):<u>Biochemistry</u>,17:3811-3817.
78. Trifaro,J.M.(1977):<u>Ann.Rev.Pharmacol.Toxicol.</u>,17:22-47.
79. Tsai,K.-H.,and Lenard,J.(1975):<u>Nature</u>,London,253:554-555.
80. Vance,D.E.,Choy,P.C.,Farren,S.B.,Lim,P.,and Schneider,W.J.(1977): <u>Nature</u>,270:268-269.
81. Waite,M.,DeChatelet,L.R.,Kuig,L.,and Shirley,P.S.(1979):<u>Biochem. Biophys.Res.Commun.</u>,90:984-992.
82. Wang,J.Y.,and, Mahler,H.R.(1976):<u>J.Cell Biol.</u>,71:639-658.
83. White, D.A.(1973):<u>In</u>"Form and Function of Phospholipids" edited by G.B. Ansell,R.M.C. Dawson and J.N. Hawthorn,pp.441-482, Elsevier,Amsterdam.
84. Zwaal,R.F.,Roelofsen,B.,and Cooley,C.M.(1973):<u>Biochim.Biophy.Acta</u>, 300:159-182.

Phospholipids in the Nervous System, Vol. 1: Metabolism, edited by L. Horrocks, et al. Raven Press, New York © 1982.

Asymmetry of Brain Microsomal Membranes: Correlation Between the Asymmetric Distribution of Phospholipids and the Enzymes Involved in Their Synthesis

L. Freysz, J. Dreyfus, G. Vincendon, *L. Binaglia, *R. Roberti, and *G. Porcellati

*Centre de Neurochimie du CNRS, U44 de l'INSERM, 67084 Strasbourg Cedex, France; *Institute of Biological Chemistry, University of Perugia, 06100 Perugia, Italy*

Phospholipids are found in relatively high concentrations in nervous tissue. In adult brain they account for about 20 to 25% of the dry weight. The distribution of these lipids differs qualitatively and quantitatively in various membrane structures (32). Studies on their metabolism have shown that the different phospholipids turned over at different rates with respect to their structure and their localization in different cells and membranes (9,11,21,22). The differences in the lipid composition of the various nerve cell membranes and the heterogeneity of their turnover raise questions on the mechanisms which control the assembly of the different membrane components and their metabolism. The distribution and the metabolism of the phospholipids in a membrane may be regulated at the level of the enzymes involved in their synthesis, during the transport from their site of synthesis to other membranes and during their incorporation into the membrane structure, where other compounds like proteins and lipids already present may exert some control. Once embedded, different enzymes involved in the redistribution of fatty acids and bases may act upon the specific distribution of the phospholipids in the various membranes.

In brain ethanolamine and choline glycerophospholipids account for about 70 to 80% of total phospholipids, and in spite of some controversial results of their intramembrane localization it is becoming more and more evident that they are distributed asymmetrically (7,8,29). The de novo synthesis of phosphatidylethanolamine and phosphatidylcholine is carried out by Kennedy's pathway (1). The last step of their synthesis is catalyzed by CDPethanolamine:1,2-diacylglycerol phosphoethanolaminetransferase (EC 2.7.8.1) and CDPcholine:1,2-diacylglycerol phosphocholinetransferase (EC 2.7.8.2) which transfer phosphoethanolamine or phosphocholine from the corresponding cytidine nucleotide to a diglyceride. Both enzymes are mainly located in endoplasmic reticulum though recent studies suggest that plasma membranes like myelin and rod outer segments may also contain these enzymes (10,33). The activities of phosphoethanolamine and phosphocholine transferases reside in different proteins, are lipid dependent and react with several species of diglycerides, indicating that these enzymes have no specificity for the lipid substrate (12).

This report deals specifically with the intramembrane localization of ethanolamine and choline phosphoglycerides in brain microsomes, of the enzymes involved in their synthesis and with the regulation of the synthesis of these lipids with respect to the availability of the diglycerides.

TOPOGRAPHICAL DISTRIBUTION OF PHOSPHOLIPIDS AND ENZYMES INVOLVED IN THEIR SYNTHESIS IN BRAIN MICROSOMES

Phospholipids

Lipid localization in biological membranes has been carried out mostly via chemical or enzymic modifications (23). These techniques provide valuable results only when the reagents react quantitatively with the lipids facing the outer side, do not penetrate the membrane and do not lyse the membranes (23). For these reasons the distribution of the phospholipids in microsomes was examined using two different methods: treatment with phospholipase C C. Welchii and with trinitrobenzene sulfonic acid (TNBS).

Chicken brain microsomes were prepared by the method described by Freysz et al. (12). Incubation of the microsomes with phospholipase C produced the hydrolysis of 50% of the phospholipids in 1 h (Table 1).

TABLE 1. Hydrolysis of chicken brain microsomal phospholipids with phospholipase C C. welchii

	% hydrolysis			
	10 min	60 min	120 min	180 min
Total phospholipids	33.0	48.5	51.1	50.7
Phosphatidylcholine	63.1	78.0	82.0	77.2
Phosphatidylethanolamine	17.5	31.3	35.7	34.2
Phosphatidylserine	2.2	14.1	20.9	21.9
Sphingomyelin	42.9	53.4	55.4	51.6

Intact microsomes (2.5 mg protein) were incubated with 3 U phospholipase C as described by Higgins and Dawson (15). Lipids were extracted at appropriate times and separated by two dimensional thin-layer chromatography (28).

The rate of hydrolysis did not increase between 1 and 3 h. However with disrupted microsomes or with a microsomal phospholipid extract more than 80% of the phospholipids were hydrolysed. Thus it can be assumed that under the conditions used the phospholipase C C. welchii does not lyse the membrane, and that 50% of the phospholipids accessible to the phospholipase C are located on the outer side of the microsomal vesicle. The determination of the extent of hydrolysis of the different phospholipids shows that 80% of the phosphatidylcholine, 54% of the sphingomyelin, 35% of the phosphatidylethanolamine and 21% of the phosphatidylserine was digested (Table 1).

TABLE 2. Percent of chicken brain microsomal aminophospholipids reacting with TNBS under non-penetrating conditions

Phospholipids	% reacted phospholipid
Diacylglycerophosphoethanolamine	34
Alkenylacylglycerophosphoethanolamine	26
Diacylglycerophosphoserine	22

Microsomes were incubated with 1.66 mM TNBS as described by Rothman and Kennedy (26) under non-penetrating conditions. Lipids were extracted and separated by two dimensional thin-layer chromatography (28).

In order to confirm the results for aminophospholipids, microsomes were incubated with TNBS in permeating and non-permeating conditions. When the TNBS was allowed to penetrate the membrane about 90% of the different aminophospholipids reacted with the reagent. However in non-penetrating conditions only 34% of the phosphatidylethanolamine, 26% of the ethanolamine plasmalogens and 22% of the phosphatidylserine were accessible to the reagent (Table 2). These results are in good agreement with those obtained with phospholipase C, and suggest that under our conditions only the phospholipids of the outer leaflet of the microsomal vesicle were available for the chemical and the enzymic reagents. Assuming that all external phospholipids were accessible, the distribution on each side of the bilayer could be evaluated (Table 3). The outer leaflet of the microsomal bilayer contains predominantly phosphatidylcholine and the inner leaflet mostly ethanolamine and serine glycerophospholipids. Sphingomyelin is nearly equally distributed between the two leaflets. Phosphatidylinositol is not hydrolysed by phospholipase C C. welchii, but since the hydrolysed lipids account for 50% of the total phospholipids, phosphatidylinositol can be tentatively assigned to the inner leaflet of the bilayer.

TABLE 3. Distribution of phospholipids on either side of the bilayer of chicken brain microsomal membranes

Phospholipids	outer leaflet	inner leaflet
Phosphatidylcholine	32.3	8.1
Phosphatidylethanolamine	5.9	11.0
Ethanolamine plasmalogen	5.2	14.8
Phosphatidylserine	2.1	7.9
Sphingomyelin	3.7	3.0

Results are expressed as mole percentage of total phospholipids

Phosphocholine and Phosphoethanolamine Transferases

Recent kinetic studies on brain microsomal phosphotransferases have suggested that they may be embedded differently in the membranes, which may explain the asymmetrical distribution of the phospholipids (12,13). In order to test this hypothetical relationship between the intramembrane localization of the enzymes and the products, the distribution of phosphoethanolamine and phosphocholine transferases in chicken brain microsomes was examined. This study was carried out by investigating

TABLE 4. Effect of proteases on phosphocholine and phosphoethanolamine transferase activities of chicken brain microsomes

		Phosphocholine transferase	Phosphoethanolamine transferase	
		- DOC	- DOC	+ DOC
Control		100	100	100
Trypsin treatment	5 min	8.0	146.1	48.4
	20 min	1.4	94.4	3.7
Pronase treatment	5 min	2.3	92.1	11.0
	20 min	1.2	62.0	13.7

Microsomes (1 mg protein) were incubated with 1 mg trypsin from bovine pancreas or 0.1 mg pronase from Streptomyces griseus in absence or presence of 0.35% deoxycholate (DOC), as described by Freysz et al. (11). Phosphocholine and phosphoethanolamine transferases were assayed as reported by Freysz et al. (12). Results are expressed as percentage of the specific activities of control microsomes.

the effect of various proteases and neuraminidase on the activities of both enzymes in intact and deoxycholate disrupted microsomes, as described previously (11).

Treatment of intact microsomes with trypsin produced a rapid and nearly complete inactivation of phosphocholine transferase (Table 4). However, a 46% stimulation of the phosphoethanolamine transferase activity was observed when microsomes were treated with trypsin for 5 minutes, followed by a slight decrease after long treatment. On the contrary incubation of deoxycholate disrupted microsomes with trypsin also entirely inactivated phosphoethanolamine transferase. Similar results were also obtained when microsomes were exposed to pronase (Table 4). Short time treatment of intact vesicles led to the inactivation of phosphocholine transferase and had no significant effect on phosphoethanolamine transferase. A slow and increasing inactivation of phosphoethanolamine transferase was observed when intact microsomes were treated with pronase for a long time. This enzyme is however inactivated within a few minutes when deoxycholate disrupted microsomes were treated with pronase as observed for trypsin.

The incubation of microsomes with neuraminidase produced a release of sialic acid from sialoglycoproteins and gangliosides. With intact microsomes about 72% of the glycoprotein and about 34% of the ganglioside sialic acid were removed (Table 5). This treatment had no significant effect on either phosphotransferases. When deoxycholate disrupted microsomes were exposed to neuraminidase nearly all sialic acid was removed from glycoproteins and about 75% of that of gangliosides. In parallel the phosphoethanolamine transferase was nearly completely inactivated. Comparable data could not be obtained for phosphocholinetransferase since this enzyme is inhibited by deoxycholate.

These data indicate that phosphocholine and phosphoethanolamine transferases are two different enzymes, in agreement with previous observations (13). Moreover the inactivation of phosphoethanolamine transferase by neuraminidase suggests that this enzyme is a glycoprotein. The treatment of microsomes with proteases did not lead to the same effects on the activities of both enzymes, indicating that the

TABLE 5. Effect of neuraminidase on phosphocholine and phosphoethanolamine transferase activities of chicken brain microsomes

	Glycoprotein sialic acid remaining		Ganglioside sialic acid remaining		Phosphocholine transferase	Phosphoethanolamine transferase	
	- DOC	+ DOC	- DOC	+ DOC	- DOC	- DOC	+ DOC
Control	100	100	100	100	100	100	100
Neuraminidase 5 min	41.5	12.3	64.8	46.7	95.7	94.5	22.3
Treatment 20 min	28.0	1.9	66.4	24.4	97.2	97.4	4.2

Microsomes (1 mg protein) were treated with 30 mU neuraminidase of Arthrobacter ureafaciens in absence or present of 0.35% deoxycholate (DOC) as described by Freysz et al. (11). Phosphotransferases were assayed as described in Table 4. Results are expressed as percentage of control microsomes.

phosphotransferases are embedded differently in the microsomal membranes. The rapid and total inactivation of phosphocholine transferase by the proteases suggests that this enzyme may be situated on the external side of the microsomal vesicle. On the contrary the very slow decrease of the activity of phosphoethanolaminetransferase by treatment of intact microsomes with proteases compared to the rapid decrease when disrupted microsomes were submitted to proteolytic digestion suggests that this enzyme may be located on the internal side of the vesicle or may have a transmembrane location. This hypothesis is consistent with the effect of neuraminidase, which inactivated the phosphoethanolamine-transferase only with deoxycholate disrupted microsomes. If we assume that phosphoethanolamine transferase has a transmembrane position, it seems likely that the sialic acid residue of this enzyme may be exposed on the internal side of the microsomal vesicles. The stimulation of this enzyme activity after treatment of microsomes with trypsin for a short time may be due to the removal of external proteins which allows a better interaction of the substrate with the enzyme, whereas the slight inactivation after treatment for a long time may be due to the penetration of the proteases into the microsomal vesicles (14).

REGULATION OF THE BIOSYNTHESIS OF CHOLINE AND ETHANOLAMINE PHOSPHOGLYCERIDES IN BRAIN MICROSOMES

In brain, phospholipids differ not only with regard to their bases but also in their fatty acid composition. Phosphatidylcholine contains high amounts of saturated and monoenoic molecular species and low amounts of polyenoic species whereas the opposite distribution is found in phosphatidylethanolamine (25,32). In vitro studies have shown that phosphocholine and phosphoethanolamine tranferases have a broad specificity for the diglyceride (for ref. see 13), which suggest that the synthesis of various molecular species of choline and ethanolamine phosphoglycerides by Kennedy's pathway may be controlled by the availability of the molecular species of diglycerides.

In order to investigate the availability of diglycerides for phosphoglyceride synthesis, a kinetic study of microsomal phosphotransferases in the presence of various amounts of endogenous diglycerides was performed. Rat brain microsomes were prepared as described by Porcellati et al. (24) and enriched in endogenous diglycerides through the glycerol phosphate pathway (3). Incubation of these microsomes with either CDP choline or CDPethanolamine showed a biphasic curve for the synthesis of phosphatidylcholine or phosphatidylethanolamine (Fig. 1). As a function of time, the rate of synthesis of both phosphoglycerides decreased rapidly in the first 10 minutes and continued at a much slower rate thereafter. Since after 10 minutes of incubation less than 15% of the endogenous diglycerides were utilized, the slower rate should not be attributed to the depletion of diglycerides, but rather to a slower interaction between the lipid substrate and the phosphotransferase. It seems likely therefore that the synthesis of phosphatidylethanolamine and phosphatidylcholine by phosphotransferases in brain microsomes may undergo two different reaction rates, a rapid one and a slow one. Similar observations were also reported in the presence of exogenous diglycerides (20).

Fig. 2 shows the fast and slow reaction rates of both phosphotransferases as a function of temperature. It is clear that during the fast synthesis of the phospholipids the Arrhenius plot differs for phosphoethanolamine and phosphocholine transferases. On the contrary identical Arrhenius plots were observed for the slow kinetic reactions. The interpretation of these results is rather difficult. However, they suggest that the synthesis of ethanolamine and choline phosphoglycerides may be regulated by the phosphotransferases during the fast kinetic reaction, while another process may be rate limiting during the slow kinetic reaction. It is possible that the two kinetics observed in the microsomal synthesis of both phospholipids may be due to the presence in microsomes of two compartments of diglycerides which differ in their interaction with the phosphotransferases and/or their localization with respect to these enzymes.

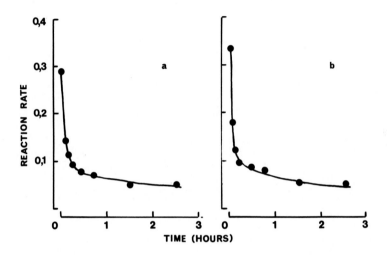

FIG. 1. Kinetics of phosphatidylcholine and phosphatidylethanolamine synthesis in rat brain microsomes. Microsomes were enriched in diglycerides, pelleted and incubated with 1 mM [^{14}C]CDPcholine or 1 mM [^{14}C]CDPethanolamine in 50 mM Tris HCl buffer (pH 8.0), 10 mM MnCl$_2$ in a final volume of 0.3 ml. Reaction rates (nmol/mg protein/min) have been calculated as the average rates between points in the time course curves. Rates of synthesis of phosphatidylcholine (a) and of phosphatidylethanolamine (b).

In order to confirm this hypothesis the effects of CDPbases on the synthesis of ethanolamine and choline phosphoglycerides were investigated. In this study microsomes enriched in endogenous diglycerides were preincubated in the absence or presence of cold CDPbases, pelleted and reincubated with labelled CDPbases. The results reported in Fig. 3 show that in control microsomes the synthesis of phosphatidylethanolamine and phosphatidylcholine proceeded according to a fast kinetic reaction followed by a slow kinetic reaction. In microsomes pretreated with unlabelled bases, the synthesis of both phospholipids occured only via the slow kinetic reaction. Similar results were obtained for the synthesis of phosphatidylcholine and phosphatidyl-

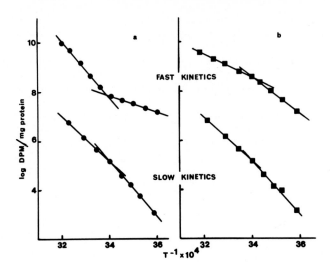

FIG. 2. Arrhenius plots for microsomal (a) phosphoethanolamine and (b) phosphocholine transferases during the fast and slow kinetic synthesis of phosphatidylethanolamine and phosphatidylcholine. In the fast kinetic reaction, microsomes were incubated with 1 mM [^{14}C]CDPcholine or 1 mM [^{14}C]CDPethanolamine for 10 min at different temperatures as described in Fig. 1. For the slow kinetic reaction microsomes were incubated with 1 mM cold CDPbase at 37° for 40 min. Membranes were pelleted and reincubated with 1 mM [^{14}C]CDPbases for 30 min at different temperatures.

ethanolamine when microsomes were preincubated either with cold CDPcholine or with cold CDPethanolamine. These data suggest that phosphocholine and phosphoethanolamine transferases utilize the diglycerides from the first compartment during the fast kinetic reaction, and once this compartment is depleted, they utilize those located in the second compartment which may react at a much slower rate with these enzymes. In a recent study Binaglia (3) using microsomes containing labelled diglycerides reached a similar conclusion.

The compartmentation of the diglyceride pool in brain microsomes raises the question of localization with respect to the phosphotransferases. Our most likely hypothesis is that the fast reacting compartment may be situated in the vicinity of the phosphotransferases, whereas the slow reacting compartment may be located in another part of the membrane. The diglycerides of this second compartment have to reach the enzymes before interaction either by lateral diffusion (4,5) and/or by transbilayer movement (19,27,30,31).

CONCLUSION

Results of the present work indicate an asymmetric distribution of phospholipids in brain microsomal membranes. The outer leaflet of the microsomal vesicles contains about 75% of the choline phospholipids and about 25% of the aminophospholipids, whereas an opposite distribution is observed for the inner leaflet. Similar results were also reported for ethanolamine phospholipids in synaptosomal plasma membrane by Fontaine

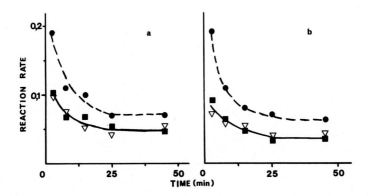

Fig. 3. Effect of the preincubation of rat brain microsomes with cold CDPbases on the phosphotransferase activities. Microsomes enriched in diglycerides were preincubated at 37° for 30 min with or without 1 mM cold CDP bases as reported in Fig. 1. Membranes were pelleted and re-incubated with (a) 1 mM [^{14}C]CDPethanolamine or (b) 1 mM [^{14}C]-CDPcholine for various times. Microsomes preincubated without CDP bases ●---● with CDPethanolamine ■---■ and with CDPcholine ▽---▽. The rate of phospholipid synthesis is expressed as nmol/mg protein/min.

et al. (7,8). Moreover the experiments performed to establish the localization of the phosphotransferases catalyzing the synthesis of ethanolamine and choline phosphoglycerides strongly suggest that the phosphocholine transferase is situated on the external side of the microsomal vesicle and the phosphoethanolamine transferase is either located on the internal side of the vesicle or has a transmembrane position. Since, under the conditions used for the preparation of the microsomal vesicles, it is not known how the vesicles seal, it is difficult to state whether the external surface of the microsomal vesicles corresponds to the cytoplasmic surface of the endoplasmic reticulum. Nevertheless, for brain microsomes the data suggest a relationship between the asymmetric localization of the phospholipids and the enzymes catalyzing their synthesis. It seems therefore likely that the phosphotransferases may participate in the formation and maintenance of the lipid asymmetry in these membranes. The phosphocholine transferase embedded in the external side synthesizes phosphatidylcholine which may be discharged into the outer leaflet. For the phosphoethanolamine transferase, an internal localization would suggest that the phosphatidylethanolamine is synthesized inside the vesicle and discharged into the inner leaflet. This hypothesis seems unlikely, since it has been reported that the CDPbases do not cross the membrane (2,6). However if we assume that the enzyme has a transmembrane position, the phosphatidylethanolamine may be synthezised on the external side of the microsomal vesicle and discharged directly into the internal leaflet. An alternative possibility is that the newly synthesized molecules are discharged into the outer leaflet and submitted to a rapid transbilayer movement. A mechanism to control this transbilayer movement is unknown.

Although there are many suggestions regarding the mechanisms involved in the regulation of phospholipid synthesis (2), little is known about the factors which control the conversion of different molecular species of diglycerides into various species of phospholipids. Recent investigations have provided some indications that ethanolamine and choline kinases and cytidylyltransferases may be the rate limiting steps (1,18). Moreover Holub (16) reported that in liver, microsomal ethanolamine and choline phosphotransferases may have some selectivity for the utilization of various molecular species of diglycerides, although no strict specificity could be observed. It is tempting to suggest that the compartmentation of the diglyceride pool in the microsomal membrane may have some influence on the synthesis of various molecular species of ethanolamine and choline phosphoglycerides. This hypothesis requires that the diglyceride composition of the compartment reacting with the phosphoethanolamine transferase differs from that reacting with the phosphocholine transferase. However both enzymes may also react with the same molecular species of diglycerides and the newly formed choline and ethanolamine phosphoglycerides may undergo a molecular rearrangement through the phospholipase, lysophospholipid, acyltransferase pathway. Obviously more data are required to understand the mechanisms which regulate the asymmetric distribution of phospholipids in cellular membranes.

ACKNOWLEDGEMENTS

This investigation was supported by grants from the Italian C.R.N. (grant CT8100125 04) and the NATO (grant 1560).

REFERENCES

1. Ansell, G.B. (1973): In: Form and Function of Phospholipids, edited by G.B. Ansell, J.N. Hawthorne and R.M.C. Dawson, pp. 377-422, Elsevier Scientific Publishing Company, Amsterdam.
2. Bell, R.M. and Coleman, R.A. (1980): Ann. Rev. Biochem., 49:459-487.
3. Binaglia, L., unpublished results.
4. Devaux, P. and McConnell, H.M. (1972): J. Amer. Chem. Soc., 94:4475-4481.
5. Fahey, P.F., Koppel, D.E., Barak, L.S., Wolf, D.E., Elson, E.L. and Webbs, W.W. (1977): Science, 195:305-306.
6. Floridi, A., Binaglia, L., Vecchini, A., Palmerini, C.A. and Porcellati, G. (1981): Ital. J. Biochem., 30:317-319.
7. Fontaine, R.N., Harris, R.A. and Schroeder, F. (1979): Life Sci., 24:395-400.
8. Fontaine, R.N., Harris, R.A. and Schroeder, F. (1980): J. Neurochem., 34:269-277.
9. Freysz, L., Bieth, R. and Mandel, P. (1969): J. Neurochem., 16:1417-1424.
10. Freysz, L., Dreyfus, H., Harth, S. and Urban, P.F. (1977): 6th ISN Meeting Copenhagen, Abstract p. 554.
11. Freysz, L., Harth, S. and Dreyfus, H. (1982): J. Neurochem., 38: 582-587.
12. Freysz, L., Horrocks, L.A. and Mandel, P. (1977): Biochim. Biophys. Acta, 489:431-439.
13. Freysz, L., Horrocks, L.A. and Mandel, P. (1978): In: Enzymes of Lipid Metabolism, edited by S. Gatt, L. Freysz, and P. Mandel, pp. 253-268, Plenum Press, New York.
14. Guarnieri, M., Cohen, S.A. and Ginns, E. (1976): J. Neurochem., 26:41-44.

15. Higgins, J.A. and Dawson, R.M.C. (1977): Biochim. Biophys. Acta, 470:342-356.
16. Holub, B.J. (1978): J. Biol. Chem., 253:691-696.
17. Horrocks, L.A., Toews, A.D., Thompson, D.K. and Chin, J.Y. (1976): In: Function and Metabolism of Phospholipids in the Central and Peripheral Nervous System, edited by G. Porcellati, L.A. Amaducci, and C. Galli, pp. 37-54, Plenum Press, New York.
18. Infante, J.P. (1977): Biochem. J., 167:847-849.
19. Kornberg, R.D. and McConnell, H.M. (1971): Biochemistry, 10:1111-1120.
20. McCaman, R.E. and Cook, K. (1966): J. Biol. Chem., 241:3390-3394.
21. Miller, S.L., Benjamins, J.A. and Morell, P. (1977): J. Biol. Chem., 252:4025-4037.
22. Miller, S.L. and Morell, P. (1978): J. Neurochem., 27:355-359.
23. Op den Kamp, J.A.F. (1979): Ann. Rev. Biochem., 48:47-71.
24. Porcellati, G., Arienti, G., Pirotta, M.G. and Giorgini, D. (1971): J. Neurochem., 18:1395-1417.
25. Porcellati, G. and Binaglia, L. (1976): In: Lipids, edited by R. Paoletti, G. Porcellati, and G. Jacini, pp. 75-88. Raven Press, New York.
26. Rothman, J.E. and Kennedy, E.P. (1977): J. Mol. Biol., 110:603-618.
27. Rothman, J.E. and Kennedy, E.P. (1977): Proc. Natl. Acad. Sci. USA, 74:1821-1825.
28. Rouser, G., Kritchevsky, G. and Yamamoto, A. (1967): In: Lipid Chromatographic Analysis, edited by G.V. Marinetti, pp. 99-162, Marcel Dekker Inc. New York.
29. Smith, A.P. and Loh, H.H. (1976): Proc. West. Pharmacol. Soc., 19:147-151.
30. Van den Besselaar, A.M.H.P., De Kruijff, B., Van den Bosch, H. and Van Deenen, L.L.M. (1978): Biochim. Biophys. Acta, 510:242-255.
31. Van Zoelen, E.J.J., De Kruijff, B. and Van Deenen, L.L.M. (1978): Biochim. Biophys. Acta, 508:97-108.
32. White, D.A. (1973): In: Form and Function of Phospholipids, edited by G.B. Ansell, J.N. Hawthorne, and R.M.C. Dawson, pp. 441-482, Elsevier Scientific Publishing Company, Amsterdam.
33. Wu, P.S. and Ledeen, R.W. (1980): J. Neurochem., 35:659-666.

Phospholipids in the Nervous System, Vol. 1: Metabolism, edited by L. Horrocks, et al. Raven Press, New York © 1982.

Biosynthesis of Phosphatidic Acid and Polyenoic Phospholipids in the Central Nervous System

Nicolas G. Bazán

LSU Eye Center, Louisiana State University Medical Center, School of Medicine, New Orleans, Louisiana 70112

Almost three decades ago, it was shown that acetylcholine stimulates the turnover of phosphatidylinositol and phosphatidic acid (38,49), and later the general pathways for the synthesis of glycerolipids were described (16,17). However, neither the detailed enzymology nor the regulation of the biosynthesis of phospholipids and neutral glycerides and the relationship with the metabolism of their long-chain, highly unsaturated acyl groups are clearly understood.

The neural tissue phospholipids are enriched with acyl chains derived from essential fatty acids. Docosahexaenoic acid (22:6 n-3) is concentrated in the phospholipids of neuronal plasma membranes (20,26,44,61) and in photoreceptor membranes (1,59) of the retina. Docosahexaenoic acid is derived from α-linolenic acid; however, it is not known if the fatty acid is formed and then acylated to the phospholipid, or if a significant proportion of docosapentaenoic acid is acylated and then converted into docosahexaenoate. Alternatively, both processes may operate. The pathways for the elongation and desaturation of α-linolenic acid involve acyl-S-CoA derivatives (42,50). Also, the direct desaturation of eicosatrienoyl-lecithin to arachidonoyl-lecithin in liver microsomes has been described (54). Another question that remains unanswered is precisely at what point in the biosynthetic pathway of phospholipids the acylation of long-chain highly unsaturated fatty acyl chains takes place. It has been suggested that these types of fatty acids are acylated predominantly by a cycle of deacylation-reacylation reactions involving a phospholipase A_2 and acyltransferases (17,25,35,38,39,52). An alternate possibility is that, prior to phosphatidic acid synthesis, at least part of the polyenoic fatty acids may be introduced into the biosynthetic route and then channeled toward phospholipids (12,13,30).

TABLE 1.   Experimentally-induced shifts in the de novo
biosynthesis of phospholipids in the retina

Experimental conditions	Animal, retinal preparation	PA	PI	PS	PC	PE	TG	Ref.
Propranolol	Cattle, toad; whole, sub-cellular	+	+	+	-	-	-	12-15, 8,41
Phentolamine	Cattle, whole	+	+	+	-	-	-	14,15
Light stimulation	Toad, whole	+	+	nd	nd	nd	nd	7
30 days;6°C	Toad, whole	+	+	+	-	-	-	9
HEPES	Toad, cell-free	+	+	+	-	nc	-	a
TRIS	Toad, cell-free	+	nc	+	+	+	nc	a
Serine	Toad, cell-free	-	nc	-	-	nc	nd	a
Ethanolamine	Toad, cell-free	-	-	-	-	nc	nd	a

aUnpublished data.   + represents labeling above control
values; - represents labeling below control values.   PA :
phosphatidic acid; PI : phosphatidylinositol; PS : phosphatidylserine; PC : phosphatidylcholine; PE : phosphatidylethanolamine; TG : triacylglycerol; nd : not determined;
nc : no change.

An increased interest in the metabolism and function of
phosphatidic acid arose in recent years because it was suggested that this lipid may be the Ca^{2+} ionophore (23,36,
56,58,65) in synaptic membranes linking depolarization with
neurotransmitter release (36).   Studies of the physical
chemical properties of model membranes have shown that
Ca^{2+} induces lateral phase separation with clustering of
phosphatidic acid into specific domains (19,48,53).   Moreover, a question has been raised about the physiological
significance of the relatively higher rates of de novo
synthesis of phosphatidic acid in retina (6-9,11-15,31) and
brain (4,6,18).   It is not likely that these enhanced rates
are involved in the proposed phosphatidylinositol cycle,
wherein diglycerides derived from this phospholipid lead to
the formation of phosphatidic acid, which, in turn, serves
as a precursor for the resynthesis of phosphatidylinositol
(49).   Phosphatidic acid may play some functional role itself, in addition to being the key precursor in the formation of phospholipids and neutral lipids.
This chapter reviews recent work on: a) the fatty acid
composition and metabolism of phosphatidic acid in the
central nervous system; b) experimentally-induced shifts in
the de novo biosynthesis of membrane lipids; c) chain elongation, desaturation, and acylation of $[1-^{14}C]$eicosa-

pentaenoic acid, and d) alternate pathways for the synthesis of polyenoic phospholipids.

BIOSYNTHESIS OF PHOSPHATIDIC ACID

The biosynthesis of phosphatidic acid from glycerol-3-phosphate or from acyldihydroxyacetone-phosphate has been documented (16,17). Glycerol kinase (43) and acyldihydroxyacetone kinase (33) are present in the central nervous system, as well as mitochondrial glycerol kinase (64). It has been shown that there is little acylation of acyl-glycerol-3-phosphate by long-chain polyenoic fatty acids, but that this is an active process in the acylation of acyl-dihydroxyacetone-phosphate (29). Diglyceride kinase can also give rise to phosphatidic acid by phosphorylating diglyceride (21). How active this pathway is in the synthesis of phosphatidic acid either from degraded glycerolipids such as phosphatidylcholine or from phosphatidylinositol has not been clearly established. The incorporation of labeled glycerol in brain and retina showed that the rate of de novo synthesis of phosphatidic acid is high both in vivo (6,21) and in vitro (6,31).

The observation that intravitreally injected $[2-^3H]$-glycerol results in rapid labeling of phosphatidic acid in several retinal subcellular fractions, as well as in the whole retina, provides further support for the idea that these highly active metabolic processes in fact take place in vivo (21).

DRUG-INDUCED SHIFTS IN THE DE NOVO SYNTHESIS OF RETINAL MEMBRANE LIPIDS

Table 1 lists several experimental conditions that modify the de novo biosynthesis of retinal glycerolipids from $[2-^3H]$glycerol. Short exposure to propranolol or phentolamine markedly redirects the pathway toward acidic phospholipids through a mechanism not involving adrenergic receptors (8,14,15,41). Hence, a stimulated synthesis of phosphatidic acid, phosphatidylinositol, and phosphatidylserine takes place. At the same time, inhibition of the formation of triacylglycerol, phosphatidylcholine, and phosphatidylethanolamine is observed.

When retinas were labeled with radioactive glycerol, exposed briefly (10-20 min) to propranolol, and fractionated, increased radioactivity was observed in lipids of all subcellular fractions, implying that a rapid distribution from the sites of synthesis (the microsomes and perhaps also the mitochondria) to other fractions took place (8). Figure 1 shows that lipid labeling in microsomal fractions increased from 20% to 33% as a result of the addition of propranolol. At the same time, an increased amount of radioactive glycerol was observed in all other fractions.

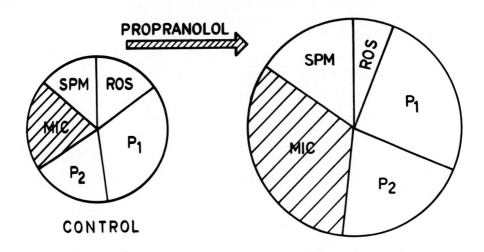

FIG. 1. Increase in [2-^{3}H]glycerol in total glycerolipids of subcellular fractions of the toad retina resulting from the addition of dl-propranolol. Retinas were
incubated for 30 min with or without 0.5 mM dl-propranolol.
Subcellular fractions were collected. SPM : postmicrosomal
supernatant; MIC : microsomes; P$_2$: mitochondrial enriched fraction; P$_1$: fraction containing mainly nuclei and
inner segments of visual cells; ROS : rod outer segments.

Light stimulation also increases retinal lipid synthesis
from radioactive glycerol (7). However, if toads are maintained for 36 days at 6°C and the profiles of glycerolipid
synthesis are examined, changes similar to those exerted by
the cationic amphiphilic drugs are seen (9). In cell-free
preparations, buffers such as HEPES and TRIS also modify the
patterns of labeling with [^{3}H]glycerol. Moreover, the
actions of added unlabeled serine or ethanolamine are also
not readily explainable by a change in the base-exchange
reaction for the synthesis of phosphatidylserine from
phosphatidylethanolamine (unpublished observations).
In conclusion, highly dynamic responses can be obtained
in the de novo biosynthesis of phosphatidic acid by subject-
ing the retina to various experimental conditions. This
indicates that the shifting and redirecting of the biosynthetic pathway may underlie neural cellular function.

NET SYNTHESIS OF PHOSPHATIDIC ACID

Short-term incubation of entire bovine (12,13,15) or toad
(8) retinas with 0.5 mM propranolol promotes accumulation of
phosphatidic acid. Combined studies assessing glycerol
labeling and mass changes in phosphatidic acid have shown

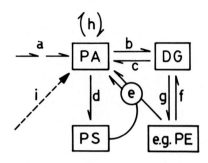

FIG. 2. Metabolic pathways involving phosphatidic acid
(PA). a : de novo synthesis; b : phosphatidate phosphohydrolase; c : diglyceride kinase; d : suggested metabolic
pathway for the synthesis of phosphatidylserine (PS) from
phosphatidic acid (15,55). e : phospholipase D; f : phospholipase C; g : cytidylnucleotide pathway for the synthesis
of phosphatidylethanolamine (PE); h : deacylation-reacylation of phosphatidic acid; DG : diacylglycerol; i : monoacylglycerol route.

that the drug, in addition to inhibiting the phosphatidate
phosphohydrolase step, stimulates conversion into phosphatidylinositol and de novo biosynthesis of phosphatidic acid.
Moreover, the increase in phosphatidic acid accumulation
induced by propranolol was reversed by reincubating the
retinas in drug-free medium. These observations add further
interest to the question of why neural tissue is able to
synthesize relatively large amounts of phosphatidic acid in
short periods of time.

DIACYLGLYCEROL POOL IN THE NEURAL TISSUE

Although the diacylglycerol pool in neural tissue is
relatively small, it displays a high turnover rate (62).
Diacylglycerol can be phosphorylated to yield phosphatidic

TABLE 2. Fatty acid composition of phosphatidic acid.

Acyl group	Microsomes		Rod outer segments
	Cerebral cortex	Retina (mole %)	
16:0	5.4	15.3	3.5
18:0	42.6	28.2	20.3
20:4 n-6	6.0	6.9	3.8
22:6 n-3	31.8	21.1	65.3

Cerebral cortex and rod outer segments (unpublished observations); retina (30).

acid (c, Fig. 2) and it can be formed from phosphatidic acid (b, Fig. 2). However, there are several pools of diacylglycerol in the central nervous system which are not directly related to phosphatidic acid metabolism. Diglycerides can arise from the back reaction of phosphocholine transferase (32) and from phosphatidylinositol degradation (49). Neural stimulation promotes rapid and transient accumulation of stearoyl-arachidonoyl glycerides in the brain (3). Although it is not likely that this diglyceride is derived from phosphatidic acid, this observation is the first in vivo demonstration of modifications in the endogenous concentration of diglycerides in the brain.

Information obtained on retinal diglycerides indicates that this lipid is a major component of the reactions that make up glycerolipid metabolism. Retinal diglyceride takes up a high proportion of labeled arachidonic acid (5), and in the toad, contains large amounts of docosahexaenoate (20). When radioactive glycerol was used, labeled diglyceride evolved after the peak of phosphatidic acid labeling. Hence, active conversion through the phosphatidic acid phosphohydrolase step was observed in vivo (6,21) and in vitro (6,31) in the retina. Inhibition of this enzyme by propranolol, however, resulted in a rapid decrease in diglyceride labeling from glycerol and then an enhancement in radioactivity. Again, this second phase may not involve phosphatidic acid to diglyceride conversion, but may take place by other routes of labeling as yet undefined (15).

FATTY ACID COMPOSITION OF PHOSPHATIDIC ACID

The outstanding feature of the fatty acid profile of phosphatidic acid from retinal microsomes, cerebral cortex microsomes, and photoreceptor membranes is the high content of docosahexaenoate (Table 2), whereas the proportion of arachidonate is similar in microsomes from retina and cerebral cortex (about 7% and 6%, respectively). In rod outer segments, however, about 65% of the fatty acid was docosa-hexaenoate. No earlier data for the retinal membranes are available, and, to the best of our knowledge, these values represent the largest amounts of docosahexaenoate found in phosphatidic acid from any particular membrane. Other studies have shown that phosphatidic acid from the whole rat brain (4), microsomes from rat brain (60), and guinea pig cerebral hemispheres (47) contains about 1.2%, 10%, and 8.8% docosahexaenoate, respectively.

The high content of docosahexaenoyl-phosphatidic acid raised the following questions: a) Is this fatty acid added by acylation during de novo biosynthesis of phosphatidic acid? (a, Fig. 2) b) Alternatively, is this hexaenoic phosphatidic acid derived from a phospholipid through the action of phospholipase D? (e, Fig. 2) c) Are precursors of docosahexaenoic acid, such as eicosapentaenoic or docosapentaenoic acid, acylated in phosphatidic acid?

In addition, two other, more general questions evolved. How is docosahexaenoic acid synthesized in neural tissue, and are the acylation and metabolism of long-chain polyenoic fatty acids coordinated with the overall metabolism of neuronal membrane phospholipids? Experiments with $[1-^{14}C]$eicosapentaenoic acid that were designed to explore these questions are described below.

ANOXIA-STIMULATED DEGRADATION OF PHOSPHATIDIC ACID
IN THE NEURAL TISSUE

Different amounts of phosphatidic acid were found in various regions of rat brain (12), and an increased accumulation of this phospholipid was seen in mouse brain from birth to adulthood (12). Ischemia triggers a selective and very rapid increase in free fatty acids in the brain; arachidonic acid is a major component of this pool (10). It has been proposed that these free fatty acids are derived from the deacylation of membrane lipids (for references, cf. 57). This fatty acid accumulation is the first change that occurs in the membrane lipids of the nervous system during blood shortage. Moreover, in the newborn mouse, anoxia resulted in the degradation of brain phosphatidic acid (57). This observation further emphasizes the active metabolism of this acidic phospholipid in the brain.

CHAIN ELONGATION, DESATURATION, AND ACYLATION
OF EICOSAPENTAENOIC ACID IN THE RETINA

Docosahexaenoic acid is synthesized from dietary α-linolenic acid as acyl-S-CoA by a series of elongation and desaturation reactions (42,50). The ability of the developing (27,28) and mature (for references, cf. 50) brain to use linolenic acid as a precursor for longer chain, highly unsaturated derivatives has been explored. In addition, the incorporation of linolenic acid in neurons (24), glial cells

(24), brain (after intracranial injection) (28), cultured retinoblastoma (40), cultured dissociated brain cells (69, 70), and brain mitochondria (68) has been studied. However, information was not available on a) the elongation and desaturation of eicosapentaenoic acid; b) acylation of eicosapentaenoic acid in individual phospholipids; c) time-course of appearance of products of eicosapentaenoic acid in individual phospholipids: and d) in vivo studies of this kind. With the use of [1-^{14}C]eicosapentaenoic acid synthesized by Dr. Howard Sprecher, we were able to observe rapid acylation in both retinal lipids and brain microsomal lipids. In addition, [^{14}C]eicosapentaenoic and [^{14}C]docosahexaenoic acids were formed, indicating the presence of the following reactions:

$$5,8,11,14,17-20:5 \quad \longrightarrow \quad 7,10,13,16,19-22:5$$

$$\longrightarrow \quad 4,7,10,13,16,19-22:6$$

Both products were found when [1-^{14}C]eicosapentaenoic acid was incubated with brain microsomes and photoreceptor membranes (unpublished observations). The same reactions may take place in vivo in the retina, since similar data were obtained following intravitreal injection of the label-ed fatty acid. In addition, all phospholipids were rapidly labeled, and proportionally higher amounts of [^{14}C]doco-sapentaenoate and [^{14}C]docosahexaenoate were formed as a function of time after injection. These results indicate that rapid acylation takes place and that elongation and Δ4 desaturation takes place in vivo in the rat retina. More-over, since significant amounts of [^{14}C]docosa-pentaenoate were found in several phospholipids, perhaps desaturases that act directly on the acyl chains of these lipids are present in the retina. Similar direct desatura-tion reactions were recently described for polyenoic acyl chains derived from linoleic acid (54).

SYNTHESIS OF DOCOSAHEXAENOYL-PHOSPHATIDIC ACID

Retinal phosphatidic acid labeling after intravitreal injections of [1-^{14}C]eicosapentaenoic acid was seen to be dependent on the concentration of the precursor and the length of the postinjection period (Fig. 3). Moreover, 3 min after injection, the highest specific activity and 16% of the incorporated activity were found in phosphatidic acid, compared with other phospholipids (data not shown). However, increasingly larger amounts of labeled docosa-hexaenoate were seen in this phospholipid during the post-injection period (Fig. 3). Other phospholipids were not labeled uniformly, which suggests that elongation and desaturation took place first, and then the products were acylated.

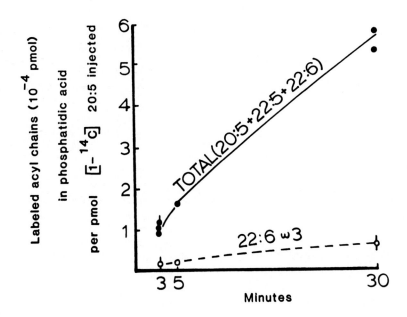

FIG. 3. Labeling of phosphatidic acid by $[1-^{14}C]20:5$ in the rat retina in vivo. The precursor was injected intravitreally into the rat eye. Labeling is depicted in relation to the amount of precursor injected and the time after injection. An increased proportion of 22:6 n-3 is seen with time.

DEACYLATION-REACYLATION CYCLE AND DE NOVO BIOSYNTHESIS AS ROUTES TO INTRODUCE POLYENOIC ACYL CHAINS IN MEMBRANE LIPIDS

Acyl chains turn over at a rate different from that of the glycerol backbone of phospholipids due to acyl-CoA:mono-acyl phospholipid acyltransferases, as was first shown in rat liver (37,45). Although there are inconsistent reports on the specificity of different fatty acids in vivo and in vitro (17), the asymmetric distribution of saturated and unsaturated fatty acids in C-1 and C-2, respectively, is thought to result from the interplay of acyltransferases (17,66) during and after phospholipid synthesis. Polyenoic fatty acids are thought to be acylated predominantly through a deacylation-reacylation cycle catalyzed by phospholipase A_2 and acyltransferases. Moreover, saturated and less unsaturated fatty acids are predominantly acylated during the de novo synthesis of phosphatidic acid (34,51,63,67). An alternative route for the synthesis of polyenoic-phosphatidic acid and, in turn, therefore, for polyenoic-phospholipids, may be through the acylation of polyenoic fatty acids during the formation of phosphatidic acid

(12,13,30). This pathway might be responsible for the synthesis of a large proportion of the highly unsaturated molecular species of membrane lipids. In addition, deacylation-reacylation reactions may operate on phosphatidic acid. In fact, rapid acylation-deacylation reactions have been seen in arachidonate of phosphatidic acid in horse neutrophils (46).

Figure 2 outlines the known pathways of phosphatidic metabolism in animal tissues. Some of the indicated reactions are hypothetical and others have not been demonstrated in the nervous system.

Alternatively the high content of docosahexaenoate in phosphatidic acid from the various membrane preparations examined may represent a degradation product of phospholipase D. In fact, this enzyme has been shown to be present in brain (22). However, labeling experiments have disclosed that a large amount of intravitreally-injected [14C]eicosapentaenoic acid and increasingly larger amounts of [14C]docosahexaenoic acid are found in retinal phosphatidic acid at 3 and 5 min after injection (Fig. 3).

CONCLUSIONS

In the study of phospholipid metabolism in the central nervous system during the past decades, the turnover of ^{32}P has been examined extensively, but only recently has the pathway of de novo biosynthesis been recognized as an active metabolic sequence both in vivo and in vitro. Although the phospholipids of neuronal membranes are richly endowed with long-chain, highly unsaturated fatty acyl groups, it is not known whether they are acylated by means of deacylation-reacylation cycles, de novo biosynthesis, or a combination of the two.

We have used vertebrate retinas and cerebral cortex to study the de novo biosynthesis of phospholipids in relation to the desaturation and chain elongation of polyenoic fatty acids. Based on the results of studies measuring net synthesis of phosphatidic acid and the flow of [2-3H]glycerol toward individual phospholipids during short-term incubation, the de novo biosynthesis of phospholipids appears to be an active metabolic process (6,21,31). This pathway can be shifted by cationic amphiphilic drugs, regardless of their pharmacological actions. The overall effect of these drugs is increased formation of acidic phospholipids and decreased synthesis of triacylglycerol, phosphatidylcholine, and phosphatidylethanolamine (8,9,11-15). The amount of labeling increased early in the incubation period in microsomal phosphatidic acid, after which it decreased in this compound and increased in phosphatidylserine and phosphatidylinositol (8,14,15). A net accumulation of phosphatidic acid was also observed. This effect, as well as the redirecting of the pathway, can be reversed by a further 5 min incubation in drug-free medium (unpublished observations).

The existence of control points where endogenous metabolites may act was explored. Retinas from toads adapted to
an environment of 6°C were compared to retinas from toads
kept at 23°C. A stimulated synthesis of acidic phospholipids which resembled the propranolol-induced changes was
observed in the retinas from the cold-adapted toads (9).
The phosphatidic acid in the microsomal fractions of the
retina and the cerebral cortex was found to be enriched in
docosahexaenoate.

[1-^{14}C]Eicosapentaenoate was used to study incorporation in individual lipids, and desaturation and further
chain elongation to [1-^{14}C]docosahexaenoate. Labeled
eicosapentaenoate was injected intravitreally in the rat
eye; rapid and non-uniform incorporation was found in all
phospholipids. The highest amount of radioactivity, based
on lipid mass, was found in phosphatidic acid at 3 to 5 min
after injection. Thirty minutes later, phosphatidic acid
labeling had decreased. Time-dependent desaturation and
elongation were seen in all phospholipids. Moreover, the
highest specific activity for docosahexaenoyl chains was
observed in phosphatidic acid; high specific activities for
docosahexaenoate were also seen in phosphatidylinositol and
phosphatidylcholine. It appears that a significant proportion of docosahexaenoate present in membrane phospholipids
is introduced through the de novo formation of phosphatidic
acid. However, in phosphatidylcholine and phosphatidylinositol, introduction of the fatty acid by a deacylation-
reacylation cycle also takes place.

In summary, the de novo synthesis of phospholipids and
neutral glycerides takes place at a high rate in the retina
in vivo and in vitro. Several experimental manipulations
indicated that rapid changes occur in the pathway for the
synthesis of lipids, producing predominantly acidic phospholipids and reducing the formation of zwitterionic lipids.
The patterns of the changes suggested that there may be
associated sets of reactions, mediated perhaps by the
association of enzymes. Moreover, in vivo modulators may
affect these pathways, redirecting them toward the formation
of a phospholipid class that may be needed in a membrane for
a specific function.

Docosahexaenoate may be acylated during the synthesis of
phosphatidic acid through a pathway committed to the synthesis of polyenoic phospholipids. In addition, direct
desaturation of essential fatty acids may occur in phospholipids from neural tissue. The rapid formation of polyenoic
molecular species of phospholipids may operate when a sudden
need arises for higher membrane fluidity. Thus, a retailor-
ing of phospholipids in a membrane area by this mechanism
may allow the replacement not only of the two preexisting
fatty acids, but also of the rest of the molecule. Hence,
changes in the polar head may also result when a complete
phospholipid molecule needs to be replaced.

The highly dynamic state of membrane molecules may be
sustained by a rapid, efficient, and specific mechanism that
synthesizes hexaenoic phospholipids and/or phosphatidic acid

to support specific membrane functions. Such pathways may underlie localized molecular plasticity changes in excitable or transducing membranes.

Supported in part by a Research Manpower Award from Research to Prevent Blindness, Inc., New York City.

REFERENCES

1. Anderson, R., and Andrews, L. (1981): In: Visual Cells in Evolution, edited by J. Westfall, (in press), Raven Press, New York.
2. Aveldano, M.I., and Bazan, N.G. (1973): Biochim. Biophys. Acta, 296:1-9.
3. Aveldano de Caldironi, M.I., and Bazan, N.G. (1979): Neurochem. Res. 4:213-221.
4. Baker, R.R., and Thompson, W. (1972): Biochim. Biophys. Acta, 270:489-503.
5. Bazan, H.E.P., and Bazan, N.G. (1975): Life Sci., 17:1671-1679.
6. Bazan, H.E.P., and Bazan, N.G. (1976): J. Neurochem., 27:1051-1057.
7. Bazan, H.E.P., and Bazan, N.G. (1977): Adv. Exp. Med. Biol., 83:489-495.
8. Bazan, H.E.P., Careaga, M.M. and Bazan, N.G. (1981): Biochim. Biophys. Acta, 666:63-71.
9. Bazan, H.E.P., Marcheselli, V.L., Careaga, M.M., and Bazan, N.G. (1981): In: New Trends in Nutrition, Lipid Research and Cardiovascular Diseases, edited by N.G. Bazan, R. Paoletti, and J.M. Iacono, pp. 101-110. Alan R. Liss, New York.
10. Bazan, N.G. (1970): Biochim. Biophys. Acta, 218:1-10.
11. Bazan, N.G. (1982): In: Handbook of Neurochemistry, edited by A. Lajtha, Vol. 3., (In press), Plenum Press, New York.
12. Bazan, N.G., Aveldano de Caldironi, M.I., Giusto, N.M., and Rodriguez de Turco, E.B. (1981): Progress in Lipid Research, 20:307-313.
13. Bazan, N.G. and Giusto, N.M. (1980): In: Control of Membrane Fluidity, edited by M. Kates and A. Kuksis, pp. 223-236. Humana Press, New Jersey.
14. Bazan, N.G., Ilincheta de Boschero, M.G., Giusto, N.M., and Bazan, H.E.P. (1976): Adv. Exp. Med. Biol., 72: 139-148.
15. Bazan, N.G., Ilincheta de Boschero, M.G., and Giusto, N.M. (1977): Adv. Exp. Med. Biol., 83:377-388.
16. Bell, R.M., Ballas, L.M., and Coleman, R.A. (1981): J. Lipid Res., 22:391-403.
17. Bell, R.M., and Coleman, R.A. (1980): Ann. Rev. Biochem., 49:459-487.
18. Binaglia, L., Roberti, R., and Porcellati, G. (1978): Adv. Exp. Med. Biol., 101:353,366.
19. Boggs, J.M. (1980): Can. J. Biochem., 58:755-770.

20. Breckenridge, W.C., Gombos, G., and Morgan, I.G. (1971): Brain Res., 33:581-586.
21. Careaga, M.M., and Bazan, H.E.P. (1981): Neurochem. Res., 6:1169-1178.
22. Chalifour, R.J., and Kanfer, J.N. (1980): Biochem. Biophys. Res. Comm., 96:742-747.
23. Clark, R.B., Salmon, D.M., and Dewhurst, S.A. (1971): J. Cyc. Nuc. Res., 6:37-49.
24. Cohen, S.R., and Bernsohn, J. (1978): J. Neurochem., 30:661-669.
25. Corbin, D.R., and Sun, G.Y. (1978): J. Neurochem., 30:77-82.
26. Cotman, C., Blank, M.L., Moehl, A., and Snyder, F. (1969): Biochemistry, 8:4606-4612.
27. Crawford, M.A., Casperd, N.M., and Sinclair, A.J. (1976): Comp. Biochem. Physiol., 54B:395-401.
28. Dhopeshwarkar, G.A. and Subramanian, C. (1976): Lipids, 11:67-71.
29. Fleming, P.J., and Hajra, A.K. (1977): J. Biol. Chem., 252:1663-1672.
30. Giusto, N.M. and Bazan, N.G. (1979): Biochem. Biophys. Res. Commun., 91:791-794.
31. Giusto, N.M., and Bazan, N.G. (1979): Exp. Eye Res. 29:155-168.
32. Goracci, G., Horrocks, L.A., and Porcellati, G. (1978): Adv. Exp. Med. Biol., 101:269-278.
33. Hajra, A.K., and Burke, C. (1978): J. Neurochem., 31:125-134.
34. Haldar, D., Tso, W.W., and Pullman, M.E. (1979): J. Biol. Chem., 254:4502-4509.
35. Harmon, C.K., and Neiderhiser, D.H. (1978): Biochim. Biophys. Acta, 530:217-226.
36. Harris, R.A., Schmidt, J., Hitzemann, B.A., and Hitzemann, R.J. (1981): Science, 212:1290-1291.
37. Hill, E.E., and Lands, W.E.M. (1970): In: Lipid Metabolism, edited by S. Wakil, pp. 185-279, Academic Press, New York.
38. Hokin-Neaverson, M. (1977): Adv. Exp. Med. Biol., 83:429-446.
39. Holub, B.J., MacNaughton, J.A., and Piekarski, J. (1979): Biochim. Biophys. Acta, 572:413-422.
40. Hyman, B.T., and Spector, A.A. (1981): J. Neurochem., 37:60-69.
41. Ilincheta de Boschero, M.G., Giusto, N.M.,and Bazan, N.G. (1980): Neurochemistry, 1:17-28.
42. James, A.T. (1977): Adv. Exp. Med. Biol., 83:51-74.
43. Jenkins, B.T., and Hajra, A.K. (1976): J. Neurochem., 26:377.
44. Kishimoto, Y.L., Agranoff, B.W., Radin, N.S., and Burton, R.M. (1969): J. Neurochem., 16:397-405.
45. Lands, W.E.M. (1960): J. Biol. Chem., 235:2232-2237.
46. Lapetina, E.G., Billah, M., and Cuatrecasas, P. (1980): J. Biol. Chem., 255:10966-10970.
47. Luthra, M.G., and Sheltawy, A. (1976): J. Neurochem., 27:1503-1511.

48. Massari, S., and Pascolini, D. (1977): Biochemistry, 16:1189-1195.
49. Michell, R.N., Jafferji, S.S., and Jones, L.M. (1977): Adv. Exp. Med. Biol., 83:464-467.
50. Naughton, J.M. (1981): Int. J. Biochem., 13:21-32.
51. Okuyama, H., Eibl, H., and Lands, W.E. (1971): Biochim. Biophys. Acta, 248:263-273.
52. Okuyama, H., Yamada, K., and Ikezawa, H. (1975): J. Biol. Chem., 250:1710-1713.
53. Patil, G.S., Dorman, N.J., and Cornwell, D.G. (1979): J. Lipid Res., 20:663-668.
54. Pugh, E.L., and Kates, M. (1977): J. Biol. Chem., 252:68-73.
55. Pullarkat, R.J., Sbaschnig-Agler, M., and Reha, H. (1981): Biochim. Biophys. Acta, 663:117-123.
56. Putney, J.W., Weiss, S.J., Van De Walle, C.M., and Haddas, R.A. (1980): Nature (London), 284:345-347.
57. Rodriguez de Turco, E.B., Cascone, G.D., Pediconi, M.F., and Bazan, N.G. (1977): Adv. Exp. Med. Biol., 83:389-396.
58. Salmon, D.M., and Honeyman, T.W. (1980): Nature (London), 284:344-345.
59. Stone, W.L., Farnsworth, C.C., Dratz, E.A. (1979): Exp. Eye Res., 28:387-397.
60. Su, K.L., and Sun, G.Y. (1978): J. Neurochem., 31:1043-1047.
61. Sun, G.Y., and Sun, A.Y. (1972): Biochim. Biophys. Acta, 280:306-315.
62. Sun, G.Y., and Horrocks, L.A. (1969): J. Neurochem., 16:181-189.
63. Tamai, Y., and Lands, W.E.M. (1974): J. Biochem., 76:847-860.
64. Tildon, J.T., Stevenson, J.H., Jr., and Ozand, P.T. (1976): Biochem. J., 157:513-516.
65. Tyson, C.A., Zande, H.V., and Green, D.E. (1976): J. Biol. Chem., 251:1362-1332.
66. Van Golde, L.M.G. (1976): Am. Rev. Resp. Dis., 144:977-1000.
67. Yamashita, S., Nakaya, N., Miki, Y., and Numa, S. (1975): Proc. Nat. Acad. Sci., 72:600-603.
68. Yatsu, F.M. and Moss, S. (1972): J. Neurochem., 19:1813-1815.
69. Yavin, E., and Menkes, J.H. (1974): Lipids, 9:248-253.
70. Yavin, E., and Menkes, J.H. (1974): J. Lipid Res., 15:152-157.

Phospholipids in the Nervous System, Vol. 1: Metabolism, edited by L. Horrocks, et al. Raven Press, New York © 1982.

Deacylation and Acylation of Phospholipids in Nervous Tissue

S. K. Fisher, F. J. Doherty, and C. E. Rowe

Department of Biochemistry, University of Birmingham, Birmingham B15 2TT, United Kingdom

Brain tissue can de-acylate diacylglycerophospholipids to form lysophospholipids. It can also acylate lysophospholipids, with long chain fatty acids both in vivo and in vitro to form diacylglycerophospholipids. For acylation in vitro ATP is an essential cofactor and the reaction is stimulated by CoA. From the results of experiments in vitro Webster and Alpern (27) postulated the existence of a deacylation-acylation cycle in brain analogous to that suggested by Lands (16) for liver. Essential features of such a cycle are shown in Fig. 1. Three enzymes are involved directly, namely phospholipase A, acyl-CoA synthetase and acyl-CoA: lysophosphatide acyl transferase. Two other

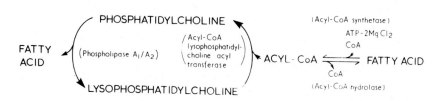

Fig. 1. Deacylation-acylation cycle

enzymes, namely acyl-CoA hydrolase and lysophospholipase (not shown), could conceivably regulate the cycle by controlling the concentrations of acyl-CoA and lysophospholipid, respectively. As pointed out by Lands (16), such a cycle could lead to independent turnover of the fatty acid esters of phospholipid molecule without extensive degradation and de novo synthesis. It would also give a simple explanation of why the distribution of fatty esters in different classes of phospholipids differ from one another, and from that of phosphatidic acid, from which phospholipids are formed by synthesis de novo by the Kennedy pathway. In order to assess the importance of the cycle, information is required about the subcellular distribution of the relevant enzymes. Could the cycle function as a multienzyme complex or would transport systems be required to carry intermediates between enzymes and between intracellular sites?

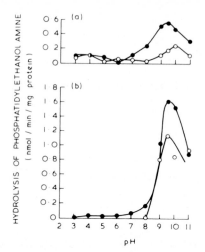

Fig. 2. (11) Comparison of the effect of pH on the activities of phospholipase A_1 in homogenate and soluble supernatant of rat brain cerebral cortex. (a) Homogenate. (b) Soluble supernatant. $\bigcirc$, release of lysophosphatidylethanolamine from 1-acyl-2-[9,10-^{3}H]oleoyl-sn-glycero-3-phosphorylethanolamine; $\bullet$, release of fatty acid from 1-[9,10-^{3}H]palmitoyl-2-acyl-sn-glycero-3-phosphorylethanolamine. Buffers (final concentration = 40 mM) were, pH 3-6, sodium acetate; pH 7-8, Tris HCl; pH 9-11, glycine-NaOH.

Deacylation

In brain, as in liver, phospholipase A_2 activity is concentrated in the mitochondrial fraction, and phospholipase A_1 activity in the microsomal fraction (4,28,29,30,31). Moreover there are phospholipases A_1 and A_2 with pH optima in the range 4-5 (6,14) suggesting, by analogy with liver, that they are of lysosomal origin. The activities of all these enzymes were determined in the presence of detergents, under conditions such that the membranes in which the enzymes are initially located were disrupted. In addition to the enzymes mentioned above, brain contains a phospholipase A_1 which is inhibited by detergent but activated by Ca^{2+} (25). The preferred substrate is phosphatidylethanolamine which is hydrolysed at a pH optimum of 9.4 as shown in Fig. 2. From Fig. 2 it can be seen that the activity is concentrated in the supernatant fraction of brain homogenate. Activation of the activity in the supernatant by Ca^{2+} is shown in Fig. 3.

The subcellular distribution of the enzyme is shown in Table 1 (11), and correlated with the distribution of the soluble cytoplasmic marker lactate dehydrogenase. It did not correlate with the subcellular distributions of the lysosomal enzyme, β-galactosidase, the microsomal enzyme, NADPH-cytochrome c reductase, or the mitochondrial enzyme succinate dehydrogenase.

Phosphatidylethanolamine changes from a lipid with a net neutral charge to one with a net negative charge as the pH is increased from 8 to 10 (2). The alkaline pH optimum with phosphatidylethanolamine may reflect the preference of the enzyme for negatively charged phospholipids. In this connection it is of interest that the negatively charged phospholipids phosphatidylinositol and phosphatidylserine are preferentially distributed on the cytoplasmic side of plasma membranes

TABLE I

The hydrolysis of phosphatidylethanolamine by subcellular fractions of rat cerebral cortex

Correlation coefficients between phospholipase A1 (release of lysophosphatidylethanolamine and fatty acid) and lactate dehydrogenase were 0.976 and 0.977 ($P < 0.001$), respectively. Correlation coefficient for release of lysophosphatidylethanolamine and lactate dehydrogenase for the tissue fractions from three independent subcellular fractionations was 0.821 (16 degrees of freedom). Correlation coefficient for the release of fatty acid and lactate dehydrogenase for tissue fractions from 6 subcellular fractionations was 0.953 (33 degrees of freedom). $P < 0.001$ in all cases.

Fraction	Protein (% recovered)	Phospholipase A1 hydrolysis of phosphatidylethanolamine (nmol/min/mg protein)		Relative specific activity					
		(a) Production of lyso-phosphatidyl-ethanolamine	(b) Production of fatty acid	Phospholipase A1		Lactate de-hydrogenase	β-Galacto-sidase	Succinate de-hydrogenase	NADPH-cytochrome c reductase
				(a)	(b)				
Homogenate	—	0.25	0.43	1.00	1.00	1.00	1.00	1.00	1.00
Crude nuclear (P1)	28.7	0.10	0.19	0.37	0.43	0.36	0.98	0.93	0.73
Light myelin (P2A)	3.1	0.00	0.00	0.00	0.00	0.04	1.10	0.00	0.76
Nerve endings (P2B)	9.5	0.00	0.08	0.01	0.18	0.42	1.06	0.32	0.82
Mitochondrial fraction (P2C)	10.4	0.00	0.05	0.09	0.10	0.61	1.95	3.96	0.89
Microsomal fraction (P3)	6.2	0.02	0.05	0.09	0.11	0.64	0.76	0.00	2.52
Supernatant (S3)	15.0	1.47	1.76	5.94	4.07	2.87	0.31	0.00	1.24

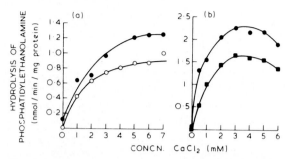

Fig. 3.   (11) Effect of CaCl$_2$ on the hydrolysis of phosphatidyl-ethanolamine by soluble supernatant.   Release of lysophosphatidyl-ethanolamine from 0.40 mM 1-acyl-2-[9,10-^{3}H]oleoyl-sn-glycero-3-phosphorylethanolamine; ●, release of fatty acid from 0.40 mM 1-[9,10-^{3}H]palmitoyl-2-acyl-sn-glycero-3-phosphorylethanolamine; ■ , release of fatty acid from 0.10 mM 1-[9,-10-^{3}H]palmitoyl-2-acyl-sn-glycero-3-phosphorylethanolamine.   Data in (a) and (b) are from different preparations of soluble supernatant.

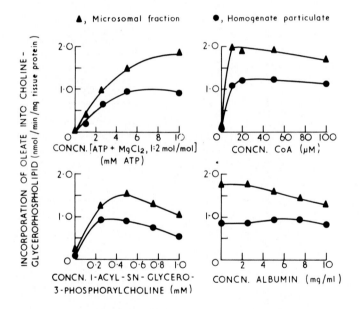

Fig. 4.   Effect of ATP plus MgCl$_2$, CoA, lysophosphatidylcholine and bovine serum albumin on acylation.

(13,21).   A cytoplasmic phospholipase might be expected to have access to all phospholipids on the cytoplasmic side of cell membranes.

Acylation

The effects of ATP + MgCl$_2$, CoA, 1-acyl-sn-glycero-3-phosphoryl-choline (LPC) and bovine serum albumin on the acylation of LPC by guinea pig brain, are shown in Fig. 4.

Under the experimental conditions used maximum rates of acylation were obtained with 10 mM ATP, 20 mM $MgCl_2$ and 10-20 μM CoA. Acylation was greatly stimulated by added LPC as found for rat brain microsomes by Baker and Thompson (3). This indicated that the acylating power of the tissue was more than sufficient to acylate endogenous LPC. Moreover it indicated that experiments in which lysophospholipid is not added give results which reflect the concentration of endogenous lysophospholipid, and therefore previous phospholipase A activity, rather than acylating potential of the tissue. Albumin was used to complex the fatty acid (0.1 μmol fatty acid/mg albumin), but acylation was relatively insensitive to the concentration of albumin. Using optimum concentrations of substrates and cofactors, acylation increased linearly with time for 20 min and approximately linearly with enzyme concentration up to a concentration of 1.5 mg protein/ml. The apparent K_m values for fatty acid for the microsomal and homogenate-particulate fractions were 51 μM and 58 μM, respectively.

All subcellular fractions acylated LPC. Fractions were characterized by enzyme markers. Since acylation was only carried out by particulate fractions, specific activities for acylation and enzyme markers were expressed relative to that of homogenate particulate from which the supernatant fraction had been removed. The relative specific activities (RSAs) for acylation with oleate of fractions are plotted against the RSAs of enzyme markers in Fig. 5. Acylation correlated with NADPH-cytochrome c reductase (Fig. 5a). For the microsomal fraction the RSA for both acylation and NADPH-cytochrome c reductase was 2.2. NADPH-cytochrome c reductase is located in the endoplasmic reticulum (18,23,24). Interest centers on whether the plasma membrane, including the synaptic plasma membrane, is capable of acylating phospholipids. The synaptic plasma membrane is of particular interest in view of its role in synaptic transmission. It was isolated by the procedure of Sun et al. (26) following osmotic lysis of synaptosomes in alkaline buffer (7). The plasma membrane marker, Na^+/K^+ activated ATPase, was concentrated 4.5 times in this fraction but the RSA for acylation was only 0.5 (Fig. 5d). When all the subcellular fractions are considered there was no correlation between acylation and Na^+/K^+ activated ATPase. Likewise there was no correlation between acylation and acetylcholinesterase (Fig. 5c) or succinate dehydrogenase (not shown). The correlation between acylation and 5-nucleotidase (Fig. 5b), an enzyme considered to be a marker for plasma membrane in liver, was poor (correlation coefficient = 0.47; P<0.05).

These experiments indicated that, with respect to oleate and lysophosphatidylcholine, and within the sensitivity of the measurements, acylation was wholly attributable to the endoplasmic reticulum. Acylation by subcellular fractions other than the microsomal fraction was due to microsomal contamination. This conclusion was tested further by adding increasing amounts of microsomes to non-microsomal fractions and determining the changes in the ratio of acylation to NADPH-cytochrome c reductase. If the acylation by a particular fraction had been entirely due to microsomal contamination the ratio should be equal to that of the microsomal fraction and independent of the amount of microsomes added. If on the other hand, the fraction itself had intrinsic acylating activity the ratio should be higher than that of the microsomal fraction, but decline asymptotically to it as microsomes were added in increasing

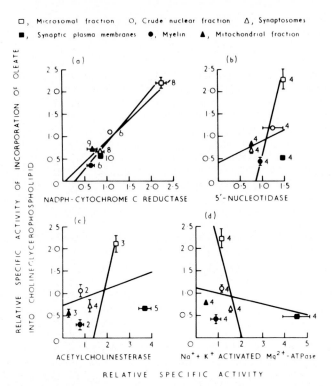

Fig. 5. Comparison of acylation of lysophosphatidylcholine by sub-cellular fractions of guinea pig brain cerebral cortex with the activities of enzyme markers. Results shown are means of determinations from independent fractionations (numbers as shown) of brain homogenate. Lines drawn are calculated regression lines. The lengths of the horizontal and vertical bars through experimental points indicate SEMs.

amount. Such plots are shown in Fig. 6. No fraction had a ratio greater than that of the microsomal fraction and thus there was no evidence of acylating activity independent of microsomal contamination.

Subcellular distributions of three other enzymes, namely acyl-CoA synthetase (fatty acid:CoA ligase EC 6.2.1.3), acyl-CoA:1-acyl-sn-glycero-3-phosphorylcholine (lysophosphatidylcholine) acyl transferase (EC 2.3.1.23) and acyl-CoA hydrolase (EC 3.1.2.2) were determined using optimum concentrations of $[1-^{14}C]$- or $[9,10^3H]$-oleate or $[1-^{14}C]$-palmitate, ATP plus $MgCl_2$, CoA and bovine serum albumin (12). With the microsomal fraction the K_m values for oleate and ATP were 45 µM and 7.1 mM, respectively. The corresponding values for unfractionated homogenate-particulate were 24 µM (fatty acid) and 1.8 mM (ATP). Formation of acyl-CoA increased linearly with time for 5 min and with tissue up to a conc of 0.4 mg protein/ml. Acyl-CoA synthetase was found in all subcellular fractions, the highest activities being in the microsomal and the mitochondrial fractions. The relative activity in the mitochondrial fraction was higher than that reported by Murphy and Spence (20). The subcellular distributions obtained using oleate and palmitate were the same confirming the conclusion of Marcel and Suzue (17) with liver that acyl-CoA synthetase is relatively non-specific for long chain fatty acids. From Fig. 7 it is clear that the mitochondrial fraction had acylating activity independent of microsomal contamination.

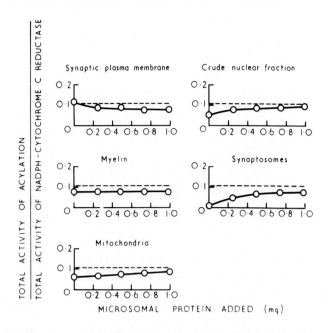

Fig. 6. Effect of the addition of microsomal fraction on the ratio of acylation to NADPH-cytochrome c reductase. Acylation was measured directly. NADPH-cytochrome c reductase was calculated from the specific activities and protein contents of microsomes and fractions respectively. Dotted line indicates ratio for the microsomal fraction.

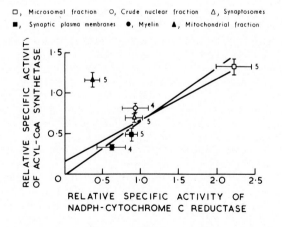

Fig. 7. Comparison of acyl-CoA synthetase with the activity of NADPH-cytochrome c reductase in subcellular fractions of guinea pig cerebral cortex. Lines, bars and numbers are as indicated for Fig. 5.

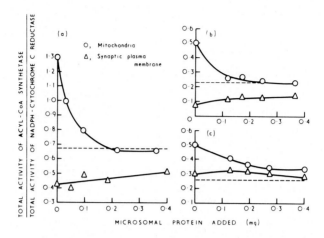

Fig. 8.   Effect of the addition of microsomal fraction on the ratio of
acyl-CoA synthetase to NADPH-cytochrome c reductase of the mitochondrial
fraction and synaptic plasma membranes.   Acyl-CoA synthetase was determined   directly.   Values   for   NADPH-cytochrome   c   reductase   were
calculated. Dotted line indicates ratio for the microsomal fraction.
Acyl-CoA synthetase was determined using [1-^{14}C]palmitate, (a); or
[9,10-^{3}H]oleate, (b) and (c).

The activities of the other subcellular fractions correlated with the
activities of NADPH-cytochrome c reductase (correlation coefficient =
0.88; P<0.001).   The effects of the addition of microsomes on the ratio
of acyl-CoA synthetase to NADPH-cytochrome c reductase of the mitochondrial fraction and synaptic plasma membranes, respectively, are
shown in Fig. 8.   Acyl-CoA synthetase activity in the mitochondria is
confirmed.   There is no evidence for acyl-CoA synthetase in the synaptic
plasma membranes.
        Acyl-CoA: lysophosphatidylcholine acyl transferase was determined
using optimum concentrations of lysophosphatidylcholine, [9,10-^{3}H]-
oleoyl-CoA, and albumin (12).   Acyl transfer increased linearly with
time for 20 min after which 20% of the oleate had been transferred.   The
correlation between acyl-CoA: lysophosphatidylcholine acyl tranferase
and NADPH-cytochrome c reductase is shown in Fig. 9.   The RSAs for
transferase and reductase for the microsomal fraction were 1.90 and
2.06, respectively, and the correlation coefficient was 0.93 (P<0.001).
This correlation agrees with the results obtained by Pik and Thompson
(22) who, using linoleoyl-CoA, concluded that lysophosphatidylcholine
acyl transferase cofractionated with NADPH-cytochrome c reductase on
subfractionation of rat brain.   Using arachidonoyl-CoA, Pik and Thompson
(22) obtained the same result for acyl transfer to lysophosphatidylinositol.
        Acyl-CoA hydrolase was found in the soluble cytosol as reported
previously (1,5).   Subcellular distribution of acyl-CoA hydrolase, determined from the hydrolysis of oleoyl-CoA or palmitoyl-CoA, correlated
with that of lactate dehydrogenase, a marker for soluble cytoplasm, as
shown in Fig. 10.   Thus hydrolase activity in particulate fractions was
due to contamination by soluble cytoplasm.   Under the conditons used for
the determination of acyl transfer, hydrolase activity of the microsomal
fraction was inhibited 81% by the albumin present.

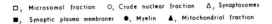

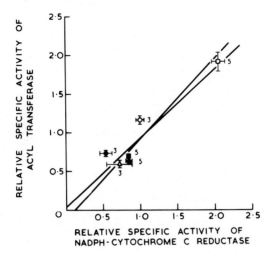

Fig. 9. Comparison of acyl-CoA:lysophosphatidylcholine acyl transferase and NADPH-cytochrome c reductase in subcellular fractions of guinea pig cerebral cortex.

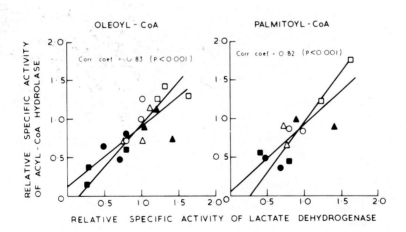

Fig. 10. Comparison of acyl-CoA hydrolase and lactate dehydrogenase of particulate subcellular fractions of guinea pig cerebral cortex. □, Microsomal fraction; ○, crude nuclear fraction; Δ, synaptosomes; ■, synaptic plasma membranes; ●, myelin; ▲, mitochondrial fraction.

TABLE 2. Comparison of acyl CoA synthetase and acyl transferase, respectively, with acylation

Tissue fraction	Acyl-CoA:lysophosphatidyl-choline acyl transferase Acylation	Acyl-CoA synthetase Acylation
Microsomes	1.1 ± 0.1 (5)	2.6 ± 0.1 (6)
Mitochondria	0.97± 0.14 (5)	8.0 ± 0.8 (6)

Values are means ± SEM. Acyl transferase was determined under the same conditions as acylation except that ATP, MgCl$_2$ and CoA were omitted and fatty acid was replaced by [9,10-^{3}H]oleoyl-CoA. Acyl-CoA synthetase was determined under the same conditions as acylation except that lysophosphatidylcholine was omitted (12).

A comparison of the rates of synthesis of acyl-CoA, and of acyl transfer, with the rates of acylation by the microsomal and mitochondrial fractions is shown in Table 2. Rates of acyl transfer and acylation are the same. This is consistent with acyl transfer being the rate-determining step in acylation, a conclusion contrary to that suggested by Murphy and Spence (19). With the microsomes the rate of synthesis of acyl-CoA was 2.6 times the rate of acylation. The high ratio of acyl-CoA synthetase to acylation of the mitochondrial fraction reflects the presence of synthetase unconnected with acylation, the latter being solely due to microsomal contamination.

The conclusions from the experiments with brain are that, within the limits of the sensitivity of the experiments described, only the microsomal fraction contained both enzymes necessary to acylate lysophosphatidylcholine. The mitochondrial fraction contained acyl-CoA synthetase but lacked the lysophosphatidylcholine acyl transferase necessary for acylation. There was no evidence for acylation by the plasma membrane, which lacked both of the essential enzymes.

TABLE 3. Correlation of acylation, acyl-CoA synthetase and acyl CoA: 1-acyl-sn-glycero-3-phosphorylcholine acyl transferase, with NADPH-cytochrome c reductase (10)

Activity	Correlation coefficient*	Slope	Intercept
Acylation of lysophosphatidylcholine	0.88[+]	0.15	0.01
Acyl-CoA synthetase	0.88[+]	0.30	-0.06
Acyl-CoA:1-acyl-sn-glycero-3-phosphoryl-choline acyl transferase	0.87[+]	0.39	-0.16
Acyl-CoA hydrolase	0.42NS	2.6	12.13

Values for the slope and intercept refer to the calculated regression line obtained from plotting acylation or enzymic activity against activity of NADPH-cytochrome c reductase.
*Values are calculated from paired data obtained from the same tissue.
[+]Correlation is significant, P<0.001. NS, Correlation is not significant. Acylation, acyl-CoA synthetase and acyl-CoA:LPC acyl transferase, but not acyl-CoA hydrolase correlated with NADPH-cytochrome c reductase.

The conclusion that acylation was wholly due to the endoplasmic reticulum was tested further by comparing brain, superior cervical ganglion, vagus nerve and sciatic nerve of rat. The nerves would be expected to contain few mitochondria and no synapses. The ratio of plasma membrane to endoplasmic reticulum is high, thus any contribution of the plasma membrane to acylation would be more easily detectable than in brain. The results are shown in Table 3.

Since phospholipase A_1 is present in the microsomal fraction the endoplasmic reticulum contains all the enzymes required for the deacylation-acylation cycle. For the cycle to operate with phosphatidylcholine and oleate in the mitochondria and plasma membrane, respectively, lipid intermediates must be transported to the endoplasmic reticulum. Modified phosphatidylcholine would have to be transported back to complete the cycle.

Blood plasma contains LPC which is formed by the cholesterol phosphatidylcholine acyl transferase in plasma. Illingworth and Portman (15), using doubly labelled radioactive LPC, demonstrated that in the squirrel monkey plasma LPC is acylated in the brain to form phosphatidylcholine. Plasma fatty acids are rapidly incorporated into phospholipids, including phosphatidylcholine, of rat brain (8,9). Thus endoplasmic reticulum of brain can synthesize phosphatidylcholine directly from plasma lipids which are derived from the diet.

ACKNOWLEDGEMENTS

Thanks are due to Miss Susan Hinks for skilled technical assistance. We are grateful to the Medical Research Council of Great Britain, which supported this work with two project grants. We thank Elsevier/North-Holland Biomedical Press for permission to reproduce Figs. 2 and 3 and Table 1, and the International Society for Neurochemistry Ltd. for permission to reproduce Table 3.

REFERENCES

1. Anderson, A.D. and Erwin, V.G. (1971): J. Neurochem., 18:1179-1186.
2. Bangham, A.D. (1968): Progr. Biophys. Mol. Biol., 18:29-95.
3. Baker, R.R. and Thompson, W. (1973): J. Biol. Chem., 248:7060-7065.
4. Bazán, N.G. (1971): Acta. Physiol. Latinoam., 21:101-106.
5. Bonser, R.W. and Lunt, G.G. (1976) Biochem. Soc. Trans., 4:321-324.
6. Cooper, M.F. and Webster, G.R. (1970): J. Neurochem., 17:1543-1554.
7. Cotman, C.W. and Matthews, D.A. (1971): Biochim. Biophys. Acta, 249:380-394.
8. Dhopeshwarkar, G.A. and Mead, J.F. (1970): Biochim. Biophys. Acta, 210:250-256.
9. Dhopeshwarkar, G.A., Subramanian, C., McConnell, D.H. and Mead, J.F. (1972): Biochim. Biophys. Acta, 255:572-579.
10. Doherty, F.J. and Rowe, C.E. (1979): J. Neurochem., 33:819-822.
11. Doherty, F.J. and Rowe, C.E. (1980): Brain Res., 197:113-122.
12. Fisher, S.K. and Rowe, C.E. (1980): Biochim. Biophys. Acta, 618:231-241.
13. Fontaine, R.N., Harris, R.A. and Schroeder, F. (1980): J. Neurochem., 34:269-277.
14. Gatt, S. (1968): Biochim. Biophys. Acta, 159:304-316.
15. Illingworth, D.R. and Portman, O.W. (1972): Biochem. J., 130:557-567.

16. Lands, W.E.M. (1960): J. Biol. Chem., 235:2233-2237.
17. Marcel, Y.L. and Suzue, G. (1972): J. Biol. Chem., 247:4433-4436.
18. Miller, E.K. and Dawson, R.M.C. (1972): Biochem. J., 126:805-821.
19. Murphy, M.G. and Spence, M.W. (1977): J. Neurochem., 29:251-259.
20. Murphy, M.G. and Spence, M.W. (1980): J. Neurochem., 34:367-373.
21. Op den Kamp, J.A.F. (1979): Ann. Rev. Biochem., 48:47-71.
22. Pik, J.R. and Thompson, W. (1978): Canad. J. Biochem., 56:765-768.
23. Possmayer, F., Meiners, B. and Mudd, J.B. (1973): Biochem. J., 132:381-394.
24. Possmayer, F., Kleine, L., Duwe, G., Stewart-DeHaan, P.J., Wong, T., MacPherson, C.F.C. and Hardin, P.G.R. (1979): J. Neurochem., 32:889-906.
25. Rooke, J.A. and Webster, G.R. (1976): J. Neurochem., 27:613-620.
26. Sun, A.Y., Sun, G.Y. and Samorajski, T. (1971): J. Neurochem., 18:1711-1718.
27. Webster, G.R. and Alpern, R.J. (1964): Biochem. J., 90:35-42.
28. Woelk, H. and Porcellati, G. (1973): Hoppe-Seyler's Z. Physiol. Chem., 354:90-100.
29. Woelk, H., Peiler-Ichikawa, K., Binaglia, L., Goracci, G. and Porcellati, G. (1974): Hoppe-Seyler's Z. Physiol. Chem. 355:1535-1542.
30. Woelk, H., Porcellati, G. and Gaiti, A. (1979): Neurochem. Res., 4:535-543.
31. Woelk, H., Rubly, N., Arienti, G., Gaiti, A. and Porcellati, G. (1981): J. Neurochem., 36:875-880.

Phospholipids in the Nervous System, Vol. 1: Metabolism, edited by L. Horrocks, et al. Raven Press, New York © 1982.

Metabolic Turnover of Arachidonoyl Groups in Brain Membrane Phosphoglycerides

Grace Y. Sun

Sinclair Comparative Medicine Research Farm and Biochemistry Department, University of Missouri, Columbia, Missouri 65201

Regulation of membrane phosphoglyceride metabolism is governed by many factors involving complex enzymic reactions (51). Not only are different types of phosphoglycerides associated with different modes of metabolic turnover within the membrane, but different parts of the phosphoglyceride molecules may also undergo distinctive metabolic profiles. Thus, an evaluation of the metabolic turnover of these phosphoglycerides may depend on the type of precursors used and the subcellular membranes isolated for the analysis (21,34). The acyl groups of phosphoglycerides are important in providing a suitable micro-environment for proper functioning of the membranes (42). In addition, some of the polyunsaturated fatty acids (PUFA) released from the phosphoglycerides can serve as precursors for prostaglandin biosynthesis. It is the purpose of this review to discuss the enzymic mechanisms which may be important in regulating the turnover of arachidonoyl groups of membrane phosphoglycerides in brain.

IN VIVO METABOLISM OF THE PHOSPHOGLYCERIDE ACYL GROUPS IN BRAIN

From results of previous *in vivo* studies in which labeled fatty acids were injected intracerebrally into mouse brain, it became evident that long chain fatty acids are readily taken up by the brain tissue and are subsequently incorporated into the membrane phosphoglycerides (46). The rate of arachidonate uptake, however, is usually more rapid than that of the saturated fatty acids (44,47). Arachidonic acid was preferentially incorporated into diacyl-glycerophosphoinositols (GPI) and diacyl-glycerophosphocholines (GPC) in both microsomal and synaptosomal fractions (50). A dynamic equilibrium between the free arachidonic acid and those esterified to the phosphoglycerides was established within one hour after intracerebral injection of the labeled precursor (61). The *in vivo* pulse-labeling technique was subsequently used for studying acyl group turnover among various membrane phos-

phoglycerides (43,47,49). The results of one study revealed
the presence of distinct patterns for metabolism of various
arachidonoyl-labeled phosphoglycerides in brain (49). In
general, turnover of arachidonoyl-GPI in the brain membranes
was more rapid than other types of phosphoglycerides. Within
each membrane fraction, the presence of two metabolic pools
was observed: a small pool with a more rapid turnover rate
giving half-life in hours and a larger pool with half-life in
days.

The rapid metabolic turnover of arachidonoyl-GPI in brain
membranes suggests a role for this phosphoglyceride in membrane functions. Although this phospholipid comprises only
4-5% of the total phosphoglycerides in brain, its acyl group
composition is highly enriched in the stearoyl-arachidonoyl
species (41). Arachidonate metabolism in brain is correlated
to factors or agents affecting neuronal activity. Thus, a
decrease in arachidonate uptake by brain synaptosomes (but
not by the microsomes) was observed in mice after stimulation
due to injection of carbamylcholine (40). The decrease in
uptake activity was attributed to an increase in endogenous
arachidonate which was liberated during stimulation. Under
the stimulated condition, there was a specific decrease in
arachidonate incorporation into diacyl-GPI which was marked
by a concomitant increase in labeling of the diacylglycerols
(DG) and triacylglycerols (40). Similar results were obtained in another study in which young rats were made convul-
sive due to acute hypoxic treatment (39). Although the
results of these in vivo studies suggest a metabolic role for
arachidonoyl-GPI in neuronal membrane function, the biochemical mechanism underlying these changes remains to be
elucidated.

DEGRADATION OF MEMBRANE PHOSPHOGLYCERIDES

In order to understand the various factors affecting membrane phosphoglyceride metabolism, it is necessary to examine
the enzymes involved in each metabolic process. A stimulated
degradation of the membrane phosphoglycerides may be the
initial response associated with membrane phosphoglyceride
turnover. This degradative event can be mediated by any one
of the following enzymic systems:

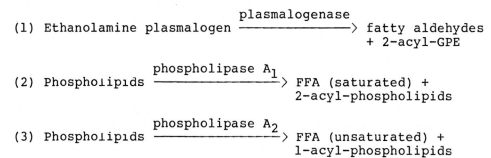

(1) Ethanolamine plasmalogen $\xrightarrow{\text{plasmalogenase}}$ fatty aldehydes + 2-acyl-GPE

(2) Phospholipids $\xrightarrow{\text{phospholipase A}_1}$ FFA (saturated) + 2-acyl-phospholipids

(3) Phospholipids $\xrightarrow{\text{phospholipase A}_2}$ FFA (unsaturated) + 1-acyl-phospholipids

```
                  phospholipase C      diglyceride lipase
(4) Diacyl-GPI ──────────────────> DG ──────────────────> FFA
```

The lysophospholipids resulting from the above reactions may be further degraded by lysophospholipases yielding more FFA:

```
                        lysophospholipase
(5) Lysophospholipids ────────────────────>  FFA  +  glycero-
                                                     phospho-base
```

A number of factors are known to regulate these enzymic processes.   Among them, agents which affect the micro-environment of the membranes are important for consideration because most of the enzymes as well as substrates are localized within the membrane. The lysophospholipids are known for their detergent properties; therefore, an accumulation may lead to alteration of other membrane functions (55). Some of the enzymes are stimulated by Ca^{++}; however, a direct involvement of the enzymes in the neuronal Ca^{++} flux mechanism remains to be elucidated.

DEGRADATION OF ETHANOLAMINE PLASMALOGENS

From results of <u>in vivo</u> studies, it is evident that the turnover of arachidonoyl group of ethanolamine plasmalogen is slower than that in its diacyl counterpart (49,61).   The slower rate of uptake is probably due to the absence of an active lysophospholipid acyltransferase system for this type of molecule (9).   The slow rate of decay may be attributed to the fact that plasmalogens are poor substrates for phospholipase A_2 (59).   Consequently, turnover of the acyl groups in plasmalogens would depend on prior hydrolysis of the alkenyl-ether side chain via plasmalogenase followed by lysophospholipase (19). Activity of the plasmalogenase in brain is apparently maintained at a low level under normal conditions and becomes elevated only in pathological conditions such as in canine distemper (13) and demyelinating human white matter (20). Degradation of plasmalogens is frequently marked by a concomitant release of PUFA, suggesting that an active lysophospholipase is present in the tissue for further degradation of the lysophospholipids.

HYDROLYSIS OF PHOSPHOGLYCERIDE ACYL GROUPS BY PHOSPHOLIPASES A_1 AND A_2

Phospholipases A_1 and A_2 are membrane-bound enzymes present ubiquitously in brain as well as in other body organs. In the rat brain, phospholipase A_1 is predominantly localized in the microsomal fraction, whereas phospholipase A_2 is largely found in the mitochondrial fraction (14). Some of the phospholipases in brain exhibit activity at more than one pH. In synaptosomes, the pH 8.4 phospholipase A_2 is localized mainly in the mitochondrial membranes, whereas the pH 4.8

enzyme is found in the synaptic vesicles (58). Other than the
fact that ethanolamine plasmalogen is a poor substrate for
phospholipase A_2 (59), the specificity of different phospholipases towards individual membrane phospholipids has not
been investigated in detail. Most in vitro assay systems for
the phospholipases require labeled phospholipids as substrates which are added exogenously to the incubation mixture. Detergents are also added to facilitate interaction of
the enzyme with the substrates. In the presence of detergents, however, a successful demonstration of an involvement
of the enzymic action in neuronal membrane functions may be
difficult. Recently, a system was developed in which phosphoglycerides (mainly diacyl-GPC and diacyl-GPI) in synaptosomes were prelabeled with arachidonoyl groups (29). Using
the prelabeled synaptosomes, we have shown that some arachi-
donoyl-phosphoglycerides are responsive to degradation due to
depolarization by high K^+ (Fig 1). The degradation of membrane phospholipids was calcium-dependent, and the stimulated
degradation of diacyl-GPI was twice as responsive as the
diacyl-GPC. In a different experiment, the arachidonoyl-
labeled synaptosomes were superfused with a Krebs-Ringer-
bicarbonate buffer containing serum albumin. Upon depolarization of the synaptosomes with 50 mM of K^+, a calcium-
dependent increase in arachidonate release was observed (Fig
2). However, the amount of arachidonate released constituted
only a very small portion of the total radioactive pool in
the fraction.

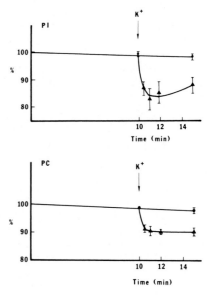

FIG. 1. Degradation of arachidonoyl-labeled diacyl-GPC
and diacyl-GPI in brain synaptosomes with respect to K^+-
depolarization (Majewska and
Sun, unpublished data).

FIG. 2. Calcium-dependent release of arachidonate from prelabeled synaptosomes due to K^+-depolarization. BSA was added to the superfusion medium (Lazarewicz et al., unpublished data).

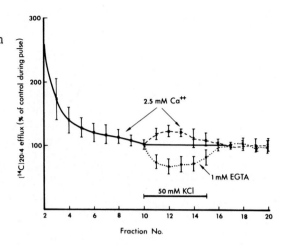

METABOLIC TURNOVER OF THE ARACHIDONOYL GROUPS OF DIACYL-GPI

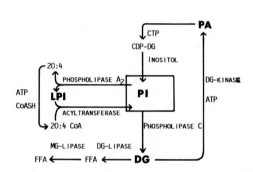

FIG. 3.
A scheme depicting the enzymic pathways for diacyl-GPI metabolism.

Since in vivo studies indicate that the arachidonoyl group of diacyl-GPI in brain membranes is more active than in other phosphoglycerides, recent in vitro experiments are directed mainly towards studying the enzymes responsible for diacyl-GPI metabolism. As shown in Fig. 3, biosynthesis of diacyl-GPI is derived from two enzymic routes: [1] via the de novo pathway through conversion of phosphatidic acids to CDP-diacylglycerols (7), and [2] via acylation of 1-acyl-GPI (3,9). Similarly, degradation of diacyl-GPI may also be mediated by two enzymic routes: [1] via phospholipase A_1 or A_2 hydrolysis, and [2] via the diacyl-GPI-specific phospholipase C action. Thus, the arachidonoyl groups of diacyl-GPI may be released directly by phospholipase A_2 action (although this enzyme is not specific for diacyl-GPI) or indirectly via a sequential hydrolysis by phospholipase C and diacylglycerol lipase. In some non-neural tissues, arachidonic acid released as a result of diacyl-GPI breakdown has been correlated with an increase in prostaglandin biosynthesis (6).

The newly synthesized prostaglandins may, in turn, play a role in the stimulus-secretion coupling process (31).

Although studies regarding metabolism of the polar head group of diacyl-GPI and its stimulated turnover by neurotransmitter substances, hormones and receptor agonists have been described in detail (16,17,18,32,33), the mechanism regulating the turnover of the arachidonoyl groups of diacyl-GPI in brain has not been investigated extensively. We have recently examined the enzymic degradation of diacyl-GPI by brain synaptosomes using arachidonoyl-labeled diacyl-GPI as substrate (11). Very little diacyl-GPI were degraded if synaptosomes were incubated with the substrate in the absence of deoxycholate. The presence of deoxycholate, however, specifically enhanced the phospholipase C activity but not the phospholipase A_2 activity. A similar study carried out by Shum et al. (38) also indicated that aside from phospholipase C, a large portion of the diacyl-GPI was also degraded by the phospholipases A_1 and A_2 in brain microsomes.

Stimulation of diacyl-GPI turnover by neurotransmitter substances is an event normally observed only with intact tissues (32). It is likely that the phospholipase C responsible for this process is dependent on membrane integrity for full expression of its physiological functions. In spite of this, the subcellular distribution of the phospholipase C in brain has not been defined. The enzyme is found in the soluble as well as the membrane fractions (1,23). In a study with brain synaptosomes, we observed differences in detergent requirement for activating the membrane enzyme as compared to the cytosolic enzyme (30). Using synaptosomes prelabeled with arachidonoyl-GPI, an attempt was made to study the factors involved in regulating the phospholipase C in brain synaptosomes (30). We found a complex relationship between the detergent concentration and enzymic activity (Fig. 4). In addition, phospholipase C activity was also activated by taurocholate (4mg/ml), but only in the presence of Ca^{++} (3.5mM) and EDTA (1mM). A number of lipophilic compounds are known to either suppress or stimulate diacyl-GPI hydrolysis by the soluble phospholipase C in brain (24,25). Testing the synaptosomes with some of these compounds indicated obvious differences in response between enzymes in the cytosolic and synaptosomal fractions (30). Unlike the soluble enzyme, phospholipase C in synaptosomes was also inhibited by a number of divalent cations other than Ca^{++}. As shown in Fig 5, complete inhibition of the synaptosomal phospholipase C (as assayed in the presence of deoxycholate and Ca^{++}) was achieved by adding 50 uM of Zn^{++} or Cu^{++} to the incubation medium.

FFA RELEASE FROM BRAIN

A rapid increase in brain FFA level is known to occur under various conditions including electroconvulsive shock and ischemia induced by post-decapitation and ligation (4,10). The release of arachidonate from brain during early

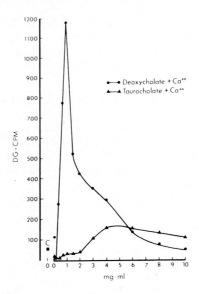

FIG. 4. Effect of detergents on DG release from synaptosomes prelabeled with arachidonoyl-GPI (30).

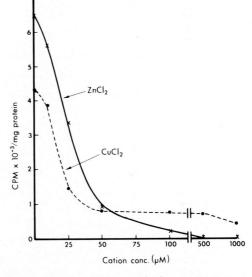

FIG. 5. Effect of Cu^{++} and Zn^{++} on PI-specific phospholipase C activity in brain synaptosomes (Manning and Sun, unpublished data).

onset of ischemia was thought to correlate with membrane permeability changes which could subsequently lead to further cellular damage and edema (5). In conjunction with the increase in FFA, there was a decrease in the PUFA content of diacyl-GPC and diacyl-GPE in rat brain synaptosomes due to ischemia induced by decapitation (48). An attempt to assay for phospholipase A_2 in brain synaptosomes, however, indicated only a slight increase in activity in the samples obtained at one min after the ischemic treatment (12,29). Apparently, successful demonstration of an involvement of the phospholipases in brain ischemia may also depend on membrane integrity. Analysis of the brain FFA released during ischemia revealed a biphasic mode of increase for both 18:0 and 20:4 with respect to time of the ischemic treatment (Fig 6). Interestingly, the endogenous level of 18:0 and 20:4 in brain was also altered after administration of psychoactive drugs, ethanol and anesthetic compounds (52). Barbiturate anesthesia (but not Ketamine) inhibited slightly the initial phase of the 18:0-20:4 increase after decapitation (Fig. 7).

LYSOPHOSPHOLIPIDS

Except for a demonstration of their presence (53,54), little is known about the lysophospholipids in brain. Analysis of the acyl group composition of lysophospholipids in tissue may yield useful information regarding the mode of

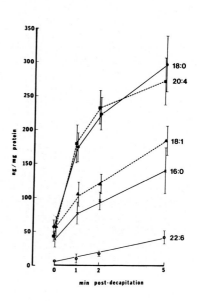

FIG. 6. FFA release from rat brain due to post-decapitative ischemia (52).

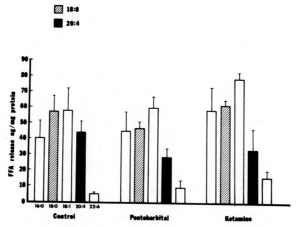

FIG. 7. Effect of pentobarbital, Ketamine on FFA level in rat brain (52).

phospholipases A_1 and A_2 action. Results of one study revealed that the lyso-GPC in normal brain tissue contain
mainly 16:0, 18:0 and 18:1, with only trace amounts of 20:4
and 22:6 (Fig. 8). In spite of the dramatic increase in FFA
during ischemia and brain stimulation, a parallel increase of
the lyso-GPC level was not observed. This observation together with the extremely low level of the lysophospholipids
present in brain tissue suggests that these compounds are
rapidly turning over. Two enzymic routes are known to be
responsible to their catabolism: [1] via degradation by lysophospholipases, and [2] by conversion to the respective
diacyl-phosphoglycerides via the lysophospholipid acyltransferase. Removal of the lysophospholipids by lysophospholipase would lead to complete degradation of the membrane
phospholipids. Lysophospholipases are present widely in
organs and tissues (26), although their biochemical action in
brain has not been correlated to physiological functions. In
a recent study by Pendley et al. (35), a lysophospholipase in
brain white matter was co-purified with a diglyceride lipase.
We have also obtained evidence for an active lysophospholipase with wide substrate specificity in brain synaptosomes
(Fig. 9).

FATTY ACID UPTAKE BY MEMBRANE PHOSPHOLIPIDS

$$\text{FFA + CoASH + ATP} \xrightarrow{\text{ligase}} \text{acyl-CoA + AMP}$$

$$\text{l-acyl-phospholipids + acyl-CoA} \xrightarrow{\text{acyltransferase}} \text{phospholipids}$$

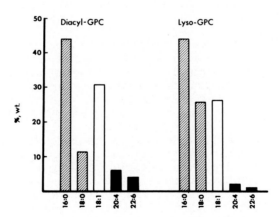

FIG. 8. Fatty acid profile of
diacyl-GPC and lyso-GPC in
rat brain (Hallett and Sun,
unpublished data).

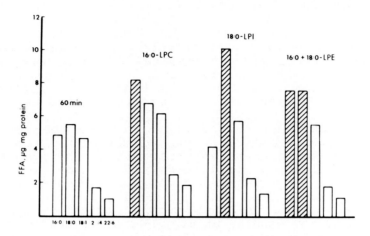

FIG. 9. Evidence for 1-acyl-lysophospholipase in brain synaptosomes. LPC: 1-16:0-GPC, LPI: 1-18:0-GPI, LPE: 1-16:0, 18:0-GPE (Huang and Sun, unpublished data).

FFA are activated to their acyl-CoA via the ATP-dependent fatty acid:CoASH ligase prior to being utilized by various acyltransferases. In the ischemic brain tissue, a decrease in activity of the fatty acid ligase may occur due to a decrease in ATP level. However, since ATP is normally not completely depleted during the initial stage of the ischemic treatment, the decrease in ligase activity can only account for the increase in FFA pool during the latter stage of the event.

The level of acyl-CoA in tissue is normally maintained at a low level because a number of the membrane transport functions, including mitochondrial adenosine nucleotide translocation and membrane ion transport mechanisms are known to be affected by this compound (2,28,60). An elevation of the acyl-CoA level in heart was correlated to myocardial ischemia and anoxia (22,37,56). However, whether this same phenomenon is occurring in brain remains to be confirmed. Recently, we obtained evidence that the fatty acid:CoASH ligase in brain microsomes is coupled to the lysophospholipid acyltransferase (Fig. 10). Thus, upon addition of 1-acyl-GPC or 1-acyl-GPI to the incubation system, there was a marked increase in the conversion of FFA to acyl-CoA which was subsequently transferred to the lysophospholipids to form the corresponding diacyl compounds. This coupling mechanism is highly desirable because it provides an intricate system for regulating the level of acyl-CoA as well as lysophospholipids within the membrane.

The phospholipase A_2-mediated deacylation coupled with lysophospholipid acyltransferase is a mechanism through which the unsaturated acyl groups of membrane phosphoglycerides can undergo specific turnover (27). Although the lysophospholipid acyltransferase in brain is present largely in the microsomal fraction, some enzyme activity is also found in the synaptosomal membranes (9). This type of enzyme tends to show great specificity towards the acyl donors as well as the lysophospholipid acceptors, and arachidonoyl group is preferentially transferred to 1-acyl-GPI and 1-acyl-GPC (3,9). Part of the substrate specificity may be due to the fact that the enzymic action is mediated through a "ping pong"-like mechanism (57). A number of detergents, psychoactive drugs, and membrane active compounds are potent inhibitors of the enzyme (15,36,45).

On account of the membrane-dependent properties of the acyltransferases, uptake of fatty acids by membrane phospholipids through this pathway is found to be regulated by a number of factors including tissue homogenization, subcellular fractionation and in vitro aging of membranes at elevated temperature (Foudin et al., unpublished data). Although the exact mechanism for the inhibitory effects is not known, there is some evidence that generation of free radicals due to peroxidation of the membrane PUFA may be involved. Thus, removing the endogenous FFA by washing the synaptosomes with serum albumin resulted in an enhancement of the acylation activity (Fig 11). Surprisingly, this enhancement of acylation activity due to the BSA-washing was preferential for incorporation of the labeled arachidonate into diacyl-GPI but not diacyl-GPC. The results suggest a difference in the

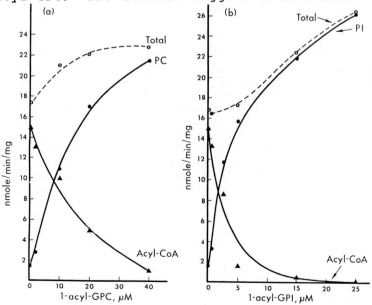

FIG. 10. Evidence for the coupling action between fatty acid: CoASH ligase and the lysophospholipids acyltransferase (Tang and Sun, unpublished data).

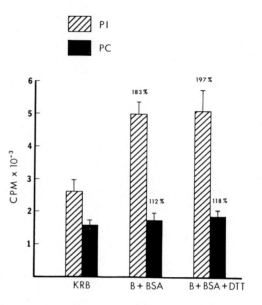

FIG. 11. Effect of BSA and BSA + dithiothreitol (DTT) washing of brain synaptosomes on arachidonate incorporation into diacyl-GPI and diacyl-GPC (Foudin et al., unpublished data).

acylation process between the two types of lysophospholipids in synaptosomes. The mechanism underlying this intriguing phenomenon is currently being investigated.

SUMMARY

It is well recognized that the acyl groups of phospholipids in brain play an important role in regulating neuronal functions (42). Metabolic turnover of these acyl groups, however, is mediated through multiple enzymic processes. In brain, arachidonoyl groups of diacyl-GPI are metabolically more active than in other phosphoglycerides. A dynamic equilibrium exists between the FFA and the acyl groups esterified to the membrane phospholipids. This equilibrium can be disturbed easily by factors such as brain stimulation, hypoxia and ischemia. Information regarding the biochemical mechanisms underlying the disturbances will be useful towards understanding the metabolic turnover of the acyl groups in membrane phospholipids.

ACKNOWLEDGMENT

Thanks to Dr. L. Foudin and to D. Torres for assistance in preparation of the manuscript. This research program is supported in part by grants NS-12960 from National Institutes of Health and BNS-79-04754 from National Science Foundation.

REFERENCES

1. Abdel-Latif, A.A., Luke, B., and Smith, J.P. (1980): *Biochim. Biophys. Acta*, 614:425-434.
2. Asimakis, G.K. and Sordahl, L.A. (1977): *Arch. Biochem. Biophys.*, 179:200-210.
3. Baker, R.R. and Thompson, N. (1973): *J. Biol. Chem.*, 248:7060-7065.
4. Bazan, N.G. (1976): In: *Function and Metabolism of Phospholipids in Central and Peripheral Nervous System*, edited by G. Porcellati, L. Amaducci, and G. Galli, pp. 317-336. Plenum Press, New York.
5. Bazan, N.G. and Rodriquez de Turco, E.B. (1980): *Adv. Neurol.*, 28:197-205.
6. Bell, R.L., Baenziger, N.C., and Majerus, P.W. (1980): *Prostaglandins*, 20:269-274.
7. Bishop, H.H. and Strickland, K.P. (1976): *Can. J. Biochem.*, 54:249-260.
8. Cooper, M.F. and Webster, G.R. (1970): *J. Neurochem.*, 17:1543-1554.
9. Corbin, D.R. and Sun, G.Y. (1978): *J. Neurochem.*, 30:77-82.
10. DeMedio, G.E., Goracci, G., Horrocks, L.A., Lazarewicz, J.W., Mazzari, S., Porcellati, G., Strosznajder, J., and Trovarelli, G.G. (1981): *Ital. J. Biochem.*, 29:412-432.
11. Der, O.M. and Sun, G.Y. (1981): *J. Neurochem.*, 36:355-362.
12. Edgar, A.D., Strosznajder, J., and Horrocks, L.A. (1980): *Fed. Proc.*, 39:1993.
13. Fu, S.C., Mozzi, R., Krakowka, S., Higgins, R.J., and Horrocks, L.A. (1980): *Acta Neuropathol. (Berl.)*, 49:13-18.
14. Goracci, G., Porcellati, G., and Woelk, H. (1978): In: *Advances in Prostaglandin and Thromboxane Research*, Vol. 3, edited by C. Galli, G. Galli, and G. Porcellati, pp. 77-84. Raven Press, New York.
15. Greenberg, J.H. and Mellors, A. (1978): *Biochem. Pharmacol.*, 27:329-333.
16. Hawthorne, J.N. and Pickard, M.R. (1977): In: *Function and Biosynthesis of Lipids*, edited by N.G. Bazan, R.R. Brenner, and N.M. Giusto, pp. 419-427. Plenum Press, New York.
17. Hawthorne, J.N. and Pickard, M.R. (1979): *J. Neurochem.*, 32:5-14.
18. Hokin-Neaverson, M. (1977): In: *Function and Biosynthesis of Lipids*, edited by N.G. Bazan, R.R. Brenner, and N.M. Giusto, pp. 429-446. Plenum Press, New York.
19. Horrocks, L.A. and Fu, S.C. (1978): In: *Enzymes of Lipid Metabolism*, edited by S. Gatt, L. Freysz, and P. Mandel, pp. 397-406. Plenum Press, New York.
20. Horrocks, L.A., Spanner, S., Mozzi, R., Fu, S.C., D'Amato, R.A., and Krakowka, S. (1978): In: *Myelination and Demyelination*, edited by J. Palo, pp. 423-438. Plenum Press, New York.
21. Horrocks, L.A., Toews, A.D., Thompson, D.K., and Chin, J.Y. (1976): In: *Function and Metabolism of Phospholipids*

in Central and Peripheral Nervous System, edited by G. Porcellati, L. Amaducci, and C. Galli, pp. 37-54. Plenum Press, New York.

22. Idell-Wenger, J.A., Grotyohann, L.W., and Neely, J.R. (1978): J. Biol. Chem., 253:4310-4318.
23. Irvine, R.F. and Dawson, R.M.C. (1978): J. Neurochem., 31:1427-1434.
24. Irvine, R.F., Hemington, N., and Dawson, R.M.C. (1979): Eur. J. Biochem., 99:525-530.
25. Irvine, R.F., Letcher, A.J., and Dawson, R.M.C. (1979): Biochem. J., 178:497-500.
26. deJong, J.G.N., van den Besselaar, A.M.H.P. and van den Bosch, H. (1976): Biochim. Biophys. Acta, 441:221-230.
27. Lands, W.E.M. and Crawford, C.G. (1976): In: The Enzymes of Biological Membranes, edited by A. Martonosi, pp. 3-85. Plenum Press, New York.
28. McMillin-Wood, J. and Bush, B. (1977): Biochem. Biophys. Res. Comm., 74:677-684.
29. Majewska, M.D., Manning, R., and Sun, G.Y. (1981): Neurochem. Res., 6:567-576.
30. Manning, R. (1981): Metabolism of Phosphatidylinositol in Brain, Univ. Missouri, M.S. Thesis.
31. Marshall, P.J., Dixon, J.F., and Hokin, L.E. (1980): Proc. Natl. Acad. Sci., 77:3292-3296.
32. Michell, R.H. (1975): Biochim. Biophys. Acta, 415:81-147.
33. Michell, R.H., Jafferji, S.S., and Jones, L.M. (1979): In: Function and Biosynthesis of Lipids, edited by N.G. Bazan, R.R. Brenner, and N.M. Giusto, pp. 447-463. Plenum Press, New York.
34. Miller, S.L., Benjamins, J.A., and Morell, P. (1977): J. Biol. Chem., 252:4025-4037.
35. Pendley, C., Singh, H. and Cox, J. (1981): Fed. Proc., 40:1708.
36. Shier, W.T. (1977): Biochem. Biophys. Res. Comm., 75:186-193.
37. Shug, A.L., Thomsen, J.H., Folts, J.D., Bittar, N., Klein, M.I., Koke, J.R., and Huth, P.J. (1978): Arch. Biochem. Biophys., 187:25-33.
38. Shum, T.Y.P., Gray, N.C.C., and Strickland, K.P. (1979): Can. J. Biochem., 57:1359-1367.
39. Strosznajder, J. and Sun, G.Y. (1981): Neurochem. Res., (in press).
40. Su, K.L. and Sun, G.Y. (1977): J. Neurochem., 29:1059-1063.
41. Su, K.L. and Sun, G.Y. (1978): J. Neurochem., 31:1043-1047.
42. Sun, A.Y. and Sun, G.Y. (1976): In: Function and Metabolism of Phospholipids in Central and Peripheral Nervous System, edited by G. Porcellati, L. Amaducci, and C. Galli, pp. 169-198. Plenum Press, New York.
43. Sun, G.Y. (1973): J. Neurochem., 21:1083-1092.
44. Sun, G.Y. (1977): Lipids, 12:661-665.
45. Sun, G.Y., Corbin, D.R., Wise, R.W., and MacQuarrie, R. (1979): Int. J. Biochem., 10:557-563.
46. Sun, G.Y. and Horrocks, L.A. (1971): J. Neurochem., 18:1963-1969.

47. Sun, G.Y. and Horrocks, L.A. (1973): J. Lipid Res.,
    14:206-214.
48. Sun, G.Y., Manning, R., and Strosznajder, J. (1980):
    Neurochem. Res., 5:1211-1219.
49. Sun, G.Y. and Su, K.L. (1979): J. Neurochem., 32:1053-
    1059.
50. Sun, G.Y. and Yau, T.M. (1976): J. Neurochem., 27:87-92.
51. Sun, G.Y., Su, K.L., Der, O.M., and Tang, W. (1979):
    Lipids, 14:229-235.
52. Tang, W. and Sun, G.Y. (1982): Neurochem. Int., in press.
53. Thompson, R.H.S., Niemiro, R., and Webster, G.R. (1960):
    Biochim. Biophys. Acta, 43:142-144.
54. Webster, G.R. and Thompson, R.H.S. (1962):
    Biochim. Biophys. Acta, 63:38-45.
55. Weltzien, H.V. (1979): Biochim. Biophys. Acta, 559:259-
    287.
56. Whitmer, J.T., Idell-Wenger, J.A., Rovetto, M.J., and
    Neely, J.R. (1978): J. Biol. Chem., 253:4305-4309.
57. Wise, R.W., Sun, G.Y. and MacQuarrie, R. (1980):
    Eur. J. Biochem., 109:201-206.
58. Woelk, H., Peiler-Ichikawa, K., Binaglia, L., Goracci,
    G., and Porcellati, G. (1974): Hoppe-Seylers Z. Physiol.
    Chem., 355:1535-1542.
59. Woelk, H., Goracci, G., Arienti, G., and Porcellati, G.
    (1978): In: Advances in Prostaglandin and Thromboxane
    Research, edited by C. Galli, G. Galli, and G.
    Porcellati, pp. 77-84. Raven Press, New York.
60. Wolkowicz, P.E. and McMillin-Wood, J. (1980):
    Biochem. J., 186:257-266.
61. Yau, T.M. and Sun, G.Y. (1974): J. Neurochem., 23:94-104.

Phospholipids in the Nervous System, Vol. 1: Metabolism, edited by L. Horrocks, et al. Raven Press, New York © 1982.

Use of HPLC to Determine the Turnover of Molecular Species of Phospholipids

Firoze B. Jungalwala, Sankar Sanyal, and *Francis LeBaron

*Department of Biochemistry, E. K. Shriver Center, Waltham, Massachusetts 02254; *Department of Biochemistry, University of New Mexico, Albuquerque, New Mexico 87131*

High performance liquid chromatography (HPLC) is now widely employed for the analysis of a variety of medium and high molecular weight substances which are non-volatile and cannot be separated by gas-liquid chromatography. A conventional HPLC system includes a high pressure solvent delivery and sample injection system, a reusable and efficient column filled with microparticulate adsorbant and a suitable detection system with low cell-volume (8-10 µl) The most commonly used detectors are variable wave-length ultra-violet and visible light monitors.

We have been interested in the application of modern tools and techniques of HPLC for the separation and quantitative analysis of phospholipids and glycosphingolipids of the nervous system. HPLC methods for the quantitative analysis of glycosphingolipids have been described elsewhere (2,8,14,15). Here we first discuss the HPLC method for the analysis of phospholipids and then describe how the method is applied for studying the metabolism of molecular species of phospholipids in the nervous system.

HPLC OF PHOSPHOLIPIDS WITHOUT DERIVATIZATION

Phospholipid molecules do not absorb significant amounts of ultra-violet or visible light. However, phospholipids do absorb light in the far ultraviolet region (< 210 nm) mainly due to $\pi \longrightarrow \pi^*$ transitions of electrons in double bonds in the fatty acid side-chains and due to functional groups such as carbonyl, carboxyl, phosphate and amino groups. The response of the detector varies with the number of functional groups mainly the number of double bonds in the phospholipid molecules. Thus direct quantitation of phospholipids with an unknown degree of unsaturation is not possible. However, the separated phospholipids can be easily collected and quantitated by independent micro-methods. The solvents to be used for HPLC of phospholipids should be transparent at 200 nm, thus commonly used chromatographic solvents such as chloroform cannot be used.

An HPLC separation of commonly occuring phospholipids is shown in Fig. 1. The separation of phosphatidylethanolamine and phosphatidyl-serine is possible with the conditions used. Analyses of phospholipids present in lipid extracts from animal tissues and body fluids such as blood and amniotic fluids were performed without interference from other

91

lipids or other ultra-violet absorbing material, after purification of
the phospholipid fraction on a short silicic acid column (7,13,18). The
sensitivity of the detection is dependent upon the degree of unsaturation
of the phospholipid. Approximately 1 nmol of a phospholipid containing
at least one double bond per molecule can be detected.

   Other solvent systems are also available for the HPLC of phospholipids. Geurts Van Kessel et al. (3) published a procedure for the
separation of erythrocyte membrane phospholipids employing a n-hexane-2-
propanol-water gradient system with detection at 206 nm. Although most
phospholipids appear to be well resolved, a clear separation of phosphatidylcholine and sphingomyelin was not achieved. Cross and Sobel (4)
separated phosphatidylethanolamine, phosphatidylcholine, their lyso-
derivatives, and sphingomyelin on a cation exchange column of benzene
sulfonate residues covalently bonded to 10 µm silica particles. However,
they were unable to resolve phosphatidylserine from phosphatidylethanolamine.

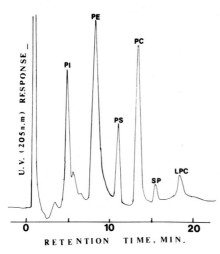

Fig. 1. HPLC separation of pig liver
phosphatidylinositol (PI), bovine brain
phosphatidylethanolamine (PE), bovine
brain phosphatidylserine (PS), egg
phosphatidylcholine (PC), bovine brain
sphingomyelin (SP) and lysophosphatidylcholine (LPC) on a Micro-pak-SI- 5 µm
column. The elution was with a 20 min
linear gradient of acetonitrile:methanol:
water:ammonium hydroxide (15 M) from
95:3:2:0.05 to 65:21:14:0.35, pumped at
2 ml/min. The rise in the base-line
at 205 nm was corrected by using a
Schoffel memory module with the monitor.

   The HPLC technique described previously by us has been used for the
preparation and purification of individual phospholipids from brain subcellular membranes (12). The method has also been employed for the
separation of sphingomyelin, phosphatidylcholine and phosphatidylethanolamine from extracts of cultured skin fibroblasts of normal controls
and patients with various types of Niemann-Pick disease and other
neurological diseases (10). A considerable increase in the ratio of
sphingomyelin to phosphatidylcholine and sphingomyelin to phosphatidylethanolamine was observed in the lipid extracts of fibroblasts from
patients with Niemann-Pick Type A disease but not in Type C disease or
in other neurological disorders when compared to normal controls. The
HPLC method was also used for the measurement of the enzyme sphingomyelinase in cultures of fibroblasts and amniotic fluid cells. The
amount of sphingomyelin was determined by HPLC before and after
hydrolysis by the enzyme (10).

HPLC OF PHOSPHOLIPIDS AFTER DERIVATIZATION

Formation of light absorbing derivatives and subsequent analysis of
the derivatized products has been the best approach for the quantitative

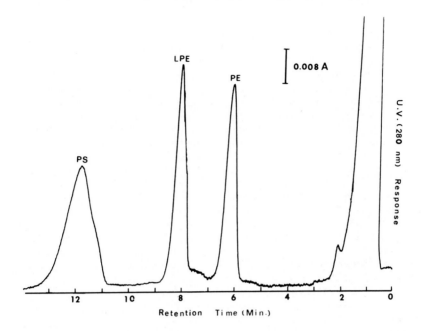

Fig. 2. HPLC separation of biphenylcarbonyl derivatives of PE, 200 ng P, lysoPE, 211 ng P and PS, 300 ng with a Lichrosorb SI 60-20 μm column (2.5 mm x 50 cm). Elution was with a 10 min linear gradient of dichloromethane:methanol: 15 M NH_4OH, 94:7:0.75 to 80:15:3, pumped at 2 ml/min.

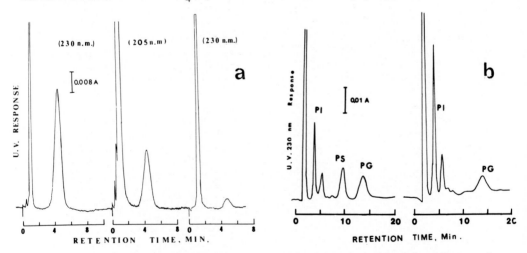

Fig. 3(a). HPLC separations of benzoylated sphingomyelin on a Micro-pak SI-10 column with acetonitrile-methanol-water (75:21:14) pumped at 1 ml/min. Left:benzoylated sphingomyelin (6.7 nmol) with detection at 230 nm. Middle: Same amount but with detection at 205 nm. Right: Detection of 0.6 nmol of sphingomyelin.

Fig. 3(b). HPLC separation of benzoylated phosphatidylinositol, phosphatidylserine and phosphatidylglycerol (PG) on a Micro-pak column. Left: standard phospholipids; Right:An acidic lipid fraction from rat lung. The elution was with a linear gradient of hexane-2-isopropanol-2N NH_4OH from 93:6.9:0.1 to 80:19.7:0.3 (v/v) pumped at 1.5 ml/min.

analysis of many lipids (13-15). We have prepared biphenylcarbonyl
derivatives of phospholipids containing amino groups for quantitative
analysis by HPLC (11). Fig. 2 shows the gradient-elution HPLC of
biphenylcarbonyl derivatives of phosphatidylethanolamine, lysophosphatidylethanolamine and phosphatidylserine. The amino phospholipids
containing vinyl ether bonds (plasmalogens) can be determined separately
from the corresponding diacyl- and alkylacyl- phospholipids by HPLC
before and after a brief exposure of the sample to HCl vapours (5,11).
The lower limit of detection by HPLC of these lipids is about 10-15 pmol
or 0.3-0.4 ng of phospholipid phosphorus.

We have assayed sphingomyelin, phosphatidylglycerol and phosphatidylinositol by HPLC after quantitative formation of their benzoyl
derivatives (Fig. 3). Quantitative analysis was performed on samples
ranging from 5-500 nmol of these lipids. Sphingomyelin was analyzed in
0.5 ml of serum from patients with various types of Niemann-Pick disease
and normal controls. It was surprising to find that the serum of
Niemann-Pick patients has sphingomyelin within the normal range (267±
90 µg/ml) although red cell sphingomyelin is known to be elevated in
Niemann-Pick Type A disease.

HPLC OF MOLECULAR SPECIES OF PHOSPHOLIPIDS

Recently, a great interest in the analysis of the molecular species
of individual phospholipids has been evident. We first attempted to
separate the molecular species of sphingomyelin, since the composition
of sphingomyelin fatty cahins in nature is relatively simple as compared
to other phospholipids (9). Most natural sphingomyelins have C_{18}-
sphingenine as the long chain base, whereas the fatty acid portion of the
molecule varies. Bovine brain sphingomyelin was resolved by reversed-
phase HPLC into ten major peaks (Fig. 4). Three separate peaks
containing 18:0 fatty acid but distinctly different long chain base
composition were identified. The major long chain base was C_{18}-sphingenine
in peak III, peak IV had mainly C_{18}-sphinganine, whereas peak V had 76%
C_{20}-sphingenine. Thus sphingomyelin species were resolved not only on
the basis of fatty acid composition but also through differences in the
long chain base.

The HPLC analysis of sphingomyelin species was made quantitative and
more sensitive by separating benzoylated sphingomyelins on a fatty acid
analysis column (Fig.5). This molecular species separation with
detection at 230 nm was similar to that observed with direct detection
at 205 nm. About 5 µg of benzoylated sphingomyelin could be separated
and quantitated in about 30 min by this method. The sphingomyelin
species were primarily resolved due to specific hydrophobic interaction
of their fatty acid and sphingoid chains with the alkyl ligand of the
stationary phase. However, sphingomyelins having a double bond in the
acyl side-chain (e.g. 24:1) were not resolved from the lipid having a
saturated fatty acid with two less carbon atoms (22:0). Separations
based on the degree of unsaturation was achieved with a commercially
prepared silica bonded silver column (17). The argentation HPLC of 3-0-
benzoylated sphingomyelin is shown in Fig. 6. The two peaks resolved
were collected and rechromatographed separately on a reversed-phase HPLC
column (Fig. 7). Sphingomyelin in peak 1 from the silver column
contained only saturated fatty acids, mainly 18:0, whereas peak 2
contained sphingomyelin with only monounsaturated fatty acids, mainly
24:1.

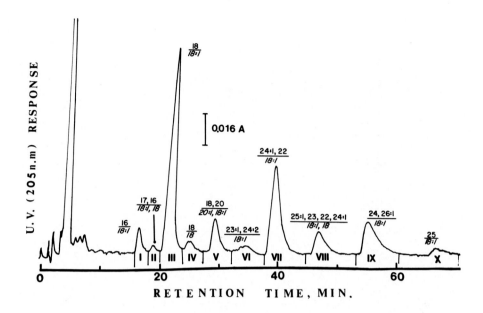

Fig. 4. HPLC analysis of bovine brain sphingomyelin on a Nucleosil-5-C_{18} column. The solvent was methanol-5 mM phosphate buffer, pH 7.4, 97:3 (v/v) with a flow rate of 1 ml/min. Sphingomyelin, 350 μg dissolved in 35 μl dichloromethane-methanol 1:1 (v/v), was injected. The major fatty acid (top lettering) and sphingoid (bottom lettering) composition of the sphingomyelin in an individual peak is given near the peak.

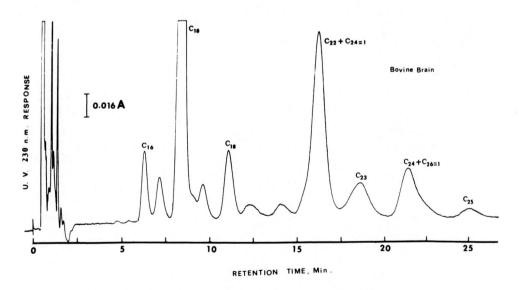

Fig. 5. HPLC of benzoylated sphingomyelins (about 50 μg) from bovine brain on a "fatty acid analysis" column (4 mm x 30 cm) with tetrahydrofuran:acetonitrile:water, 25:35:50 (by volume) pumped at a flow rate of 2 ml/min.

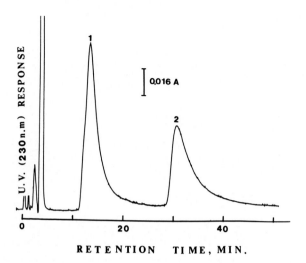

Fig. 6. Argentation HPLC of 3-0-benzoylated sphingomyelin (50 µg) on a
Chrompak silver column with methanol-2-isopropanol 8:2 (v/v) as the
solvent. The flow rate was 1 ml/min. Peaks 1 and 2 were collected and
analyzed by reversed-phase HPLC (see Fig. 7 B and C).

   Reversed-phase HPLC separation of egg phosphatidylcholine is shown in
Fig. 8 (16). The major fatty acid species separated are listed in
Table 1. It is known that the elution pattern of lipids from a reversed-
phase column is dependent upon the magnitude of hydrophobic interaction
which is determined by the contact area. The contact area is determined
by the molecular structure and conformation of the ligand and the
solute (6). In the case of phospholipids with the same base (choline,
ethanolamine, serine etc.), differences in the magnitude of the hydrophobic interaction are determined mainly by the number of carbon atoms
and double bonds in the two side chains (16). The retention time and
therefore the hydrophobic interaction of acyl chains of PC species
increased logarithmically as the total number of carbon atoms in the
chains increased in the homologous series (Fig. 9). The retention times
decreased nonlinearly as the number of double bonds in the fatty chains
increased. Introduction of the first double bond in the side chain
reduced the retention time to the greatest extent. From the
chromatography data the reduction in the retention time was calculated
to be equivalent to 1.8 carbon atoms compared to the fully saturated PC.
Further introduction of 2, 3, 4, 5, and 6 double bonds in the same side
chain reduced the retention time additionally, equivalent to 1.4, 1.2,
1.0, 1.0, and 1.0 less carbon atoms. Each molecular species of PC was
assigned a "Hydrophobic Carbon Number" (HCN) based upon the total number
of carbon atoms and double bonds in the side chain. PC molecules with
the same HCN had the same retention time. HCN presents a simple measure
of relative hydrophobicity of each phosphatidylcholine molecule (16).
   The molecular species of phosphatidylethanolamine and phosphatidylserine as their biphenylcarbonyl derivatives were also separated and
quantitated by reversed-phase HPLC.

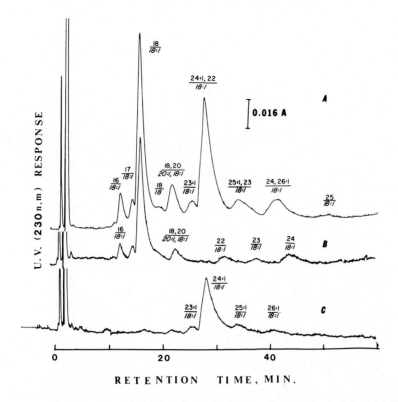

Fig. 7. Reversed-phase HPLC analysis of bovine brain 3-0-benzoylated sphingomyelin on a Nucleosil-5-C$_{18}$ column. The solvent was methanol-acetonitrile-phosphate buffer, pH 5.4, 5 mM (100:20:1, by volume) pumped at a flow rate of 2 ml/min. A, benzoylated sphingomyelin, 100 μg; B, peak 1 (Fig. 6); and C, peak 2 (Fig. 6) from the silver column. The major fatty acid (upper lettering, "numerator") and the long chain base (lower lettering, "denominator") composition of the sphingomyelin is given near each peak.

The separation of individual phospholipids based upon the degree of unsaturation was achieved on a silver coated silica-gel column. The separation of rat brain microsomal phosphatidylcholine according to degree of unsaturation is shown in Fig. 10. Peaks 3 and 4 display a partial resolution of molecular species containing 18:0 and 16:0. In the case of the hexaenoates (peak 6) the former peak was mostly phosphatidylcholine containing 18:0-22:6, whereas the later peak was the species with 16:0-22:6. We have also separated other individual naturally occurring phospholipids according to degree of unsaturation by slight modifications in the eluting solvents. Thus by the combined use of argentation and reversed-phase HPLC it has been possible to completely resolve major molecular species of intact phospholipids.

TURNOVER OF MOLECULAR SPECIES OF PHOSPHOLIPIDS

It has been known that the biological properties of membranes such as transport of small molecules, cell membrane integrity, enzymic activity etc. can be manipulated by changing the acyl group composition of lipids in the membrane (1). The membrane fluidity is mostly determined by the

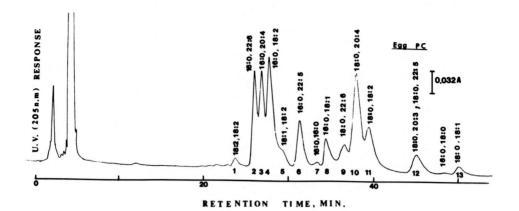

Fig. 8. HPLC analysis of egg phosphatidylcholine on a Nucleosil-5-C$_{18}$ column. The solvent was methanol-1 mM phosphate buffer, pH 7.4, 9.5:0.5 (v/v) at a flow rate of 1 ml/min. PC, 500 μg dissolved in dichloro-methane-methanol 1:1, 10 μl, was injected. The PC species eluted were collected as indicated in the figure by numbers and analyzed (see Table 1). The major fatty acid composition of the PC in an individual peak is given near the peak.

acyl group composition of the membrane lipids. It is not known if there is any relationship between membrane lipid fluidity and metabolic activity (turnover) of the lipids. If such a relationship exists, then we expect that lipids which are more fluid (shorter chain and unsaturated acyl groups) should have faster metabolic turnover rates. Conversely, membrane lipids that have a higher transition temperature and are closely packed in a membrane (long chain and saturated) should be relatively inaccessible to metabolic enzymes and should have a slower turnover rate. In order to test this possibility, turnover rates of molecular species of sphingomyelin and phosphatidylcholine in microsomal and myelin membranes of adult rat brain were determined after an intracerebral injection of 100 μCi of [Me-^{3}H]choline (12). Myelin and microsomal membrane sphingomyelin and phosphatidylcholine were isolated and purified by HPLC as described previously (7). The molecular species of benzoylated sphingomyelin were resolved on a reversed-phase HPLC column as previously described (Fig. 11). The major fatty acid of the microsomal sphingomyelin was 18:0 (70%), whereas myelin sphingomyelin contained only 30% of 18:0, with the rest mostly long chain fatty acids, such as 24:1 (35%) (12). The specific radioactivity of various molecular species of the microsomal sphingomyelin declined at similar rates after reaching a maximum (Fig. 12). There was no significant difference in the rate of decline between sphingomyelins containing short chain and long chain fatty acids. A similar result was obtained for the molecular species of sphingomyelin from myelin.

Microsomal and myelin phosphatidylcholine was resolved by argentation HPLC as shown in Fig. 10. In both cases, the monoenoic PC fraction at each time point had 50-60% of the total radioactivity. The PC dienes of the microsomal and myelin fraction had about 25% and 10% respectively of the total radioactivity of phosphatidylcholine. However, at each time point the specific radioactivity of the various unsaturated fatty

TABLE 1. Percentage composition of fatty acid species of egg phosphatidylcholine fractions obtained by HPLC

Peak No.	Fatty Acid									Probable Major Molecular Species of PC	Percent Composition of PC	HCN
	16:0	18:0	18:1	18:2	18:3	20:3	20:4	22:5	22:6			
1	8		9	70	13					18:2–18:2;16:0–18:3;18:1–18:3	0.4	29.6,29.9
2	40		12						48	16:0–22:6;18:1–22:6	1.7	30.4,30.6
3	37		18	48			45			16:0–20:4;18:1–20:4	2.8	30.6,30.7
4	47		2	48			3			16:0–18:2	18.9	30.8
5	22		30	48						16:0–18:2;18:1–18:2	3.2	30.8,31.1
6	43		8	8		10		31		16:0–22:5, 16:0–20:3, 18:1–18:2	2.0	31.5,31.6
7	95		5							16:0–16:0	0.5	32
8	47		53							16:0–18:1	37.0	32.2
9	36	6	52						6	16:0–18:1;18:1–18:1;18:0–22:6	9.3	32.3,32.6
10		35	27				38			18:1–18:1;18:0–20:4	6.3	32.3,32.6
11		50		50						18:0–18:2	7.3	32.8
12		45				25		30		18:0–22:5;18:0–20:3	0.6	33.6
13		49	51							18:0–18:1	10.0	34.2

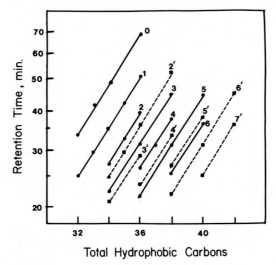

Total Hydrophobic Carbons

Fig. 9. Semilogarithmic plots of total hydrophobic carbons versus retention time of PC species on Nucleosil-5-C_{18} reversed-phase column. ● --- ●, indicates PC species with either saturated fatty acids, 0; or PC with one saturated and one unsaturated fatty acid. The number of double bonds in the unsaturated fatty acid is given near the lines, ■ --- ■ indicates PC species with both unsaturated fatty acids. The numbers with primes near the lines indicate the total number of double bonds in both unsaturated fatty acids of PC species.

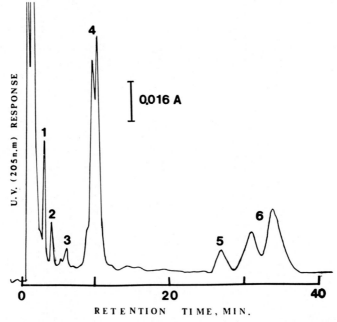

RETENTION TIME, MIN.

Fig. 10. HPLC analysis of rat brain microsomal phosphatidylcholine on a Nucleosil 10 sulfonic acid Ag+ (Chrompak) column with methanol as the eluting solvent pumped at 2 ml/min. The temperature of the column was maintained at 45°C. The number near each peak represents the total number of double bonds in the fatty acids of phosphatidylcholine.

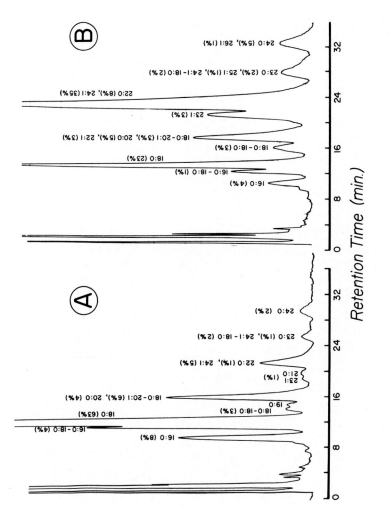

Fig. 11. Reversed-phase HPLC analysis of molecular species of benzoylated sphingomyelin from microsomal (A) and myelin (B) fractions on a
Nucleosil-5 μm-C$_{18}$ column. Amounts injected were 73 and 80 nmol
respectively. The fatty acid (first number) and the sphingoid base
(second number) components of the resolved molecular species are listed
near each peak. The sphingoid base composition is not listed if C$_{18}$
sphingenine is the sphingoid base. The percentage distribution of the
molecular species is given in parenthesis. The detection was at 230 nm.

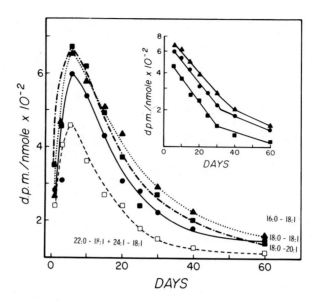

Fig. 12. Specific radioactivity of various molecular species of sphingomyelin of the microsomal fraction of rat brain after an intracerebral
injection of [Me-3H] choline. The symbols are ▲, 16:0 fatty acid and
sphingenine;●, 18:0 and sphingenine; ■ , 18:0 and C_{20}-sphingenine plus
20:0 and sphingenine; □, 22:0 + 24:1 and sphingenine. The inset shows
specific radioactivity of sphingomyelin on a semi-logarathmic plot.
The symbols for the inset are, ▲, 16:0 and sphingenine; ● 18:0 and
sphingenine and ■ , 22:0 + 24:1 and sphingenine. Each point represents
an average of two separate determinations.

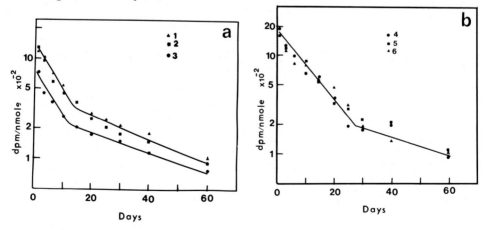

Fig. 13. Specific radioactivity of various fractions from microsomal
phosphatidylcholine from rat brain after an intracerebral injection of
[Me-3H] choline. Fig. (a) includes monoene, diene and triene species
resolved by argentation HPLC. Fig. (b) includes tetraene, pentaene and
hexaene species of phosphatidylcholine.

acid containing PC was similar, suggesting no specific incorporation into particular unsaturated fatty acid containing phosphatidylchòline. The specific radioactivity in various species of phosphatidylcholine also declined at a similar rate in both myelin and microsomal fractions (Fig. 13) suggesting that at least in the long term studies the turnover rates in vivo are not affected by the acyl-group composition of the lipids in the membranes.

Acknowledgements: Sincere thanks are due to Dr. Robert H. McCluer for his kind interest in the HPLC of phospholipids. This work was supported in part by USPHS grants NS 10437, HD 05515 and CA 16853. Dr. LeBaron was a visiting professor from the University of New Mexico, Albuquerque, New Mexico.

REFERENCES

1. Chapman, D. (1975): Q. Rev. Biophys., 8: 185-235.
2. Chou, K.H. and Jungalwala, F.B. (1981): J. Neurochem., 36: 394-401.
3. Geurts Van Kessel, W.S.M., Hax, W.M.A., Demel, R.A. and DeGier, J. (1977): Biochim. Biophys. Acta, 486: 524-530.
4. Gross, R.W. and Sobel, B.E. (1980): J. Chromatog., 197: 79-85.
5. Horrocks, L.A. (1968): J. Lipid Res., 9: 469-472.
6. Horvath, C. and Melander, W. (1978): Chromatographia., 11: 262-273.
7. Jungalwala, F.B., Evans, J.E. and McCluer, R.H. (1976): Biochem. J. 155: 55-60.
8. Jungalwala, F.B., Hayes, L. and McCluer, R.H. (1977): J. Lipid Res., 18: 285-292.
9. Jungalwala, F.B., Hayssen, V., Pasquini, J.M. and McCluer, R.H. (1979): J. Lipid Res., 20: 579-587.
10. Jungalwala, F.B. and Milunsky, A. (1978): Pediat. Res., 12: 655-659.
11. Jungalwala, F.B., Turel, R.J., Evans, J.E. and McCluer, R.H. (1975): Biochem. J., 145: 517-526.
12. LeBaron, F.N.. Sanyal, S. and Jungalwala, F.B. (1981): Neurochem. Res., 10:1075-1083.
13. McCluer, R.H. and Jungalwala, F.B. (1976): In: Current Trends in Sphingolipidoses and Allied Disorders, edited by B.W. Volk and L. Schneck, pp. 533-554. Plenum Publishing Corp. New York.
14. McCluer, R.H. and Jungalwala, F.B. (1979): In: Biological/Biomedical Application of Liquid Chromatography, edited by J. Hawk, pp. 7-30. M. Dekker, Inc. New York.
15. McCluer, R.H. and Ullman, M.D. (1980): In: Cell Surface Glycolipids, edited by C.C. Sweeley, pp. 1-13. American Chemical Society.
16. Smith, M. and Jungalwala, F.B. (1981): J. Lipid Res., 22: 697-704.
17. Smith, M., Monchamp, P. and Jungalwala, F.B. (1981): J. Lipid Res., 22: 714-719.
18. Vance, D.E. and Sweeley, C.C. (1967): J. Lipid Res., 8: 621-630.

Phospholipids in the Nervous System, Vol. 1: Metabolism, edited by L. Horrocks, et al. Raven Press, New York © 1982.

Investigations on the Lipid Turnover of Brain Tissue at a Cellular and Subcellular Level

H. Woelk and G. Porcellati

Neurochemistry Unit, Department of Psychiatry, University of Gießen, 6300 Gießen, Federal Republic of Germany; Department of Biochemistry, The Medical School, University of Perugia, Perugia, Italy

Marked differences in phospholipid metabolism have been observed between glial and neuronal cell enriched fractions as well as between the different subcellular fractions. Evidence was obtained for a faster turnover of glycerophospholipids in neurons than in glial cells, since neurons contained a considerably higher phospholipase A_1 and A_2 activity when compared to the glial cell enriched fraction (4). Furthermore the neuronal cell bodies were found to possess a much higher rate of exchange of both serine and ethanolamine into the phospholipids than the glial cell enriched fraction (2) and Freysz et al. (1) showed in their extensive investigation on the kinetics of the biosynthesis of phospholipids in neurons and glial cells, isolated from rat brain cortex, the neuronal phospholipids had a faster turnover than glial phospholipids. Further results, presented by Woelk et al. (5), indicated that phosphatidylinositol and phosphatidylcholine had the fastest and ethanolamine plasmalogen the slowest turnover in both cell populations.

Measuring the phospholipid content and composition in fractions enriched in neuronal cell bodies and in glial cells, we found that glial cells contained approx. one-third more phospholipids per unit protein than the neuronal cell bodies. The distribution and pattern of phospholipids, relative to the total amount, was rather similar in both cell types. However, a slightly larger relative concentration of phosphatidylcholine was observed in the neuronal cell bodies. Estimates of the exact cellular localization of the phospholipids between glia and neurons are necessary to understand more about their physiological function. In this connection it is interesting that the content of ethanolamine plasmalogen is rather similar in the neuronal and glial cell enriched fractions. The association of the major part of the ethanolamine plasmalogen with the myelin sheath suggested a predominantly glial localization of the ethanolamine plasmalogen since the myelin sheath derives from the plasma membrane of the oligodendrocyte in the central nervous and of the Schwann cell in the peripheral nervous system. The presence of relatively large amounts of ethanolamine plasmalogen in the neuronal cell bodies indicates however, that ethanolamine plasmalogen might also be associated with neuronal function.

Taking into account this localization a study on the enzymic properties of the de novo mechanism for phospholipid biosynthesis both in neuronal and glial cell fractions seems to be of value. As a first step we have used neurons and glia to investigate the activity of CDPethanolamine: 1,2-diacylglycerol ethanolamine phosphotransferase (EC 2.7.8.1), which catalyses the last step in the synthesis of phosphatidylethanolamine. Table 1 shows that, in the absence of any lipid acceptor, the neuronal cell fraction possessed a higher rate of ethanolamine phosphoglyceride (EPG) synthesis, when compared to glia. In terms of specific activity, the neurons displayed threefold higher activity for both phosphatidyl-ethanolamine and ethanolamine plasmalogen synthesis. Furthermore, both neurons and glial cells displayed a higher synthesis of 1,2-diacyl-sn-glycerol-3-phosphoethanolamine (diacyl-GPE) compared to that of 1-alkenyl-2-acyl-sn-glycero-3-phosphoethanolamine (alkenylacyl-GPE). The addition of 4 mM diacylglycerol caused a 5-fold and a 3-fold stimula-tion of cytidine-5'-diphosphate ethanolamine (CDPE) incorporation into diacyl-GPE in glia and neurons, respectively, whereas a corresponding 20-fold and 25-fold stimulation of ethanolamine plasmalogen synthesis was observed on adding a similar concentration of alkenylacylglycerol. On ad-ding diacylglycerol or alkenylacylglycerol, the neuronal fraction display-ed a noticeably higher activity, compared to glia (2-fold and 3.5-fold in-creases for diacyl-GPE and alkenylacyl-GPE, respectively). The increased uptake of radioactive CDPE into the two distinct phospholipid moieties following diglyceride addition was not completely specific, because a small but consistent stimulation of alkenylacyl-GPE synthesis was obtained on adding diacylglycerol, and a smaller one vice versa (Table 1).

Recently we have studied some aspects of lipid metabolism in the aging brain. Aging in the nervous system is a complex process characterized by a number of morphologic and neurochemical alterations in man and other mammalian species. The process involves biochemical changes in neural substrates, membranes, molecules, and ions correlated to behavior during aging. The more important task in the study of these changes is to deter-mine their function in terms of those mechanisms responsible for aging.

Table 1. Rate of synthesis of EPG subclasses in neurons and glia

Synthesized lipid	Fraction	Type of added diglyceride	Activity[a]	Ratio[b]
Diacyl-GPE	Neurons		1.36	
	Glia		0.43	3.1
Alkenylacyl-GPE	Neurons		0.76	
	Glia		0.28	2.7
Diacyl-GPE	Neurons	Diacylglycerol	4.00	
	Glia	Diacylglycerol	1.98	2.0
Alkenylacyl-GPE	Neurons	Diacylglycerol	1.21	
	Glia	Diacylglycerol	0.50	2.4
Diacyl-GPE	Neurons	Alkenylacylglycerol	1.97	
	Glia	Alkenylacylglycerol	0.68	2.9
Alkenylacyl-GPE	Neurons	Alkenylacylglycerol	19.0	
	Glia	Alkenylacylglycerol	5.4	3.5

[a] nmol/mg protein/30 min
[b] neuronal/glial ratio

The rate of de novo synthesis of choline and ethanolamine phosphoglycerides (CPG and EGP) was tested by incubating brain microsomes from
rats of different ages with labelled CDPethanolamine or CDPcholine without the addition of diacylglycerols. The activity of both phosphotransferases significantly decreases during the first part of the rat
lifespan, whereas a large scattering of data was found after this age, at
least in microsomes.

Based on these results, the next study focused on the biochemical
phenomena occurring at 18 months of age (aged animals), comparing these
changes with the data at 2 months of age (adult animals). The age of 18
months represents about the middle, or more than the middle, of the normal
rat lifespan; it is generally accepted that at this age the initial aging
phenomena processes have already begun.

The rate of conversion of water-soluble intermediates to CPG and EPG
subclasses was reduced in the brain microsomes of the 18-month-old rats
(aged rats). As shown in Table 2, the difference between the 2-month-old
rats and the aged rats was highly significant.

Table 2. Rate of synthesis of CPG and EPG subclasses in brain microsomes
of adult and aged male Wistar rats

Lipid subclasses	Adult rats[a]	Aged rats[b]	Decrease (%)
Diacyl GPC	1.13 (9)	0.70 (5)[d]	-38
Alkenylacyl GPC	0.33 (9)	0.17 (5)[c]	-49
Diacyl GPE	1.01 (5)	0.59 (5)[d]	-41
Alkenylacyl GPE	0.13 (5)	0.06 (5)[c]	-54

[a]56-day-old rats; [b]18-month-old rats; [c]$p < 0.001$; [d]$p < 0.01$. Data
reported as nmol/mg protein/40 min; number of experiments in brackets.

These differences found in whole brain microsomes during aging may be due
to a decrease of the neuronal populations, where the rate of the de novo
phospholipid biosynthesis is higher, and/or to an increase of glia, where
this biosynthesis is lower. Consequently, the previous findings have been
improved by studying the biosynthesis of CPG and EPG from rat brains at
different ages. A significant decrease of neuronal activity takes place
up to about 18 months of age, when the choline phosphotransferase activity
is tested by incubating neuronal cell homogenates with labelled CDPcholine
and without adding diglycerides. After 18 months of age, no significant
changes occur in neuronal or glial homogenates. In contrast, the decrease
of the rate of EPG synthesis in neurons is not as significant as that of
CPG synthesis, because of the large scattering of data found at 2 months.
Interestingly, the decrease in the rate of synthesis continues beyond 18
months, this sharper decrease giving more significance to the earlier but
variable data. No changes were found in glial activity. Although the
rate of neuronal EPG synthesis decreases over the 18 month cycle, the
study of the 18-month-old rats was undertaken in order to compare EPG synthesis with that of CPG. Separate experiments confirmed that the decrease
of the neuronal population measured as DNA content could not account for
the difference in the rate of synthesis in terms of cell reduction alone.

The decrease during aging of the rate of conversion of cytidine derivatives into corresponding phosphoglycerides in neurons may be attributable to different causes, such as variation of enzyme kinetics and/or
availability of essential lipid substrates. Because of the variation of
fatty acid composition of microsomal diglycerides, the lipid substrate may

play an important role in changing the rate of phosphoglyceride synthesis in neurons during aging. On the contrary, glial ethanolamine and choline phosphotransferases are not significantly affected by aging; this may be related to the lesser influence of glia in phospholipid biosynthesis.

Phospholipases A play an important role in the degradation of brain phospholipids and hydrolytic cleavage of one of the two fatty acid ester linkages in various glycerophospholipids yielding free fatty acids and lysoglycerophospholipids by phospholipases A_1 and A_2 is a well-established reaction. Together with the action of acyl-transferases, the phospholipases A are responsible for the fatty acid pattern of the glycerophospholipids. An investigation of the distribution of phospholipase A_1 and A_2 in rat brain subcellular particles showed that the phospholipase A_1 activity is almost exclusively located in the microsomal and plasma membrane fraction, whereas phospholipase A_2 activity predominates in mitochondria with a little activity being present in the synaptosomes (3).

Glia and neuronal-cell enriched fractions have been shown to contain phospholipase A_1 and A_2 activities (4). Neuronal and glial phospholipase A_1 had optimal activities at pH 7.2 and 5.4 respectively, whereas phospholipase A_2 activities in neurons and glial cells were optimal at pH 5.4 and 8.0, respectively. Pronounced differences in the enzyme activities of phospholipase A_1 and A_2 were found in neurons and glia, phospholipase A_1 activity being 8-fold and A_2 activity 5-fold higher in neurons than in glia. Determination of kinetic constants (K_m and V) of the neuronal phospholipase A_1 acting on specifically labelled phosphatidylcholine, phosphatidylethanolamine and phosphatidylserine showed that the enzyme was most active with phosphatidylcholine, whereas phosphatidylserine was less extensively hydrolyzed. Studies with phosphatidylserine, specifically labelled with palmitic, oleic or linoleic acid at the 1 position, demonstrated that the rate of hydrolysis of the substrate by neuronal phospholipase A_1 readily increased if the fatty acid residue in position 1 was saturated. Choline plasmalogen competitively inhibited the hydrolysis of labelled phosphatidylcholine by the neuronal phospholipase A_1 (4).

Subsequently, glycerophospholipids, specifically labelled either in the 1 or in the 2 position, were used to further characterize the neuronal phospholipase A_1 and to investigate the subcellular distribution of the enzyme. The microsomes were found to contain the bulk of enzyme activity, but an appreciable enzymic activity could still be observed in the plasma membranes isolated from the neuronal-enriched cell fraction. In another investigation the characterization of phospholipases A_1 of plasma membranes prepared from neuronal- and glial- enriched fractions of the rabbit brain was examined. As compared to the glial plasma membrane, the neuronal membrane contains more phospholipids, whereas the opposite distribution is observed for galactolipids.

Phospholipase A_1 activity occurs in the plasma membranes of both cell types. The action of neuronal and glial plasma membranes on specifically labelled phosphatidylcholine was examined over a pH range from 4.0 to 10.0 and the production of labelled lysophosphatidylcholine measured. The formation of 2-[^{14}C]oleoyl-sn-glycero-3-phosphocholine from the corresponding 1,2-diacyl derivative, representing phospholipase A_1 activity, was maximal at pH values ranging between 8.0 and 9.0 for the plasma membranes obtained from both neurons and glial cells.

As a subsequent step, the hydrolysis of the labelled phosphatidyl-choline by neuronal and glial subfractions was examined at the pH optimum found for the plasma membrane phospholipase A_1 (Table 3).

Table 3. The distribution of phospholipase A_1 activity in subcellular fractions prepared from neurons and glial cells from rabbit brain

Subfraction	Neurons	Glia	Neuronal/glial ratio
Homogenate	5.3	3.8	1.4
Nuclei	1.8	0.4	4.5
Mitochondria	4.2	2.8	1.5
Membranes I + II	9.1	5.3	1.7
Membranes III	8.7	5.7	1.5
Plasma membranes	15.6	7.9	2.0
Microsomes	38.3	19.6	2.0

Phospholipase A_1 activity was most abundant in the microsomal fraction of both cell types, with a neuronal/glial ratio of 2. The plasma membranes displayed about one-half the enzymic activity of the microsomal fraction, whereas only small amounts of activity were present in the neuronal and glial mitochondria. In order to further characterize the plasma membrane phospholipase A_1, the substrate specificity of the enzyme was investigated by the use of different glycerophospholipids. As shown in Table 4, the enzyme from the neuronal plasma membranes showed the highest activity for phosphatidylcholine, whereas the lowest specific activity was observed with the acidic phospholipids, phosphatidylserine and phosphatidylinositol. Phosphatidylethanolamine was cleaved at an intermediate rate. A completely different pattern was found for the specific activity of the glial plasma membrane enzyme tested with the same glycerophospholipids (Table 4). The plasma membrane phospholipase A_1 from glia displayed in fact the highest activity towards phosphatidylinositol and the lowest towards phosphatidylserine whereas phosphatidylcholine and phosphatidylethanolamine were hydrolysed at intermediate rates.

Table 4. The substrate specificity of phospholipase A_1 from neuronal and glial plasma membranes

Substrate	Neurons	Glia
	specific activity (nmol/mg x h)	
1-acyl-2-[^{14}C]oleoyl-GPC	16.1	8.2
1-acyl-2-[^{14}C]oleoyl-GPE	12.6	8.7
1-acyl-2-[^{14}C]oleoyl-GPS	7.5	5.2
1-acyl-2-[^{14}C]oleoyl-GPI	7.2	10.4

Although the significance of phospholipases A in cellular physiology remains to be elucidated, there is good evidence that phospholipases A are involved in the renewal and turnover of membrane phospholipids. Experiments are in progress to examine whether plasma membranes from neuronal and glial origin are able to reacylate lysophospholipds and whether a monoacyl-diacyl phospholipid cycle is present in neuronal and glial plasma membranes.

REFERENCES

1. Freysz, L., Bieth, R., and Mandel, P. (1969): J. Neurochem., 16:1417-1424.
2. Goracci, G., Blomstrand, C., Hamberger, A., and Porcellati, G. (1973): J. Neurochem., 20:1167-1180.
3. Woelk, H., and Porcellati, G. (1973): Hoppe-Seyler's Z. Physiol. Chem., 354:90-100.
4. Woelk, H., Goracci, G., Gaiti, A., and Porcellati, G. (1973): Hoppe-Seyler's Z. Physiol. Chem., 354:729-736.
5. Woelk, H., Kanig, K., and Peiler-Ichikawa, K., (1974): J. Neurochem., 23:1057-1063.

Phospholipids in the Nervous System, Vol. 1: Metabolism, edited by L. Horrocks, et al. Raven Press, New York © 1982.

Metabolism of Fatty Acids in Brain Membrane Phosphoglycerides During Normoxia and Hypoxia

J. Strosznajder and *G. Y. Sun

*Medical Research Center, Polish Academy of Sciences, 00-784 Warsaw, Poland; *Sinclair Comparative Medicine Research Farm, University of Missouri, Columbia, Missouri 65201*

Due to the presence of stringent regulatory mechanisms, the FFA pool in brain is maintained under a dynamic equilibrium. A disturbance of this equilibrium may result in an accumulation of the FFA. Two types of cyclic events are known to regulate the metabolism of brain fatty acids: (a) ATP-dependent activation of fatty acids to their acyl-CoA via the fatty acid:acyl-CoA ligase (EC 6.2.1.3) and subsequent hydrolysis of acyl-CoA by acyl-CoA hydrolase (EC 3.1.2.2), and (b) release of polyunsaturated fatty acids (PUFA) from membrane phosphoglycerides via phospholipase A_2 and subsequent reacylation of the lysophosphoglycerides via the acyl-CoA:lysophospholipid acyltransferases (29). Since the brain contains highly active acyl-CoA ligase and hydrolase (1,19), it is important to consider regulation of fatty acid metabolism by the first cyclic event. Activation of long chain fatty acids to acyl-CoA by fatty acid:acyl-CoA ligase is the initial obligatory step common to almost all metabolic sequences involving fatty acids (11,18,29). Nevertheless, excess acyl-CoA in cells may be detrimental to the cell membranes due to its potent detergent properties. Consequently, the acyl-CoA hydrolases in cellular systems are important to protect the cells from acyl-CoA accumulation.

The importance of the acyl groups of phosphoglycerides for membrane structure and functions is well recognized, although the exact mechanism regulating the metabolism of the phospholipids acyl groups is not well understood. Previous studies have shown that when synaptosomes were incubated in the presence of ATP, Mg^{2+} and CoA, exogenous fatty acids were incorporated into the synaptosomal membrane phospholipids (5). In the brain, ischemia, hypoxia and electroconvulsive shock are known to result in an increase in the FFA pool (2,3,19,21,22). Under this condition, PUFA such as arachidonate were preferentially released. The metabolism of arachidonate in brain is of special interest, because this fatty acid is metabolically very active, and it also serves as a precursor for prostaglandin biosynthesis. Among different phospholipids, the diacyl-GPI is shown to contain a high level of the arachidonic acid (10,24). The aim of this study was to examine the fatty acid metabolism of brain phospholipids under normal and oxygen deficient conditions.

MATERIALS AND METHODS

Wistar and Sprague Dawley rats were used for this study. Acute ischemia was induced by first decapitating the rat and then incubating the head at $37^{\circ}C$ for 1, 2 or 5 min. After this treatment, brain cortices were quickly removed and placed in ice. Control rats were decapitated, and the brains were removed immediately.

Acute hypoxic-hypoxia treatment was produced by keeping the animals for 1 min in a chamber of 12 l volume through which 1% O_2 in N_2 was passed with a flow rate of 2 l per min. The chamber was flushed with the gas mixture for 15 min prior to the experiments. Body temperature of animals was kept close to $37^{\circ}C$ by means of a heating pad. All animals subjected to this type of acute hypoxic treatment developed convulsions which lasted for 15-20 sec (23).

For the in vivo studies, $1-[^{14}C]$arachidonic acid (specific radioactivity 58 mCi/mmol) was emulsified in 0.32 M sucrose, 50 mM Tris-HCl pH 7.4 containing 1% bovine serum albumin. Each rat received 1.5 μCi of the label in 10 μl via intracerebral injection. Subsequently, the rats were submitted to an acute hypoxia treatment. The control group was injected intracerebrally with labeled arachidonate, except that the hypoxic treatment was omitted. These animals did not develop any signs of neurological symptoms. At 3,6,12 min after injection of $1-[^{14}C]$arachidonic acid, including 1 min of hypoxic treatment, groups of 4 rats were decapitated and brains were removed. Each brain was homogenized immediately in chloroform-methanol (2:1, v/v) and the lipids were extracted (23).

Isolation of brain cortex synaptosomes

For isolation of subcellular fractions, the brain tissue was homogenized in 0.32 M sucrose with 50 mM Tris-HCl, pH 7.4. Synaptosomes were isolated by differential and discontinuous sucrose gradient centrifugation as described by Sun and Samorajski (25) or by the method of Lai and Clark (12) with some modification as described by Strosznajder (22). The purity of synaptosomal fraction was monitored by electron microscopy and by assay of lactate dehydrogenase (9) and NADPH-cytochrome c reductase (15). In some experiments, synaptosomes were resuspended and washed with three different solutions: (a) Krebs-Ringer-bicarbonate (KRB) (b) KRB medium with 0.5% bovine serum albumin (BSA, essentially fatty acid free), and (c) the KRB medium with BSA and 3 mM dithiotreitol (DTT). In some cases, synaptosomal pellets were suspended in 5 mM Tris-HCl buffer (pH 7.4) at 4°C for 60 min and were lysed by hypotonic shock (28). Protein concentration was assayed by the method of Lowry et al. (14).

Lipid extraction and analysis

Lipids were extracted according to Folch et al. (7) with the extraction procedure performed at $0^{\circ}-4^{\circ}$C. Free fatty acids (FFA) were extracted using the procedure described by Dole and Meinertz (6), and the level of FFA was determined using gas chromatography. FFA were methylated with diazomethane after addition of C17:0 as internal standard. The brain lipid extract was applied to TLC plates coated with silica gel G and was separated by the procedure of Horrocks and Sun (8). In some instances, the less polar lipids were separated by TLC using a solvent system of petroleum ether-diethyl ether-acetic acid (90:10:1, by vol). Individual lipid spots were scraped from the plates into scintillation vials containing 10 ml of scintillation fluid. Radioactivity of samples was measured in a Nuclear Chicago Isocap 300 liquid scintillation counter. The acyl-CoA which remained in the Folch upper phase was also taken for measurement of radioactivity.

Assay of labeled arachidonate incorporation into glycerophospholipids

Activity of the fatty acid incorporation was assayed by incubation of synaptosomal fraction (1.0 mg protein) in a system containing 0.32 M sucrose in 50 mM Tris-HCl (pH 7.4), 2.5 mM ATP, 10 mM $MgCl_2$, 0.1 mM CoA, 0.1 mM DTT and 0.05 μCi of 1-[^{14}C]arachidonic acid (1 nmole) bound to BSA. The total incubation volume was 0.5 ml and samples were incubated at 37°C for 0-30 min in a shaking incubator. Enzymic reactions were terminated by addition of chloroform-methanol (2:1, v/v).

Incorporation of labeled oleoyl-CoA into phospholipids

Incorporation of labeled oleoyl-CoA into phosphoglycerides was assayed in the incubation system which contained 1-[^{14}C]-oleoyl-CoA (0.1 μCi in 10 nmole), disrupted synaptosomes equivalent to 0.4-0.6 mg protein, and 0.32 M sucrose with 50 mM Tris-HCl pH 7.4 to make a total volume of 0.5 ml. Samples were incubated in the presence of 2 mM $CaCl_2$ or 2 mM EDTA. Incubations were carried out in a shaking incubator at 37°C for 10 min, after which reactions were terminated by adding chloroform-methanol (2:1, v/v) (29).

Assay of oleoyl-CoA hydrolase activity in synaptosomes

Incubation conditions were the same as for the oleoyl-CoA incorporation study except that more oleoyl-CoA (40 μM) and less synaptosomes (50 μg proteins) were added to the incubation mixture. A one dimensional TLC system containing hexane-diethyl ether-acetic acid (70:30:3.5, by vol) was used to separate the phospholipids from the FFA. The FFA (Rf 0.7) were transferred to vials for counting of radioactivity. In some instances, the FFA formed was extracted into the heptane layer using a Dole's (6) extraction solvent mixture. Non-enzymic hydrolysis was assessed by measuring the radioactivity of FFA in the sample without incubation.

RESULTS

Uptake of arachidonate by synaptosomal phospholipids: effect of BSA washing

When synaptosomes isolated from brain cortex were incubated with labeled arachidonate in the presence of ATP, Mg^{++} and CoA, radioactivity was incorporated into various glycerolipids. After washing the synaptosomes with 0.5% BSA (essentially fatty acid free), there was a 1-fold increase in arachidonate incorporation into phosphatidylinositol (PI), but only a 12% increase into phosphatidylcholines (PC) (Fig. 1). The increase in arachidonate incorporation into PI is probably due to an increase in the acyl transfer activity. A similar increase in PI-acylation due to BSA washing is consistent with respect to incubation time (Fig. 2).

The incorporation of arachidonate into synaptosomal phosphatidylinositol (PI) was 30% lower in samples isolated from rat brains after an acute hypoxic treatment (1% O_2 in N_2) as compared to controls. On the other hand, the incorporation activity into phosphatidylcholine (PC) after hypoxic treatment was not appreciably altered (Fig. 3). After washing the synaptosomes with the BSA medium, incorporation of arachidonate into PI in both hypoxic and control samples was enhanced by 80%, but the incorporation into PC was not altered (Fig. 3). The decrease in arachidonate incorporation into PI in the hypoxic sample correlated well with *in vivo* findings in which labeled arachidonate was administered intracerebrally (23). However, the mechanism underlying this inhibitory effect is not yet understood.

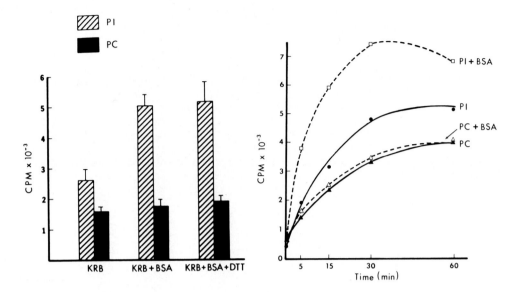

FIG. 1.   Incorporation of arachidonate into synaptosomal phospholipids after washing the membrane
with: (a) Krebs-Ringer-bicarbonate (KRB) (b) KRB
with 0.5% BSA, and (c) KRB with 0.5% BSA plus 3 mM
dithiothreitol (DTT).   PI - phosphatidylinositol,
PC - phosphatidylcholine.   Each value represents
the mean ± S.D. of 3 brain samples.

FIG. 2. Effect of BSA washing on incorporation of
arachidonate into synaptosomal phospholipids as a
function of incubation time.

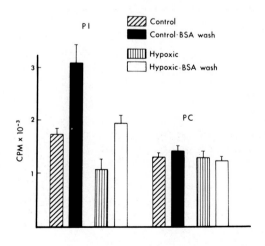

FIG. 3   Incorporation of
arachidonate into rat brain
synaptosomal phospholipids
(PI and PC) after acute
hypoxic treatment.   Each
value represents the mean ±
S.E.M. from 4 control and 4
hypoxic brains.

In vivo incorporation of arachidonate into brain phospholipids: effect of acute hypoxia

In an **in vivo** study, the effects of 1 min of acute hypoxic treatment (1% O_2 in N_2) on arachidonate metabolism was investigated at 3, 6, 12 min after intracerebral injection of 1-[^{14}C]arachidonic acid (23). When radioactivity of the aqueous upper phase was measured, there was a decrease in the upper phase radioactivity (with respect to total radioactivity of the FFA) in brain samples which were subjected to acute hypoxic treatment (Fig. 4). The labeled metabolite of arachidonate in the aqueous upper phase was later shown to be comprised mainly of arachidonoyl-CoA which is an obligate intermediate for incorporation of the arachidonate into glycerolipids.

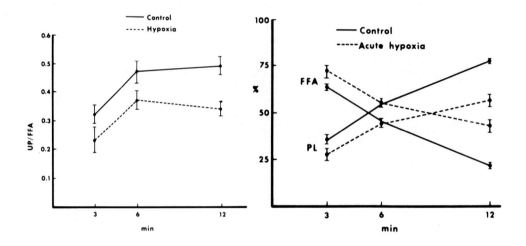

FIG. 4. The ratio of radioactivity between Folch upper phase (UP) and free fatty acids (FFA) in rat brain versus time after intra-cerebral injection of 1-[^{14}C]arachidonate. Each value represents the mean ± S.D. of 4 brain samples.

FIG. 5. Percent distribution of radioactivity between phospholipids (PL) and free fatty acids (FFA) in rat brain after intracellular injection of 1-[^{14}C]arachidonic acid. Each value represents the mean ± S.D. of 4 brain samples.

The hypoxic samples had a decreased incorporation of labeled arachidonate into the phospholipids. Furthermore, the rate of decay for the labeled precursor was slower in the hypoxic samples as compared to controls (Fig. 5). Among the phospholipids, there was also a specific decrease in incorporation of radioactivity into diacyl-GPI in the hypoxic samples (Table 1). On the other hand, the proportion of radioactivity into the neutral lipid fraction was increased. Upon further separation of the neutral lipid components by TLC, the increase in radioactivity was due mainly to labeling of the diacylglycerols. Therefore, the ratio of radioactivity between diacyl-GPI and diacylglycerols was lower in the hypoxic samples as compared to controls (Fig. 6).

TABLE 1. Effects of acute hypoxia on the incorporation of 1-[^{14}C]arachidonate into glycerolipids of rat brain

Glycerolipid	Time min	% of total glycerolipids	
		Control	Hypoxia
Diacyl-GPI	3	14.58 ± 0.72 (4)	12.53 ± 0.58 (3) *
	6	14.98 ± 0.92 (5)	12.72 ± 0.37 (3) *
	12	15.67 ± 3.31 (5)	11.08 ± 0.94 (4) *

Each value represents the mean ± S.D. with the number of samples indicated in parentheses. Values that are significantly different from controls by Student's t test are designated by asterisk (*), p>0.05.

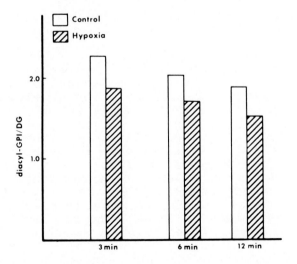

FIG. 6. The ratio of radioactivity of diacyl-GPI versus diacylglycerols (DG) in rat brain after intracerebral injection of 1-[^{14}C]arachidonate. Each value represents the mean of 4 brain samples.

Metabolism of long chain acyl-CoA in brain

Long chain fatty acids are activated to their acyl-CoA via an energy dependent fatty acid:CoA ligase prior to incorporation into the glycerolipids. Consequently, there is an intimate relationship between conversion of FFA to their acyl-CoA and incorporation of acyl-CoA into the phospholipid fraction. When rat brain synaptosomes were incubated in a system containing labeled acyl-CoA, over 85% of the label appearing in the organic phase was recovered as FFA and the remaining as phospholipids. Among the phospholipids, radioactivity was incorporated mainly into diacyl-GPC and diacyl-GPE, but other phosphoglycerides such as diacyl-GPI and diacyl-GPS were also labeled to a small extent. With synaptosomes isolated from brain samples after a 5 min post-decapitative ischemic treatment, incorporation of labeled oleoyl-CoA into diacyl-GPC and diacyl-GPE was increased by 16 to 24% (Table 2). The increase in acylation activity suggests that some lyso-compounds are generated during the ischemic treatment.

TABLE 2. Incorporation of $[^{14}C]$-oleoyl-CoA into phospholipids of rat synaptosomes

Phospholipids	Control	Ischemia (5 min)	% change
	(pmol/mg protein/10 min)		
Phosphatidate	25.2 ± 6.7	25.9 ± 5.3	–
Diacyl-GPS	19.8 ± 5.4	22.9 ± 9.2	–
Diacyl-GPI	42.7 ± 4.2	42.0 ± 6.8	–
Diacyl-GPC	191.1 ± 14.0	237.7 ± 43.5	+24.4
Diacyl-GPE	79.2 ± 3.6	92.1 ± 25.1	+16.3

Results represent the mean ± S.E.M. of radioactivity incorporated into synaptosomal lipids from 3 controls and 3 ischemic samples. The changes in incorporation of oleoyl-CoA into diacyl-GPC and diacyl-GPE were significant with p>0.001.

The oleoyl-CoA hydrolase activity in brain synaptosomes increased linearly with time for the initial 5 min of incubation and with synaptosomal protein up to about 200 µg. When calcium was added to the incubation system containing labeled oleoyl-CoA and synaptosomes, there was a decrease in the amount of FFA released. The decrease in oleoyl-CoA hydrolysis was maximum around 2 mM Ca^{2+} and the inhibitory action was not complete, even at higher concentration of the inhibitor (Fig. 7). The inhibition of oleoyl-CoA hydrolase activity by Ca^{2+} could be readily reversed by adding EDTA to the incubation mixture (Fig. 8).

When synaptosomes prepared from ischemic brain samples were incubated with oleoyl-CoA, there was less FFA released from these samples as compared to controls (Fig. 9). The decrease in oleoyl-CoA hydrolysis could be shown as early as 1 min after the post-decapitative ischemic treatment.

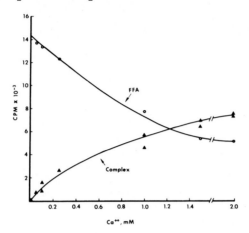

FIG. 7. Effect of calcium on hydrolysis of oleoyl-CoA by the synaptosomes. Incubation mixture contained 400 μg of protein, [^{14}C]-oleoyl-CoA (0.1 μCi in 10 nmoles).

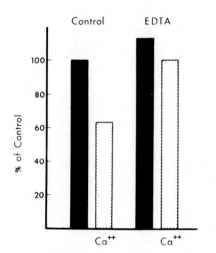

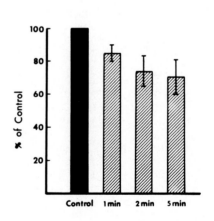

FIG. 8. The effect of Ca^{++} (2 mM) and EDTA (2 mM) on oleoyl-CoA hydrolase in synaptosomes. Results are means of duplicate assays from a typical experiment.

FIG. 9. Effect of postdecapitative ischemia on oleoyl-CoA hydrolase in brain synaptosomes. Data are means ± S.E.M. of 3 experiments.

DISCUSSION

Results from these experiments indicate that acute hypoxia and ischemia are associated with events leading to changes in brain fatty acid metabolism. These events include: (1) a decrease in the conversion of labeled fatty acids to their acyl-CoA, (2) a decrease in the rate of incorporation of labeled fatty acid into phospholipids, (3) a specific decrease in the incorporation of labeled fatty acid into inositol phospholipids, (4) an increase in labeling of the diacylglycerols, (5) an increase of acyl-CoA incorporation into membrane phospholipids, and (6) an inhibition of acyl-CoA hydrolysis.

In the presence of ATP, Mg^{++} and CoA, FFA are incorporated into the glycerolipids in synaptosomes (5,22). In general, washing the synaptosomes should diminish the microsomal contamination and remove endogenous inhibitors of phospholipid acylation. However, we found that when BSA is included in the washing procedure, there is a specific increase in arachidonate incorporation into phosphatidylinositol (PI). The differences in response towards acylation of the lyso-substrates by the BSA-washed synaptosomes suggest that the acyl transfer mechanism towards PI and PC is different. The exact mechanism underlying the change in acylation activity due to BSA washing remains to be explored.

Acute hypoxic treatment (1% O_2 in N_2) gave rise to a decrease in arachidonate incorporation into synaptosomal PI. Similar changes in linoleic acid incorporation were observed after mild hypoxic and post-decapitative ischemic treatment (22). When arachidonate was injected intracerebrally into the brain during acute hypoxic treatment, a specific decrease in incorporation of the precursor into PI was observed (23). Simultaneously, there was an increase in labeling of the diacylglycerols (23). Results here are in line with others showing an altered metabolism of diacyl-GPI and diacylglycerols in other tissues during stimulation and in response to stimulus-secretion coupling mechanism (17).

Fatty acid incorporation into phospholipids is influenced by many factors. The decrease in available energy source may affect the FFA activation process and subsequent incorporation of fatty acids into phospholipids. FFA activation in vivo may be affected by the endogenous pool which increases during stimulation and after acute hypoxic and ischemic treatment. However, Marion et al. (15) showed that the exogenous and endogenous arachidonic acid pools in brain tissue slices may not be freely interchangeable. Some FFA are also liberated during homogenization of brain tissue and preparation of synaptosomes. Since FFA liberated under these conditions specifically influences incorporation of arachidonate into PI, arachidonic acid accumulation may occur due to this disturbance.

The increase in uptake of fatty acids and their CoA derivatives by brain phospholipids in the presence of lyso-phospholipids suggests that incorporation is due mainly to acylation via the lysophospholipids:acyl-CoA acyltransferase action. Therefore, when no exogenous lysophospholipid was added to the samples, the extent of acyl transfer activity is limited to the amount of endogenous lysophospholipids which are derived from the action of phospholipase A. The presence of phospholipase A-mediated deacylation activity and subsequent reacylation by the acyltransferase in subcellular membranes is important for maintaining a steady turnover of the acyl groups of the membrane phospholipids (13). The increase in oleoyl-CoA incorporation into synaptosomal phospholipids after acute ischemic treatment is attributed largely to an increase in endogenous lysophospholipids in the membranes. However, due to the highly active acyltransferase present in the tissue, a large portion of the lysophospholipids produced during ischemia is probably immediately reacylated instead of accumulating.

In the brain tissue, acyl-CoA is probably maintained at a very low level because excess acyl-CoA are likely to be hydrolyzed by the acyl-CoA hydrolases. The acyl-CoA hydrolase activity in brain post-mitochondrial supernatant is inhibited by calcium (4). Calcium also exerts a similar inhibitory effect on acyl-CoA hydrolysis in the synaptosomes. Nevertheless, metabolism of acyl-CoA in the synaptosomes is further complicated by the tendency of this compound to bind with Ca^{++} and membrane phospholipids (27). Apparently, the membrane-bound acyl-CoA are not readily accessible to hydrolysis by the acyl-CoA hydrolase. The presence of excess acyl-CoA in membranes would also inhibit membrane transport activity. Since metabolism of acyl-CoA is related to that of lysophospholipids and FFA through two cyclic events, a disturbance of the brain FFA pool during oxygen deficient conditions may result in other changes in membrane phospholipid metabolism and alterations of neuronal membrane functions.

REFERENCES

1. Anderson, A.D. and Erwin, V.G. (1971): *J. Neurochem.*, 18:1179-1186.
2. Bazan, N.G. (1970): *Biochim. Biophys. Acta*, 218:1-10.
3. Bazan, N.G. (1971): *J. Neurochem.*, 18:1379-1385.
4. Bonser, R.W. and Lunt, G.G. (1976): *Biochem. Soc. Trans.*, 4:321-324.
5. Corbin, D.R. and Sun, G.Y. (1978): *J. Neurochem.*, 30:77-82.
6. Dole, V.P. and Meinertz, H. (1960): *J. Biol. Chem.*, 235:2595-2599.
7. Folch, J.M., Lees, M. and Sloane-Stanley, G.H. (1957): *J. Biol. Chem.*, 226:497-509.

8. Horrocks, L.A. and Sun, G.Y. (1972): In: <u>Research Methods in Neurochemistry</u>, edited by R. Rodnight, N. Marks, pp. 223-231, Plenum Press, New York.

9. Johnson, M.K. (1960): <u>Biochem. J.</u>, 77:610-618.

10. Keough, K.M.W., MacDonald, G. and Thompson, W. (1972): <u>Biochim. Biophys. Acta</u>, 270:337.

11. Kornberg, A. and Pricer, W.E., Jr. (1953): <u>J. Biol. Chem.</u>, 204:329-343.

12. Lai, J.C.K. and Clark, J.B. (1976): <u>Biochem. J.</u>, 154: 423-432.

13. Lands, W.E.M. and Crawford, G.G. (1976): In: <u>The Enzymes of Biological Membranes</u>, edited by A. Martonosi, Vol. 2, pp. 3-85, Plenum Press, New York.

14. Lowry, O.H., Rosebrough, N.J., Farr, A.L. and Randall, R.J. (1951): <u>J. Biol. Chem.</u>, 193:265-275.

15. Marion, J., Pappius, H.M. and Wolfe, L.S. (1979): <u>Biochim. Biophys. Acta</u>, 573:229-237.

16. Masters, B.S.S., Williams, C.H., Jr. and Kamin, H. (1967): <u>Methods Enzymol.</u>, 10:563-565.

17. Michell, R.H. (1975): <u>Biochim. Biophys. Acta</u>, 415:81-147.

18. Murpny, M.G. and Spence, M.W. (1977): <u>J. Neurochem.</u>, 29: 251-259.

19. Porcellati, G., DeMedio, G.E., Fini, C., Floridi, A., Goracci, G., Horrocks, L.A., Lazarewicz, J.W., Palmerini, C.A., Strosznajder, J. and Trovarelli, G. (1978): In: <u>Proceedings of the European Society for Neurochemistry</u>, edited by V. Neunoff, pp. 285-302.

20. Srere, P.A., Seubert, W. and Lynen, F. (1959): <u>Biochim. Biophys. Acta</u>, 33:313-319.

21. Strosznajder, J., Gromek, A. and Lazarewicz, J.W. (1972): <u>Neuropat. Pol.</u>, 10:447-455.

22. Strosznajder, J. (1980): <u>Neurochem. Res.</u>, 5:1265-1277.

23. Strosznajder, J. and Sun, G.Y. (1981): <u>Neurochem. Res.</u>, 6:767-774.

24. Strosznajder, J., Tang, W., Manning, R., Lin, A.Y.-T., MacQuarrie, R. and Sun, G.Y. (1981): <u>Neurochem Res.</u>, 6: 1231-1240.

25. Su, K.L. and Sun, G.Y. (1978): <u>J. Neurochem.</u>, 31:1043-1049.

26. Sun, A.Y. and Samorajski, T. (1970): <u>J. Neurochem.</u>, 17: 1365-1372.

27. Sun, G.Y. and Sun, A.Y. (1972): <u>Biochim. Biophys. Acta</u>, 280:306-315.

28. Sun, G.Y., Su, K.L., Der, O.M. and Tang, W. (1979): <u>Lipids</u>, 14:229-235.

29. Van Tol, A. (1975): <u>Molecular Cell Biochem.</u>, 7:19-31.

Phospholipids in the Nervous System, Vol. 1:
Metabolism, edited by L. Horrocks, et al. Raven
Press, New York © 1982.

Control of Lipid Metabolism in Ischemic Brain by CDPamines

R.V. Dorman, Z. Dabrowiecki, *G.E. DeMedio, *G. Trovarelli, *G. Porcellati, and L.A. Horrocks

*Department of Physiological Chemistry, The Ohio State University, Columbus, Ohio 43210; *Istituto di Chimica Biologica, Universita di Perugia, 06100 Perugia, Italy*

INTRODUCTION

CDPcholine and CDPethanolamine (CDPamines) are involved in the final step of choline and ethanolamine glycerophospholipid synthesis via their respective phosphotransferase reactions. These are the only established biochemical functions for the CDPamines. However, the effects of the CDPamines on the metabolism and function of the CNS go beyond the confines of phospholipid metabolism. We shall discuss some of the diverse effects of the CDPamines in the CNS and report our efforts to use these compounds to control the disturbed lipid metabolism observed in ischemic brain.

Ethanolamine phosphotransferase (EC 2.8.7.1) and choline phosphotransferase (EC 2.8.7.2) catalyze the last step in the synthesis of the choline and ethanolamine glycerophospholipids. The reactants are the respective CDPamine and a diglyceride molecule and the products are the complex phospholipid and CMP. Thus, the synthesis of 80% of the CNS phospholipids can be controlled by altering the concentrations of the CDPamines or the diglycerides. The synthesis of the CDPamines depends on the production of CTP, which is used by a cytidylyltransferase to form the CDPamine. This energy consuming reaction is thought to be rate-limiting (36). The diglycerides are derived from phosphatidic acid.

The CDPamines are able to regulate the de novo synthesis of phosphatidic acid in rat brain preparations (27) and presumably control the availability of diglycerides. Therefore, the CDPamines are involved in the final step of choline and ethanolamine glycerophospholipid synthesis and they are also capable of controlling the entire de novo pathway. Possmayer (28) has suggested that the rate of de novo phospholipid synthesis in the CNS depends on the state of the cytidine nucleotide pool. He found that CTP and CMP can inhibit the incorporation of glycerol-3-phosphate into phospholipids and CDPcholine can overcome this inhibition.

The CNS effects of the cytidine nucleotides are not limited to phospholipid synthesis. Miyake et al. (25) were able to shorten the time for awakening of chloralhydrate anesthetized cats and they also suggested this compound might have some beneficial effects on recovery from CNS trauma. The arousal effects of the CDPcholine were also observed by Ogashiwa et al. (26) and Shimamoto et al. (32) found that CDPcholine increased EEG activity in rabbits, much like dopamine did. In fact, they showed that CDPcholine enhanced the cholinergic blocking effects of tri-hexylphenidyl hydrochloride and improved bulbocapnine catalepsia and akin-esis. These responses are similar to those induced by dopa administra-tion. We have also observed hyperactivity due to CDPcholine treatment.

The dopamine-like effects of CDPcholine have led to the effective use of this compound for the treatment of Parkinson's disease. CDPcholine raises the concentration of dopamine in the CNS (12,20). The physio-logical effects of CDPcholine have been reviewed (40). CDPcholine stimulates the uptake of tyrosine and activates tyrosine hydroxylase activity in rat brain (21-23). The ultimate result is that CDPcholine increases dopamine synthesis and release in the CNS.

CDPcholine may be useful for the control of CNS trauma. Watanabe et al. (37) presented CDPcholine to perfused cat brain and found that glucose incorporation into amino acids increased, as did oxygen consumption and GABA synthesis. The CDPcholine also caused a decline in lactate pro-duction. It has been suggested that CDPcholine may be useful for the treatment of brain damage by restoring mitochondrial function (32). This hypothesis was supported by the work of Rigoulet et al. (31). They re-ported that CDPcholine could reverse the spreading edema and restore the lost ATPase activities associated with cold-induced trauma in cat cortex. From these reports it appears that CDPcholine does have a beneficial ef-fect in traumatized CNS.

There should be a common denominator for the diverse effects of CDPcho-line on the CNS. Membrane association is the only property shared by the affected functions. Membrane transport is required for the uptake of tyrosine, the release of dopamine, cation fluxes and the passage of water. Many enzymes affected by CDPcholine are membrane-associated including ATPases, phosphotransferases and acyltransferases. It is reasonable to assume that any event which can alter membrane structure can alter CNS function, and CDPcholine appears to improve disturbed CNS function, pro-bably by stimulating phospholipid synthesis and membrane assembly.

We have examined some details of the effects of CDPcholine and CDP-ethanolamine on brain lipid metabolism (7). This includes the use of the CDPamines in a situation that compromises cerebral function and membrane structure. The traumatic episode we have employed is that due to cerebral ischemia.

Cerebral ischemia is known to have drastic effects on membrane com-position and structure, as well as on CNS function. Bazan (2) showed that decapitation ischemia causes a rapid rise in free fatty acid concentra-tions, especially arachidonate. The ischemia-induced release of fatty acids is more severe in gray matter than white matter (3) and corres-ponds to a decline in cerebral energy charge and the loss of mitochondrial function (13,15). Cerebral ischemia in the gerbil causes a rapid accum-ulation of free fatty acids; primarily 16:0, 18:0, 18:1, 20:4 and 22:6 and a transient increase in diglyceride concentrations, an increase in CMP concentrations, the inhibition of calcium flux and a 2-fold increase of unesterified fatty acids in the mitochondrial fraction (27).

Some non-ischemic traumas also raise cerebral levels of unesterified fatty acids. Electroconvulsive shock and convulsion induced by bicuculline raise the levels of free fatty acids (2,4). Noradrenaline and 5-hydroxytryptamine increase free fatty acid levels in nerve endings (30) and hypoxia and anoxia also raise cerebral free fatty acid levels (33). Gardiner et al. (9) reported that mild or moderate hypoxia did not alter free fatty acid concentrations. However, severe hypoxia caused a loss of ATP and accumulation of free fatty acids at the time when all EEG activity was lost. Insulin-induced hypoglycemia caused a decline in the choline and ethanolamine glycerophospholipid concentrations in brain along with a concomitant increase in the free fatty acid pool (1). Thus, a wide variety of CNS traumas result in the accumulation of unesterified fatty acids.

The free fatty acids which accumulate in traumatized brain can cause damage to the membranes, the cells and the organ. The accumulated fatty acids are invariably rich in polyunsaturated species. The availability of these fatty acids for peroxidation and associated reactions has been clearly established. Strosznajder and Dabrowiecki (34) found increased peroxidation of unsaturated fatty acids in ischemic brain preparations. Malonyl dialdehyde is also formed (19,41). The arachidonate released in ischemic brain is also converted to prostaglandins (10,11) and prostaglandins can be found in the CSF of patients suffering from epilepsy, meningitis or cerebral accident (39). It is likely that both free fatty acids and related oxidized compounds can alter cerebral function.

Free fatty acids can derange mitochondrial function. In a highly oxidative organ, such as brain, mitochondrial dysfunction may be critical. Cerebral ischemia not only decreases the the energy charge and raises the free fatty acid concentration, but it also causes the uncoupling of mitochondrial oxidative phosphorylation. This effect of ischemia on mitochondrial function can be mimicked by exogenous free fatty acids (13). Bilateral ligation of the carotid arteries in the rat uncouples cerebral mitochondria and induces edema. These processes are preceded by the increase in free fatty acid concentrations, especially 16:0, 18:0, 18:1, 20:4 and 22:6 (14). The uncoupling of oxidative phosphorylation and the swelling of mitochondria due to free fatty acids had been previously reported (24). Majewska et al. (18) found that cerebral ischemia caused an increase in the mitochondrial free fatty acid pool and a corresponding loss of mitochondrial phospholipids. Exogenous Ca^{2+} enhanced these alterations and barbiturate anesthesia depressed them. Mitochondrial effects are not limited to free fatty acids, since fatty acylCoA can inhibit adenine nucleotide transport in mitochondria (38).

Our investigations have been concerned with the use of the CDPamines to control lipid metabolism in ischemic brain. Preliminary results have shown that these compounds might stimulate the synthesis of cerebral phospholipids and in the process remove the accumulated free fatty acids (7). The results of this reutilization might be the amelioration of membrane and mitochondrial changes associated with cerebral ischemia.

RESULTS

The simplest model for cerebral ischemia is decapitation. The resulting ischemia is complete and free fatty acids are known to accumulate. Male Sprague-Dawley rats (21-25 days old) were given intracerebral injections of [^{3}H]acetate (37 nmol; 136 Ci/mol). The acetate was allowed to label the cerebral fatty acids for 2 h. Control and ischemic animals were given intracerebral injections of 10 μl 0.9% NaCl 5 min prior to decapitation. Treated controls and treated ischemic animals received 10 μl of

CDPamine mixture (0.6 μmol each of CDPcholine and CDPethanolamine) 5 min prior to decapitation. Control and treated-control animals were decapitated directly into liquid N_2. The entire heads of the ischemic and treated-ischemic animals were incubated at 37°C for 5 min before freezing. The cerebral lipids were separated and counted for radioactivity.

After two hours, radioactivity was incorporated into the phospholipid classes in proportions similar to that of the phospholipid content in the CNS (Table 1). The presence of exogenous CDPamine for 5 min increased the phospholipid labeling in non-ischemic animals. This supports Possmayer and Mudd's (29) observation of enhanced lipid acylation due to the presence of CDPamines. The labeling of choline glycerophospholipids was increased 43% over the non-treated controls and ethanolamine glycerophospholipid labeling increased 51%. The minor phospholipids also had increased labeling. Five min of complete ischemia caused the loss of radioactivity from the cerebral phospholipids. Such a rapid loss of radioactivity suggests that the [^{3}H]acetate has labeled a metabolically active pool of phospholipids. The effects of the CDPamines on the ischemia-induced phospholipid changes were striking. The phospholipids of the treated animals retained radioactivity equal to that found in control animals despite five min of ischemia.

Table 1. [^{3}H]Acetate labeling of rat brain lipids: effects of ischemia and CDPamine pre-treatments[d]

Conditions	dpm/g brain ± SEM		
	Sph,IGP,SGP	CGP	EGP
Control	18,400 ± 1,400	112,800 ± 9,400	31,800 ± 2,500
+ CDPamines	27,400 ± 3,000	160,900 ± 9,900	48,100 ± 4,900
Ischemia	17,400 ± 1,400	88,500 ± 5,500	21,900 ± 2,000
+ CDPamines	20,000 ± 2,200	116,800 ± 9,500	32,500 ± 3,600

[d]All animals received an intracerebral injection of [^{3}H]acetate 2 h prior to treatments. CDPamine treated animals received 0.6 μmol each of CDPcholine and CDPethanolamine 5 min prior to decapitation. Ischemic heads were incubated at 37°C for 5 min. Sph,IGP,SGP= sphingomyelin, inositol and serine glycerophospholipids; CGP=choline glycerophospholipids; EGP=ethanolamine glycerophospholipids.

Correlated with the loss of radioactivity from the phospholipid was the accumulation of label in the free fatty acid and diglyceride pools (Table 2). The radioactivity in the free fatty acids increased 123% and that in the diglyceride fraction increased 260%. The CDPamine treatment of ischemic brain caused an increased labeling of the triglyceride and diglyceride fractions. Again, this relates to the stimulation of acyl group incorporation into cerebral lipids. More important was the ability of the CDPamines to block the accumulation of radioactivity in the free fatty acid pool.

Table 2. [3]Acetate labeling of rat brain non-polar lipids: effects of
ischemia and CDPamine pre-treatments[a]

	dpm/g brain ± SEM		
Conditions	Free Fatty Acids	Diglycerides	Triglycerides
Control	6,400 ± 400	6,300 ± 2,000	8,100 ± 700
+ CDPamines	5,000 ± 900	25,800 ± 3,300	10,700 ± 700
Ischemia	14,300 ± 1,500	22,600 ± 2,900	7,000 ± 800
+ CDPamines	2,600 ± 300	30,900 ± 3,700	8,300 ± 700

[a]Animals were treated as described in the legend for Table 1.

Since the accumulation of free fatty acids in ischemic brain may be
intimately involved in the damage processes we examined the content and
composition of this pool (Table 3). Five min of ischemia caused a 3-fold
increase in the mass of the free fatty acid pool as others have shown.
Arachidonate is enriched in this fraction. The effects of the CDPamine
treatments on the free fatty acid pool were remarkable. The total free
fatty acid fraction was reduced to 60% of the control value and 20% of the
ischemia value. This was similar to the results we obtained with [3H]-
acetate labeling. It is apparent that the CDPamines prevented the
ischemia-induced release of fatty acids, especially arachidonate.

Table 3. Content and composition of free fatty acids in rat brain:
effects of ischemia and CDPamine pre-treatment[a]

	Composition (%)			Content as % Control	
Fatty Acid	Control	Ischemia	Ischemia +CDPamines	Ischemia	Ischemia +CDPamines
16:0	36.2	21.4	14.0	180	20
18:0	15.3	26.9	16.4	520	60
18:1	9.2	14.9	13.3	480	90
18:2	13.8	9.6	19.5	210	80
20:4	8.6	17.2	8.6	580	60
			Total	300	60

[a]Animals were treated as described in the lengend for Table 1.   GLC
values were derived from peak areas and comparison to control values.

The effects of the CDPamines on free fatty acid accumulation in traumatized brain may explain the beneficial effects of CDPcholine observed by
Rigoulet et al. (31) in cold-induced trauma in cat cortex. We might also
assume that mitochondrial functions may be enhanced by this procedure. In
fact, we examined the effects of treatment on (Na^+, K^+)-ATPase and
(Ca^{2+}, Mg^{2+})-ATPase activities following decapitation ischemia.
Unlike the cold-trauma experiment, we were unable to find a beneficial
effect of treatment on the ischemia-induced loss of (Na^+, K^+)-ATPase
activity (Table 4). We interpret this to indicate that free fatty acids
are not directly responsible for the observed loss of activity. However,
we did find a beneficial effect of treatment on the (Ca^{2+}, Mg^{2+})-ATPase
activity of striatum, most of which is considered to be of mitochondrial
origin (Table 5).

Table 4. (Na^+,K^+)-ATPase activities in rat striatum and cortex: effects of ischemia and CDPamine pre-treatments

Region	nmol P_i formed/min/mg protein		
	Control	Ischemia	Ischemia + CDPamines
Striatum	113 ± 5	85 ± 4	60 ± 5
Cortex	85 ± 7	59 ± 7	66 ± 4

[a]Animals were treated as described in the legend for Table 1. (Na^+, K^+)-ATPase activities are those which are sensitive to ouabain.

The CDPamine effect on the (Ca^{2+},Mg^{2+})-ATPase activity is probably related to the increased oxygen consumption and decreased lactate production observed in perfused cat brain in the presence of CDPcholine (37). It also supports the suggestion of Shimamato et al. (32) that CDPcholine may be useful for treating brain damage by restoring mitochondrial function. Clendenon et al. (5) have reported that CDPcholine can prevent and reverse the loss of (Ca^{2+},Mg^{2+})-ATPase activity observed in acute spinal cord trauma. Certainly any treatment which can protect mitochondrial function in a traumatized tissue should be of benefit.

Table 5. (Ca^{2+}, Mg^{2+})-ATPase activities in rat striatum and cortex: effects of ischemia and CDPamine pre-treatment[a]

Region	nmol P_i formed/min/mg protein		
	Control	Ischemia	Ischemia + CDPamines
Striatum	308 ± 8	260 ± 11	295 ± 13
Cortex	200 ± 7	211 ± 12	203 ± 13

[a]Animals were treated as described in the legend for Table 1.

We have employed a mixture of CDPcholine and CDPethanolamine in order to maximize the effects on lipid metabolism. Other laboratories have used only CDPcholine, due to their interest in cholinergic mechanisms, or to the prohibitive expense of the CDPethanolamine. In order to determine if both compounds are necessary for controlling lipid metabolism, we examined their individual effects. Non-ischemic, [^{3}H]acetate-labeled rat brains were given either CDPcholine or CDPethanolamine 1, 3 and 5 min prior to decapitation into liquid N_2. We found that both compounds were able to reduce the labeling of the free fatty acid pool in non-ischemic brains (Table 6). This does not necessarily mean they are equally potent, but they both exert some control of lipid metabolism in vivo.

The ability of the CDPamines to prevent the release of fatty acids in ischemic brain is clear. However, the potential for these compounds to reverse this damage process is an important consideration. In order to investigate this possibility, we began to use a model of cerebral ischemia employing the gerbil. Ligation of the carotid arteries in the gerbil causes complete ischemia of the anterior portion of the gerbil brain due to the incomplete circle of Willis (16) and reperfusion occurs when the ligations are removed (17). We have modified existing methods so that the ligations are performed without general anesthesia. This is an important

Table 6.   Effects of CDPcholine and CDPethanolamine on free fatty acid levels in normal rat brain[d]

| | dpm/g brain | | | |
| | μmol CDPethanolamine | | μmol CDPcholine | |
Time	0.25	1.0	0.25	1.0
0	1,600	1,600	1,600	1,600
1	1,100	650	700	700
3	800	700	900	600
5	600	1,200	800	1,100

[a]Rat brains were labeled for 2 h with [^{14}C]acetate. Free fatty acids were separated and counted 0, 1, 3 and 5 min following injections of CDPcholine or CDPethanolamine.

consideration since Flamm et al. (8) have shown that anesthesia can slow the release of fatty acids in ischemic brain.

Ischemia induced the release of fatty acids in gerbil brain (Fig. 1). There was a significant increase in free fatty acids after 30 sec of ligation with continued accumulation through 5 min of ischemia. Ischemia for 5 min also caused a 70% decrease in ATP and 250% increase in lactate concentrations. Concomitant with the observed changes, we noted a loss of cerebral phospholipids due to 5 min of ischemia (Table 7) and of arachidonate from glycerophospholipids (Fig. 2).

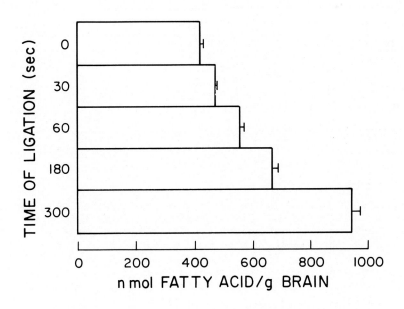

Fig. 1. Free fatty acid levels in ischemic gerbil brain (6).

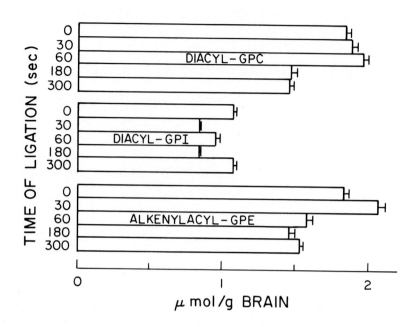

Fig. 2. Arachidonate content in glycerophospholipids in ischemic gerbil brain (6).

Table 7. Changes in polar lipid concentrations due to ischemia in the gerbil brain[d]

Polar Lipid	Control	Ischemia
Total Polar Lipids	47.1 ± 1.9	43.4 ± 1.5
Diacyl-GPS	5.9 ± 0.2	5.3 ± 0.4
Diacyl-GPC	17.1 ± 0.6	14.6 ± 0.2
Diacyl-GPE	9.0 ± 0.4	8.7 ± 0.1
Alkenylacyl-GPE	8.5 ± 0.3	8.8 ± 0.2
Diacyl-GPI	1.8 ± 0.1	1.4 ± 0.1

[d]Data are expressed as μmol/g brain ± SEM. The values are calculated from phosphorus content. Total lipids were extracted from sham-operated controls and gerbils exposed to 5 min of ischemia (6).

Treatment of gerbil brains with 0.6 μmol CDPcholine altered the course of ischemia-induced lipid changes when given before the trauma (Table 8). CDPcholine treatments 5 min prior to the onset of 10 min of ischemia reduced the levels of the free fatty acids to 72% of the non-treated ischemic values. These reductions were observed in all major fatty acids. However, CDPcholine alone was not as useful for preventing fatty acid release in gerbil brain as the mixture of CDPamines was in ischemic rat brain.

Reversal of the effects of ischemia on cerebral lipid metabolism by CDPamines was tested with the gerbil stroke model. Gerbil brains were pre-labeled with [^{14}C]arachidonate for two hours. Control animals were sham-operated prior to freezing the brains in liquid N_2. Ischemia was induced by clamping both carotid arteries for 5 min. The clamps were removed to allow for 6 min of reperfusion before freezing. Treated animals received an intracerebral injection of either a mixture of CDPamines (1.0 µmol each CDPcholine and CDPethanolamine) or 1.0 µmol of each alone. The injections were given 3 min into the reperfusion period. Radioactivity measurements and GLC analyses were performed.

Table 8. Effect of CDPcholine pre-treatment on free fatty acid concentrations in ischemic gerbil brain

| | nmol fatty acid/g brain | | |
Fatty Acid	Control	Ischemia	Ischemia +CDPcholine
Total	369 ± 30	969 ± 20	702 ± 27
16:0	92 ± 9	226 ± 16	168 ± 9
18:0	97 ± 6	264 ± 12	228 ± 6
18:1	66 ± 9	166 ± 18	103 ± 6
20:4	74 ± 6	234 ± 8	133 ± 6
22:6	10 ± 1	28 ± 2	18 ± 2

[a]Controls were sham-operated; ischemics were ligated for 10 min; CDPcholine treated animals were given 0.6 µmol CDPcholine 5 min prior to ligation of the carotid arteries. Ligations were carried out for 10 min (35).

Carotid blockage for 5 min followed by 6 min of reperfusion caused almost a 3-fold increase in the mass of the free fatty acid pool (Table 9). Again free arachidonate is enriched in this pool. When the CDPamines were given separately, CDPcholine was able to reduce the concentration of free fatty acids to 66% of the non-treated value and CDPethanolamine had a similar effect. The CDPethanolamine treatment reduced the level of free arachidonate better than the CDPcholine. This may be related to the specificities of the respective phosphotransferase enzymes for diglyceride molecular species. Ischemia and CDPamines also altered the [^{14}C]-arachidonate labeling of cerebral lipids. Ischemia caused a loss of radioactivity from the phospholipids (Table 10). The injection of a mixture of CDPamines 8 min after the onset of trauma restored the labeling to values close to those of non-ischemic controls. The CDPamines did not reverse the ischemia induced loss of triglyceride labeling and increased the radioactivity in the diglyceride fraction. Most important was the ability of the CDPamine mixture to reduce the free arachidonate to about 30% of that observed in non-treated ischemic brains. Thus, we found that the CDPamines are able to reverse some of the lipid alterations observed in ischemic gerbil brain and that a mixture of CDPcholine and CDP-ethanolamine is more beneficial for reducing free fatty acid levels than either compound alone.

Table 9. Free fatty acids in gerbil brain: effects of ischemia and post-ischemia CDPamine treatments[a]

| | μg/brain | | | |
Fatty Acid	Control	Ischemia	Ischemia +CDPcholine	Ischemia +CDPethanolamine
16:0	25.2	37.9	29.3	36.5
18:0	14.2	47.1	41.3	35.2
18:1	14.8	30.8	14.5	19.9
18:2	4.7	37.1	3.2	8.3
20:4	0.9	30.7	23.0	13.4
22:6	1.5	6.2	2.4	2.6
Total	99.7	237.2	149.6	161.2

[a]Controls were sham-operated. Ischemia was induced by clamping both carotid arteries for 5 min, followed by 6 min reperfusion. CDPamine treatments (either 1.0 μmol CDPcholine or CDPethanolamine) were given 3 min after the start of the 6 min reperfusion period.

Table 10. [14C]Arachidonate labeling of gerbil brain lipids: effects of ischemia and post-ischemia CDPamine treatments[a]

Lipid	dpm/g brain		
	Control	Ischemia	Ischemia + CDPamines
IGP	8,050	6,100	8,570
CGP	15,710	8,950	13,590
EGP	5,210	4,030	5,340
TAG	880	530	520
DAG	480	430	850
FFA	70	380	150

[a]Gerbil brain lipids were labeled for 2 h with [14C]arachidonate. Ischemia was induced by ligating carotid arteries for 5 min followed by 6 min reperfusion. Treated animals received 1.0 μmol each of CDPcholine and CDPethanolamine 3 min into the 6 min reperfusion period. IGP=inositol, CGP=choline and EGP=ethanolamine glycerophospholipids; TAG=triglycerides; DAG=diglycerides; FFA=free fatty acids.

DISCUSSION

Ischemic insult to the CNS alters the microenvironment of the neurons and supportive cells. Alterations which begin the processes of tissue necrosis and death must be transmitted into the cell via the membranes. The traumatic signal may be oxygen depletion or lack of energy substrates. Both circumstances have been shown to alter the structure of CNS membranes. We believe that trauma-induced changes of CNS membranes are closely related to the ensuing tissue damage.

A consistently observed membrane change associated with cerebral trauma is the accumulation of unesterified fatty acids. These compounds can be detrimental to normal bilayer structure and are increased in ischemic, hypoxic, anoxic and hypoglycemic brains. We found that decapitation ischemia raised the levels of the free fatty acids as previously reported.

We also found that ligation of the carotid arteries in gerbils stimulated free fatty acid accumulation. In both cases the glycerophospholipids were the major source of the free fatty acids.

The membrane changes associated with cerebral ischemia are not limited to unesterified fatty acids. Diglycerides are not compatible with normal bilayer structure and they also accumulate at the onset of trauma. Possibly more significant is the ensuing metabolism of the accumulated poly-unsaturated fatty acids. These compounds are converted to peroxides, prostaglandins and related compounds. The effects of these oxygenated compounds on membrane structure and function may be dramatic.

Normal brain function depends on intact and functional membranes. Sound mitochondrial membranes are required for cerebral energy production. Fatty acids can uncouple mitochondria. The accumulation of free fatty acids may be part of the reason for increased lactate production in ischemic brain, since the tissue would be forced from aerobic to anaerobic glycolysis. The energy produced in the mitochondria is needed for a variety of membrane-related processes. These includes neurotransmitter synthesis and release, transport of energy substrates, cation fluxes and electrical conductance. All of these energy consuming processes are adversely affected by ischemia. The observed beneficial effects of the CDPamines on these functions are probably mediated by membrane changes.

SUMMARY

The effects of CDPamines on cerebral membranes are mediated, at least in part, through effects on lipid metabolism. The CDPamines are able to prevent and reverse the accumulation of unesterified fatty acids observed in ischemic brain. Consequently, the production of peroxides and prostaglandins may also be diminished or prevented. This may be particularly important for tissue survival. The mechanism of action of the CDPamines is the stimulation of phospholipid synthesis. These compounds are able to increase lipid synthesis in non-ischemic brains, but more importantly, they are able to stimulate phospholipid synthesis in the energy deficient ischemic brains.

Many uses for the CDPamines in treatment of cerebral dysfunction are apparent. CDPcholine has already been used for the treatment of Parkinson's disease. It has also been shown to reduce trauma-induced edema and stimulate EEG activity. The CDPamines may prove useful for correcting CNS malfunctions due to altered membrane structure. This would include acute impact traumas as well as stroke. The importance of functional membranes to brain, heart, kidney and all other tissues cannot be overemphasized. If lipid precursors, such as the CDPamines, are able to protect membrane structure from trauma-induced alterations, then the tissue should have an improved chance for survival.

REFERENCES

1. Agardh, C.-D., Chapman, A.G., Nilsson, B. and Siesjö, B.K. (1981): J. Neurochem., 36: 490-500.
2. Bazan, N.G. (1970): Biochim. Biophys. Acta, 218: 1-10.
3. Bazan, N.G. (1971): Lipids, 6: 211-212.
4. Bazan, N.G., Morelli de Liberti, S. and Rodriguez de Turco, E.B. (1981): Trans. Amer. Soc. Neurochem., 12: 283.
5. Clendenon, N.R., Palayoor, S.T. and Gordon, W.A. (1981): Trans. Amer. Soc. Neurochem., 12: 116.

6. DeMedio, G.E., Goracci, G., Horrocks, L.A., Lazarewicz J.W., Mazzari, S., Porcellati, G., Strosznajder, J. and Trovarelli, G. (1980): Ital. J. Biochem., 29: 412-432.
7. Dorman, R.V., Dabrowiecki, Z., De Medio, G.E., Porcellati, G. and Horrocks, L.A. (1982): In "Head Injury", edited by R.G. Grossman and P.L. Gildenberg, in press, Raven Press, New York.
8. Flamm, E.S., Demopoulos, H.B., Seligman, M.L. and Ransohoff, J. (1977): Acta Neurol. Scand., 56 (Sup. 64):150-151.
9. Gardiner, M., Nilsson, B., Rehncrona, S. and Siesjö B. (1981): J. Neurochem., 36: 1500-1505.
10. Gaudet, R.J. and Levine, L. (1979): Biochem. Biophys. Res. Commun., 86:893-901.
11. Hsueh, W., Isakson, P.C. and Needleman, P. (1977): Prostaglandins, 13: 1073-1091.
12. Kinoshita, Y., Tanaka, K., Sasaki, A., Nosaka, H. and Kimishima, K. (1974): J. Yonaga Med. Assoc., 25: 296-299.
13. Kuwashima, J., Fujitani, B., Nakamura, K., Kadokawa, T., Yashida, K. and Shimizu, M. (1976): Brain Res., 110: 547-557.
14. Kuwashima, J., Nakamura, K., Fujitani, B., Kadokawa, T., Yashida, K. and Shimizu, M. (1978): Jap. J. Pharmacol., 28: 277-287.
15. Lazarewicz, J.W., Strosznajder, J. and Gromek, A. (1972): Bull. Acad. Sci. Polon., 20: 599-606.
16. Levine, S. and Payan, H. (1966): Exp. Neurol., 16: 255-262.
17. Levy, D.E., Brierley, J.B. and Plum, F. (1975): J. Neurol. Neurosurg. Psych., 38: 1197-12054.
18. Majewska, M.D., Lazarewicz, J.W. and Strosznajder, J. (1977): Bull. Acad. Sci. Polon., 25: 125-13.
19. Majewska, M.D., Strosznajder, J. and Lazarewicz, J.W. (1978): Brain Res., 158: 423-434.
20. Manaka, S., Sano, K., Fuchinoue, T. and Sekino, H. (1973): Experientia, 30: 179-180.
21. Martinet, M., Fonlupt, P. and Pacheco, H. (1978): Experientia, 34: 1197-1199.
22. Martinet, M., Fonlupt, P. and Pacheco, H. (1979): Arch. Int. Pharmacol., 239: 52-61.
23. Martinet, M., Fonlupt, P. and Pacheco, H. (1981): Biochem. Pharmacol., 30: 539-541.
24. Mellors, A., Tappel, A.L., Sarvant, P.L. and Desai, I.D. (1967): Biochim. Biophys. Acta, 143: 299-309.
25. Miyake, H., Hayakawa, I. and Takakura, K. (1964): Brain Nerve (Tokyo), 16: 77-82.
26. Ogashiwa, M., Takeudi, K., Hara, M., Tanaka, Y. and Okada, J. (1975): Int. J. Clin. Pharmacol., 12: 327-335.
27. Porcellati, G., DeMedio, G.E., Fini, C., Floridi, A. Goracci, G. Horrocks, L.A., Lazarewicz, J.W., Palmerini, C.A., Strosznajder, J. and Trovarelli, G. (1979): Proc. Eur. Soc. Neurochem., 1: 285-302.
28. Possmayer, F. (1974): Biochem. Biophys. Res. Commun., 61: 1415-1426.
29. Possmayer, F. and Mudd, J.B. (1971): Biochim. Biophys. Acta, 239: 217-233.
30. Price, C.J. and Rowe, C.E. (1972): Biochem. J., 126: 575-585.
31. Rigoulet, M., Guerin, B., Cohadon, F. and Vandendreissche, M. (1979): J. Neurochem., 32: 535-541.
32. Shimamoto, K., Hirano, T. and Aramaki, Y. (1975): J. Takeda Res. Lab. 34: 440-448.

33. Siesjö B.K. and Rehncrona, S. (1980): In "Biochemistry of Dementia", edited by P.J. Roberts, pp. 91-120. John Wiley and Sons Ltd., London, pp. 91-120

34. Strosznajder, J. and Dabrowiecki, Z. (1975): Bull. Acad. Sci. Polon., 23: 647-652.

35. Trovarelli, G., DeMedio, G.E., Dorman, R.V., Piccinin, G.L., Horrocks, L.A. and Porcellati, G. (1981): Neurochem. Res., 6:821-833.

36. Vance, D.E. and Choy, P. (1979): Trends Biochem. Sci., 4: 145-148.

37. Watanabe, S., Kano, S., Mitsunubu, K., Suzuki, T. and Otsuki, S. (1971): Brain Nerve (Tokyo), 25: 721-725.

38. Woldegiorgis, G. and Shrags, E. (1979): Biochem. Biophys. Res. Commun., 89: 837-844.

39. Wolfe, L.S. and Mamer, O.A. (1975): Prostaglandins, 9: 183-192.

40. Yasuhara, M. and Naito, H. (1974): Eur. Therap. Res., 16: 346-374.

41. Yoshida, S., Inoh, S., Asano, T., Sano, K., Kubota, M., Shimazuki, H. and Ueta, N. (1980): J. Neurosurg., 53: 323-331.

Phospholipids in the Nervous System, Vol. 1: Metabolism, edited by L. Horrocks, et al. Raven Press, New York © 1982.

Choline Transport and Metabolism in the Brain

G. Brian Ansell and Sheila Spanner

Department of Pharmacology, University of Birmingham, Medical School, Birmingham B15 2TJ, United Kingdom

In recent years there has been considerable research into the metaboism of brain choline in relation to: (a) its incorporation into choline-containing phospholipids, (b) its transport and release from the brain, (c) the immediate source of choline for acetylcholine synthesis and (d) neurological disorders in which choline metabolsim (particularly acetylcholine metabolism) may be affected. The levels of choline compounds in the brain are given in Table 1 and their metabolic inter-relationships in Fig. 1.

TABLE 1. <u>Choline compounds in brain tissue of the rat</u>

Compounds	Concentration (μmol/g fresh tissue)	Reference
Choline	0.024 (cerebrum)	13
Acetylcholine	0.070 (whole brain)	22
Phosphocholine	0.38	
Glycerophosphocholine	0.40	
CDP-choline	0.05	authors'
Phosphatidylcholine	14.70 (whole brain)	laboratory
Choline plasmalogen	0.60	
Sphingomyelin	3.70	

Clearly the cellular heterogeneity of the brain implies an infinite number of metabolic pools within that organ but in this brief review only some more general features are discussed.

THE CAPACITY TO SYNTHESISE CHOLINE DE NOVO

Earlier studies (12,2) had indicated that the capacity of the brain to synthesise choline by the stepwise methylation of phosphatidyl-ethanolamine, which is the only mechanism available to animal tissues, was negligible; this had interesting implications (vide infra). In the last three years however, there have been reports from different laboratories that formation of choline in the brain by this pathway can take place and the results are summarised in Table 2. These observations stem from the findings of Axelrod and his co-workers (24) that two

TABLE 2. Formation of phosphatidylcholine in brain tissue by methylation in vitro

	(pmol/mg protein/h)		
	Endogenous	+ Phosphatidyl-dimethylaminoethanol	Reference
Homogenate	0.11	1.1	31
Synaptosomes	10.3	122.0	14
Synaptosomes	2.6	–	9
	(Liver = ca 2700)		

methyltransferases are found in a variety of tissues. One of these (methyltransferase I) is dependent upon Mg^{2+} ions and can convert phosphatidylethanolamine to phosphatidylmonomethylaminoethanol. The other (methyltransferase II) introduces two further methyl groups to yield phosphatidylcholine and is independent of metallic cations. It is obvious from Table 2 however that the capacity of brain to synthesise choline in this way is very limited, as it is in all tissues except liver. The question arises therefore whether one of the functions of this pathway is to provide choline to supplement that formed in the liver or deriving from the diet or whether this stepwise methylation is only an expression of the capacity of cells to 'respond' to cell surface stimuli as investigated in detail by Hirata and Axelrod (23). In experiments in which [1,2-^{14}C]dimethylaminoethanol was injected intra-cerebrally into rats this was hown to be phosphorylated and incorporated into phosphatidyldimethylaminoethanol which was formed at a rate of about 5 nmol/g brain/h (7). However, only a negligible amount of this was methylated to phosphatidylcholine in 7 h.

Several workers have shown that there is an efflux of unesterified choline from the brain which can be as high as 12 nmol/min/g brain in the rat (11). Recent experiments on the rabbit (Garden, Key, Spanner and Ansell unpublished) have shown that, if [Me-^{3}H]choline was introduced into the lateral ventricle there was an initial rapid release of labelled choline into the transverse venous sinus. This was presumably a transfer from ventricle to sinus via the arachnoid villi. The choline was also, however, taken up into the brain and there was a continuous loss of labelled choline into the sinus, an efflux which was inhibited by hemicholinium-3 (cf. Ansell and Spanner (4)). It is clear that the efflux of choline from the brain is a real phenomenon though it cannot as yet be rationalised. Since the maximum estimated capacity for choline synthsis is no higher than 0.02 nmol/g brain/min (Table 2) it seems likely that in this species at least, the choline level in the brain needs to be maintained from an extra-cerebral supply.

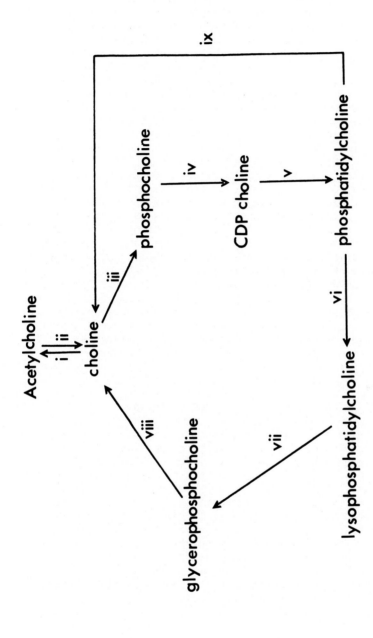

FIG. 1. Major pathways for choline metabolism in brain tissue. (i) choline acetyltransferase, (ii) acetylcholinesterase, (iii) choline kinase, (iv) cholinephosphate cytidylyltransferase, (v) choline phosphotransferase, (vi) phospholipase A$_2$, (vii) lysophospholipase, (viii) glycerophosphocholine phosphodiesterase, (ix) Ca^{2+} mediated base exchange reaction. Pathways including choline plasmalogen and sphingomyelin are less well established and are excluded.

THE TRANSPORT OF CHOLINE TO THE BRAIN

Though the choline lost from the brain cannot be replaced by synthesis within the brain it also seems unlikely that replacement occurs from unesterified choline in the plasma. This is normally at a very low level and although it can enter the brain from the arterial blood supply it is unlikely to be the major source (for a summary of the evidence see Ansell and Spanner (5)). Furthermore massive doses of choline by a variety of routes (eg. 9 μmol/min by intracarotid perfusion) do not raise the free choline levels in the brain by much more than twice the endogenous level (for a summary of these observations see Ansell and Spanner (6) and Flentge et al. (19)).

There is considerable evidence, however, that lipid-bound choline, particularly lysophosphatidylcholine, can transport choline to tissues (34). When lipid-bound choline was synthesised in the liver from labelled ethanolamine, choline lipids in the plasma were heavily labelled compared with free choline (3) and the specific radioactivity of lysophosphatidylcholine in plasma was ten times higher than free choline after an injection of labelled ethanolamine (29). One pool of lysophosphatidylcholine in the plasma of the monkey has a half life of only 12 min (32) and Illingworth and Portman (25) showed that albumin-bound doubly-labelled lysophosphatidylcholine introduced into the blood stream of the squirrel monkey was rapidly assimilated by the brain and acylated to phosphatidylcholine. Its labelled choline also appeared rapidly in the free choline, phosphocholine and acetylcholine of the brain. Jope and Jenden (26) have shown that if rats were fed deuterated choline then there were similar amounts of labelling of free choline, lysophosphatidylcholine (+ choline plasmalogen) and phosphatidylcholine in the plasma of rats from birth to three weeks. However, in the cerebral cortex and striatum the labelling of lysophosphatidylcholine was always higher than that of all other choline compounds, including acetylcholine, suggesting that the former is a primary choline donor in the brain.

THE RELEASE OF CHOLINE FROM LIPID-BOUND CHOLINE IN THE BRAIN

Although there have been many experiments on the turnover of phosphatidylcholine in the brain measured by the incorporation of labelled precursors administered by various routes, there is not, as far as we know comparable measurements of turnover by the determination of the labelling of catabolic products. In the liver there is little doubt that the major pathway is one by which fatty acids are removed by phospholipase A_1 (EC 3.1.1.32), A_2 (EC 3.1.1.4) and/or lysophospholipase (EC 3.1.1.5) and the resultant glycerophosphocholine hydrolysed by a diesterase (glycerophosphocholine phosphodiesterase (EC 3.1.4.38)). Dawson (15) clearly showed that glycerophosphocholine is on the pathway of phosphatidylcholine catabolism in the liver in vivo but as yet there has been no such study to indicate product-precursor relationships between phosphatidylcholine and its breakdown products in the brain. Glycerophosphocholine is present in brain tissue at the relatively high concentration of 0.4-0.6 μmol/g fresh weight (Table 1; refs 17 and 26) and could well yield choline by the action of the phosphodiesterase (8) but choline could also be released from phosphatidylcholine by the action of phospholipase D (EC 3.1.4.4) also known to be present (27).

It is clear from the work of Freeman and Jenden (20) that there is a

rapid rise in brain free choline post-mortem <u>in</u> <u>vitro</u> (2.3 μmol/g/h in
the striatum).   <u>In</u> <u>vivo</u> the level of free choline is very low (Table 1)
so that if the rate of production is as high <u>in</u> <u>vivo</u> as <u>in</u> <u>vitro</u> in
intact brain then it is either lost to the venous return or phosphory-
lated by the active choline kinase (EC 2.7.1.32).   Phosphocholine levels
are relatively high in brain (Table 1) and it could serve as a choline
'sink'.
      Recently Jope and Jenden (26) have drawn up a 'balance sheet' showing
changes in choline compounds in whole intact brain incubated at 37°.
Their observations are presented in a graphic form in Fig. 2. which

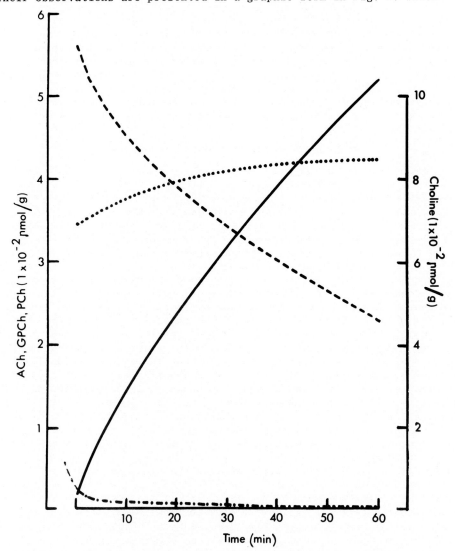

FIG. 2.   Post-mortem changes in the levels of choline compounds
in rat brain.   (———)choline,   (.....)phosphocholine,   (-----)
glycerophosphocholine,   (-.-.-.-.-)acetylcholine.   Adapted from
values given in ref. 26.

shows that the rise in free choline levels cannot be accounted for by the
hydrolysis of acetylcholine or phosphocholine. A significant amount can
be accounted for by the hydrolysis of glycerophosphocholine. Significant
losses of phosphatidylcholine but not lysophosphatidylcholine were
apparent but stoichiometric relationships cannot be deduced because, as
glycerophosphocholine and lysophosphatidylcholine were hydrolysed during
the incubation they were presumably replaced by further hydrolysis of
phosphatidylcholine. While it is by no means certain that the activity of
glycerophosphocholine diesterase is responsible for all this choline production it seems reasonable to assume that it plays a significant part.
The observation by Zeisel (35) that choline production in brain homogenates was stimulated by Mg^{2+}ions might, however, suggest a less significant role for the diesterase. Although the activity of the enzyme is
dependent upon a divalent cation, only very low concentrations are
required, e.g. <18 μM Ca^{2+} for maximal activity in subcellular fractions
(8), concentrations which would certainly be present in brain homogenates.
Thus, if choline is brought to the brain in a lipid-bound form and
assimilated within the lipid-choline pool of the brain, the mechanisms by
which it is released and eventually transferred to the venous return are
still unknown.

THE LOCALISATION OF CHOLINE RELEASE

The release of choline from a lipid-bound form can occur in all areas
of the brain though the process is more active in vitro in the striatum
compared with cortex (26). If choline release is an important factor in
producing choline for acetylcholine synthesis then the striatum, which
is rich in cholinergic activity, would be expected to show a high capacity for release and, if the diesterase is involved, this might also be
expected to show high activity. Although levels of glycerophosphocholine
are high in that region (26) the activity of the diesterase is not (8).
No well-documented information is available on the distribution of the
release mechanisms between neurones and glial cells. Certainly, lesions
of the septum leading to the destruction of cholinergic neurones did not
affect the release of choline on subsequent incubation of the hippocampus (20). The diesterase activity of the synaptosomes prepared from
the caudate nucleus was low when compared with whole brain (8). On the
other hand Blusztajn and Wurtman (9) have shown that a synaptosomal preparation from rat brain could synthesise phosphatidylcholine from added
phosphatidyldimethylaminoethanol and this bound choline liberated as the
free base (a neuronal generating system). According to Droz et al. (18),
however, axonal transport seems to account for most of the phosphatidylcholine in nerve endings and it is too early to decide whether any
choline liberated at nerve endings is that formed by a methylation pathway located there.

In so far as intraterminal acetylcholine synthesis is concerned,
there is good evidence that this is dependent on choline supplied exter-
nally to the plasma membrane of the terminal. If the uptake of this
choline into the terminal is inhibited by hemicholinium-3 the synthesis
of acetylcholine largely ceases (eg. Guyenet et al. (21)). There is indeed
considerable evidence which suggests that the formation of acetylcholine
is dependent upon a high affinity system for choline uptake though this
has been disputed (28). On this basis it is possible that choline is
liberated from adjacent glial cells ready for re-uptake by nerve terminals. This would supplement choline made available by the hydrolysis of
acetylcholine released from cholinergic terminals, the efficiency of

whose recapture is unknown.

CONCLUSION

The mechanisms associated with intermediary choline metabolism in the brain are complex and ill-defined. Though the form in which choline is delivered to the brain may well be predominantly lysophosphatidylcholine, this may vary from species to species and it is not at all obvious where this phospholipid is primarily metabolised. There is evidence that lyso-phosphatidylcholine is rapidly acylated but whether this occurs predominantly in glial cells or neuronal perikarya is unknown. This acylation may yield a pool of phosphatidylcholine which rapidly mixes with the rest of the phosphatidylcholine in the cells or it may not. There must be countless pools of this phospholipid in an organ such as the brain. It has been noted that phosphatidylcholine rapidly moves down axons so it would appear that neuronal perikarya have an active phosphatidylcholine metabolism.

The relationship between the water-soluble choline compounds in the brain is also incompletely understood except for the clear immediate relationship between acetylcholine and free choline. However there are difficulties in assessing the relationship between even these two components in vivo (1). The acetylcholine is mainly in cholinergic terminals and occurs in both free and bound forms (see discussion by Marchbanks (30)) but it is not possible to determine the free choline level in terminals because a long period of time elapses before nerve endings can be isolated postmortem, by which time it will have been released from bound sources other than acetylcholine (20,26). The turnover of phosphocholine can be determined in nerve endings (16) because it is relatively stable (33). To what extent its turnover is 'divided' between a requirement for phosphatidylcholine synthesis and the control of free choline levels is, as yet, another unanswered question.

REFERENCES

1. Ansell, G.B. (1980): In: Central Neurotransmitter Turnover, edited by C.J. Pycock and P.V. Taberner, pp 81-104, Croom Helm, London.

2. Ansell, G.B. and Spanner, S. (1967): J. Neurochem., 14: 873-885.

3. Ansell, G.B. and Spanner, S. (1971): Biochem. J., 122: 741-750.

4. Ansell, G.B. and Spanner, S. (1975): Biochem. Pharmacol., 24: 1719-1723.

5. Ansell, G.L. and Spanner, S. (1975): In: Cholinergic Mechanisms, edited by P.G. Waser, pp 117-129, Raven Press, New York.

6. Ansell, G.B. and Spanner, S. (1978): In: Cholinergic Mechanisms and Psychopharmacology, edited by D.J. Jenden, pp 431-445, Plenum Press, New York.

7. Ansell, G.B. and Spanner, S. (1979): Zh. Evol. Biokhim. Fiziol., 15: 249-253.

8. Ansell, G.B. and Spanner, S. (1981): In: Cholinergic Mechanisms: Phylogenetic Aspects, Central and Peripheral Synapses, and Clinical Significance, edited by G. Pepeu and H. Ladinsky, pp 393-403, Plenum Press, New York.

9. Blusztajn, J.K. and Wurtman, R.J. (1981): Nature, 290: 417-418.

10. Blusztajn, J.K., Zeisel, S.H. and Wurtman, R.J. (1979): Brain Res. 179: 319-327.

11. Choi, R.L., Freeman, J.J. and Jenden, D.J. (1975): J. Neurochem.,
     24: 735-741.

12. Chojnacki, T., Korzybski, T. and Ansell, G.B. (1964): Biochem. J.,
     90: 18-19P.

13. Cohen, E.L. and Wurtman, R.J. (1976): Science, 191: 561-562.

14. Crews, F.T., Hirata, F. and Axelrod, J. (1980): J. Neurochem., 34,
     1491-1498.

15. Dawson, R.M.C. (1955): Biochem. J., 59: 5-8.

16. Dowdall, M.J., Barker, L.A. and Whittaker, V.P. (1972): Biochem. J.,
     130: 1081-1094.

17. Dross, K. (1975): J. Neurochem., 24: 701-706.

18. Droz, B., Brunetti, M., Koenig, H.L., di Giamberardino, L. and
     Porcellati, G. (1982): In this volume.

19. Flentge, F. and Van den Berg, C.J. (1979): J. Neurochem., 32: 1331-
     1333.

20. Freeman, J.J. and Jenden, D.J. (1976): Life Sci., 19: 949-962.

21. Guyenet, P., Lefresne, P., Rossier, J., Beaujouan, J.C., and
     Glowinski, J. (1973): Brain Res., 62: 523-529.

22. Haubrich, D.R., Wang, P.F.L., Clody, D.E. and Wedeking, P.W. (1975):
     Life Sci., 17: 975-980.

23. Hirata, F. and Axelrod, J. (1980): Science, 209: 1082-1090.

24. Hirata, F., Viveros, O.A., Diliberto, E.J. Jr. and Axelrod, J.
     (1978): Proc. Natl. Acad. Sci. U.S.A., 75: 1718-1721.

25. Illingworth, D.R. and Portman, O.W. (1972): Biochem. J., 130: 557-
     567.

26. Jope, R.S. and Jenden, D.J. (1979): J. Neurosci. Res., 4: 69-82.

27. Kanfer, J.N. (1980): Canad. J. Biochem., 58: 1370-1380.

28. Kessler, P.D. and Marchbanks, R.M. (1979): Nature, 279: 542-544.

29. Kewitz, H. and Pleul, O. (1976): Proc. Natl.Acad.Sci.U.S.A., 73:
     2181-2185.

30. Marchbanks, R.M. (1977): In: Synapses, edited by G.A. Cottrell and
     P.R. Usherwood, pp 81-101, Blackie, Glasgow.

31. Mozzi, R. and Porcellati, G. (1979): FEBS Lett. 100: 363-366.

32. Portman, O.W., Soltys, P., Alexander, M. and Osuga, T. (1970):
     J. Lipid Res., 11: 596-604.

33. Spanner, S. and Ansell, G.B. (1979): Biochem. J., 178: 753-760.

34. Stein, Y. and Stein, O. (1966): Biochim. Biophys. Acta., 116: 95-
     107.

35. Zeisel, S.H. (1982): In this volume.

Phospholipids in the Nervous System, Vol. 1: Metabolism, edited by L. Horrocks, et al. Raven Press, New York © 1982.

The Effects of Carbamylcholine on Extrasynaptic Phosphatidylcholine Biosynthesis in Grey Matter of Cerebral Cortex

M. Giesing and U. Gerken

Labor für Nervengewebekultur, Institut für Physiologische Chemie der Universität, D-5300 Bonn, Germany

The initial observations of a regulatory effect of acetylcholine on the metabolism of some acidic phospholipids (PL) by Hokin and Hokin (17) and by Durell and Sodd (7) took some time to make an impact. Since then fundamental evidence for the role of phosphatidic acid (PA), diacylglycerol (DG) and phosphatidylinositol (PI) in synaptic transmission has emerged from the work of various groups. The whole field has been comprehensively reviewed by Hawthorne and Pickard (14). The use of a phosphate label in the lipids and the availability of nerve ending preparations served as experimental tools in many of these investigations. On the basis of these investigations it seems likely today that the neurotransmitter receptor is somehow associated with a phospholipase C type enzyme leading to the degradation of PI ("PI-breakdown"). The enigma of pre- or postsynaptic localization, however, remains for obvious reasons (14).

Because synaptosomal pellets are not homogeneous and contain only a small part of the post-synaptic structure and because we have found that ingrowing synapses affect PL other than PI in total CNS tissues in explant culture without chemical or electrical manipulation (10, 12,13), we decided to start our experiments with living material. The development and the maintenance of a complex pattern of cell specific traits that is unique for the explant system led our attention to the cellular relationship of zwitterionic lipids - mainly phosphatidylcholine (PC) - that appeared to be affected by cholinergic stimuli under certain conditions (10) as will be described here in detail. In order to obtain a preliminary structural specificity the experiments were carried out in grey matter of cerebral cortex (CC) representing a "concentrate" of nerve cells during early culture periods. A broad spectrum of biochemical and cellular analysis of the cultures allows the localization of the lipid effects in cholinergic neurons. It is known that norepinephrine stimulates the biosynthesis of zwitterionic lipids via the methylation pathway in reticulocytes (16). We have used various radioisotopes that were incorporated into lipid classes of viable cells by

---

Part of this work originates from the "Habilitationsschrift" presented to the Faculty of Medicine, University Bonn, 1978.

the activity of either the endoplasmic reticulum or the plasma membrane. Extrasynaptic enzymes involved in the formation of PC have been measured under standard conditions. And finally, an attempt was made to demonstrate the biological significance of our findings with respect to the functioning of neuronal circuits.

METHODS

Explant Culture Technique

Fragments were dissected from CC of two days old rats yielding approximately 70 tissue specimens per donor animal. Up to 12 explants were layered on a collagen covered coverslip and maintained in Petri dishes (13). Delipidation of the nutrient solution was achieved by extraction in chilled ether (18). In some experiments white matter explants were prepared. The tissue was devoid of nerve cell material and served therefore, as a glial cell model. Cell growth measurements were performed with a computerized high-speed scanning photometer light microscope (Zeiss).

Subcellular Fractionation

Nerve endings, microsomes and cytosol were obtained from homogenates (10) (4 mg protein in 5 ml sucrose solution) after the method of Kurokawa et al. (20). Cytosol, i.e. the 100000 x g supernatant was concentrated by ultrafiltration (Amicon 8MC; PM-10 filters) until appropriate accumulation of enzyme proteins was achieved.

Incubation Solutions

Viable cells were incubated after removal of the nutrient solution and repeated rinses in buffer with [2-^{3}H]glycerol or with S-[^{3}H-Me]-adenosyl-L-methionine (SAM) as indicated. The radioisotopes were dissolved in Medium M-199, a buffer solution containing a variety of auxiliary compounds. Subcellular fractions were incubated with [^{14}C]-glycerol-3-phosphate (spec.radioactivity:260 dpm/pmol) using the method of Possmayer and Mudd (30).

Lipid Analysis

Cellular lipids were extracted from culture homogenates (13) after Yavin and Menkes (37). For separating neutral lipids from PL the crude lipid extract was fractionated on Florisil columns (13). Neutral lipids were chromatographed on silica gel plates in an appropriate solvent system (30). Total PL were separated by two-dimensional chromatography (1). Chromatographic separation of PL labelled from exogenous SAM was carried out after Hirata et al. (16). Lipid phosphorus was measured after the method of Bartlett (2).

Enzyme Assays

Carbonic anhydrase (EC 4.2.1.1)
The glial specific enzyme (32) was determined essentially according to Rickli et al. (31). The shift of the indicator color was read at 610 nm.

Phospholipase A

The enzyme was measured in pulse chase experiments from lyso-PC bound radioactivity stemming from endogenously labeled [2-^{3}H-glycerol]-PC. Differentiation between A_1 and A_2 activity (EC 3.1.1.32 and 3.1.1.4) was not possible.

CTP:cholinephosphate cytidylyltransferase (EC 2.7.7.15)

The formation of CDPcholine from [^{14}C]phosphocholine (spec. radioactivity:27.5 mCi/mmol) was measured after Borkenhagen and Kennedy (3) by the modification of Fiscus and Schneider (8). The reaction product was extracted from charcoal suspensions in formic acid followed by chromatography on silica gel plates (CH$_3$OH/0.6% NaCl/NH$_4$OH; 50/50/5; by volume). Lipids were previously added in the form of emulsions (29).

CDPcholine:1,2-diacylglycerol cholinephosphotransferase (EC 2.7.8.2)

Enzyme activity was determined in microsomal fractions after Whiting et al. (35). PC-bound radioactivity originated from CDP[Me-^{14}C] choline (spec. radioactivity:0.53 mCi/mmol) in the presence of different DG as indicated.

Gamma-Aminobutyric Acid (GABA) Binding to Receptors and Carriers; GABA Transport

Binding and transport studies were carried out under isothermal equilibrium conditions either in postnuclear homogenates (binding) or in living cells (transport). Some kinetic data and pharmacological specifications have been reported recently (11). The bimolecular rection occurs according to:

$$R + GABA \xrightleftharpoons[K_{-1}]{K_{+1}} R \cdot GABA$$

in which R=receptor or carrier protein; R·GABA=receptor or carrier complex; k=rate constant for association (+) and dissociation (-). The velocity of R·GABA formation follows the equation:

$$R \cdot GABA = R_0 \cdot (1 - e^{-(k_{+1} \cdot GABA_0 \cdot t)})$$

On the basis of this equation we found under experimental conditions a half maximum occupancy time of 4 min at a ligand concentration of 25 nmol/L, of 2 min at 5 μmol/L and of 6 sec at 100 μmol/L. Two rate constants were calculated, one of $k_{+1}=7 \times 10^6$ M^{-1}min^{-1} at $K_D/10$ of the receptor binding and the other one of $k_{+1}=2.6 \times 10^4$ M^{-1}min^{-1} at approximately $K_d/2$ of the carrier binding. The data were obtained from viable cells.

The maximum receptor or carrier density (B_{max}) and the dissociation constant (K_D) was determined after the Scatchard equation. Binding and transport is expressed in specific terms as calculated from total cellular bound (transported)[^{3}H]GABA radioactivity minus binding or transport in the presence of 1000-fold excess unlabeled GABA. If not otherwise stated kinetic studies were performed in the form of association experiments for:

GABA-receptor binding:
Na$^+$-independent receptive sites (22) at ligand concentrations of 10, 20, 40, 80, 120, 160 and 240 nmol/L for 30 min at 4°C.

GABA-carrier binding:
Na$^+$-dependent receptive sites (25) at ligand concentrations of 0.2, 2,5, 10, 15, 20 µmol/L for 30 min at 4°C as measured in both cases in 0.2 ml culture protein plus 0.2 ml ligand in HEPES buffer (10 mmol/L). The reaction was terminated by glass filter assays (Whatman GF/A; 2.4 cm in diameter).

GABA-transport:
Na$^+$-dependent uptake (11) of the ligand dissolved in M-199 at a final concentration of 5, 10, 20, 30, 40, 60, 80 and 100 µmol/L given to viable cells for 4 min at 37°C in a volume of 0.2 ml per coverslip.

Radioactivity Measurement

The composition of the scintillation cocktails has been given elsewhere (10,13). Quench correction was made by the automatic external standardisation procedure for homogenates and filters and by the channel ratio method for silica gel material.

RESULTS AND DISCUSSION

De Novo Biosynthesis of Phosphatidylcholine

The de novo biosynthesis of PC was studied from exogenously applied [2-^{3}H]glycerol as a function of the culture period, the incubation time, the concentration of cholinergic stimuli and with respect to subcellular activities. Cholinergic stimulation was achieved by application of either acetylcholine (ACh) in the presence of eserine (ES), an inhibitor of acetylcholinesterase, or by carbamylcholine (CaCh).

Fig. 1 comprises the developmental sequence of two different component cells in CC explants with regard to the formation of PC. Nerve cells, astroglia and oligodendroglia showed a stepwise development that followed virtually the same pattern as reported in vivo (26). Within the first 10 days in vitro (DIV) the tissue fragments generated highly differentiated synapses (Fig. 1,a). Synaptogenesis was obviously occurring at that early stage since preparation of submitochondrial fractions on a discontinuous sucrose-Ficoll gradient (20) yielded highly purified nerve ending particles (10). The synaptosomes could be characterized by the presence of a CaCh induced "PI-breakdown" (Giesing and Gerken, in preparation).

From DIV 10 to 20 protoplasmic and fibrous astrocytes increased in size (Fig. 1,b). The growth was based on a rise in total cell volume with constant nuclear number. From DIV 20 onwards oligodendrocytes matured as could be seen in the light microscope (Fig. 1,c) and from galactolipid formation (10). After 4 to 5 weeks in vitro the tissue depicted the typical patterns of a heterogenous population of mature component cells (Fig. 1,d).

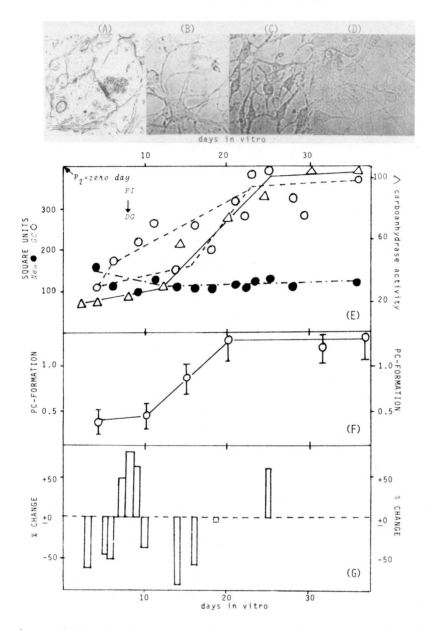

FIG. 1. Cell development in cerebral cortex explants. The morphological characteristics are: synapse formation (1,a) in phase I (days in vitro (DIV) 1-10); astroglia- (1,b) and oligodendroglia growth (1,c) in phase II,a and II,b (DIV 11-30); mature tissue depicting the typical cellular heterogeneity thereafter for extremely long periods of culture of more than 150 DIV (1,d). Quantitation of cell development is shown in i,e as measured from light microscopic scanning of viable protoplasmic astroglia (GC) and unipolar neurons (NEU).

Results are given in arbitrary square units. The glial pattern is accompanied by the activity of carbonicanhydrase and by the de novo biosynthesis of phosphatidylcholine (PC). Formation of PC is given in mol x 10^{-2} incorporated $[2-^3H]$-glycerol/nmol PC $(1,f)$ arising from a 2.5 h incubation of the label (spec.radioactivity: 200 mCi/mmol). Each coverslip was incubated with 0.2 ml of the radioisotope (1.1×10^6 dpm). The effects of cholinergic stimulation on PC biosynthesis is given in $1,g$. The cultures were simultaneously incubated with the label and acetylcholine (100 µmol/L) in the presence of eserine (100 µmol/L). Phase I can be divided into phase I,a (inhibition of PC) and phase I,b (stimulation of PC formation). Each individual result is expressed as the average value from at least four independent determinations.

The de novo biosynthesis of PC changed in parallel with the cellular development (Fig. 1,f). A stationary phase was observed during the neuronal phase I. Between DIV 10 and 20 (neuronal-glial phase II,a) the molar radioactivity increased several fold as did the glial cell master enzyme carbonic anhydrase (Fig. 1,e). Neither oligodendroglia activity (phase II,b) nor maturity was expressed by any further change in PC-formation. Control experiments in glia cell explants that were completely devoid of neuronal cell material confirmed this result suggesting that stimulation of PC biosynthesis in phase II,a is the expression of membrane production in astroglial cells.

On the basis of these results we studied the effects of cholinergic stimuli (ACh plus Es) on PC formation (Fig. 1,g). The results allowed us to divide phase I into phase I,a (DIV 2-5) in which PC biosynthesis is reduced and phase I,b (DIV 6-9) in which the stimulus enhanced the incorporation of glycerol. In phase II,a PC formation was reduced again followed by another increase in phase II,b.

An attempt was made to explain the "sigmoidal" effects by application of either hexamethonium, a blocker of the nicotinic receptor, or by atropine which antagonizes the muscarinic receptor. As can be seen in Table 1 the cholinergically induced effects on PA, DG and PC in phase I,b could be selectively abolished by hexamethonium whereas in phase II,a both blockers were inoperative. Only PA radioactivity was affected by atropine rather than by hexamethonium.

These results indicate that only neuronal PC is stimulated through activation of the nicotinic receptor. The narrow range of culture time in which this effect was observed is concomitant with the period of synaptogenesis (DIV 6-9) during which the receptor might be synthesized or activated. Even if the receptor is not operating in phase II which is unlikely an unspecific reaction of glial cells would dominate any neuronal activity since that neuron-glia ratio is then at least 1:10. With respect to the difference in cell size only 5% of the protein in the culture can be attributed to nerve cells. The distribution of neuronal protein in phase I,b would be much more in favour of nerve cells. Hence, phase II results might be less specific as suggested already by Abdel-Latif et al. (1). For that reason all experiments designed to elucidate the PC-effect were carried out in phase I,b cultures.

A major argument against our findings is the long period during which the stimulus might be in contact with the receptor. In view of the msec range in which a cholinergic neuron transmits electrical signals via its synapses application of the stimulus for only one minute would be very artificial and a shorter period is not possible for practical reasons. We conclude from these considerations that our findings are most likely not the reflection of neuronal bioelectricity. It seems more likely that the PC-effect is the expression of a neuromodulatory activity. In this context we felt that it would be useful to study the incorporation of glycerol into cellular PC as a function of time. Results are set out in Fig. 2.

TABLE 1. Effect of atropine and hexamethonium on PC formation during cell differentiation[a]

CELL LIPID CULTURE PERIOD	PA	DG	PC	PA	DG	PC
		phase I,b			phase II,a	
			CHANGE			
acetylcholine +eserine	+ 50	+ 84	+99	+600	± 0	-57
carbamylcholine	+100	+ 94	+99	+233	-49	-61
acetylcholine +hexamethonium	± 0	± 0	± 0	+100	-61	-64
acetylcholine +atropine	+75	+139	+80	± 0	-27	-57

[a] [2-^{3}H]glycerol (spec. radioactivity:6.4 Ci/mmol) was added to viable CC explants in 0.2 ml Medium M-199 per coverslip containing 10 µCi for 3 h at 34.5°C. Radioactivity in cellular phosphatidic acid (PA), diacylglycerol (DG) and phosphatidylcholine (PC) was determined in quadruplicate from previously stimulated cultures. Each additive had a final concentration of 100 µmol/L. Average values are given. Insignificant changes are expressed as ± 0%.

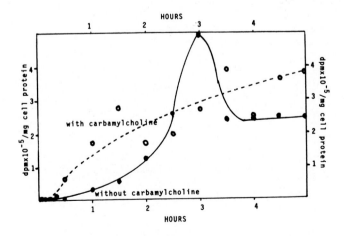

FIG. 2. Effect of time on PC formation. Carbamylcholine was incubated at 100 µmol/L in the presence of [2-^{3}H]glycerol as described in Table 1. Averages from six individual assays are given.

The stimulus was given to viable cultures for periods between 5 min
and 5 h in the presence of the radiolabel. Two different effects could
be seen, namely a "short-term" inhibition and a "long-term" stimulation
of PC biosynthesis. Both effects were dependent on the concentration of
the stimulus and also on the incubation modalities. The "short-term"
effect, i.e. incubation of the label for 30 min, could only be seen in
the range of 10^{-4}mol CaCh/L when the stimulus was given in the
presence of the label. A decrease in PC-radioactivity was found after
preincubation with the stimulus at a higher concentrations (Fig. 3).
The "long-term" effect, i.e. a 3 h incubation with [2-^{3}H]glycerol, was
different with respect to the concentration of the stimulus. The
maximum stimulation of PC formation was observed at 10^{-7} mol/L.
Preincubation with carbamylcholine for 30 min gave less incorporation
into PC than did a 3 h incubation with CaCh.

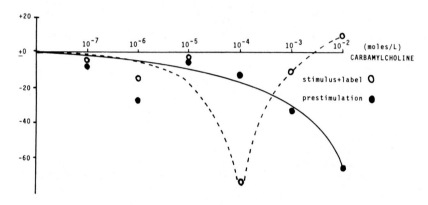

FIG. 3.   "Short-term" effect of carbamylcholine on PC-formation.
Averages from 4 determinations are given in % change.

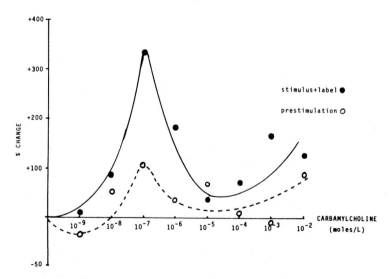

FIG. 4. "Long-term" effect of carbamylcholine on PC-formation. The results are expressed as averages from quadruplicates.

TABLE 2. Regulation of "short-term" and "long-term" effects of cholinergic stimuli on biosynthesis of PC de novo by muscarinic and nicotinic blockers[d]

[2-^{3}H-glycerol]-PC	"short-term"	"long-term"
	CHANGE	
acetylcholine +eserine	-16	+99
carbamylcholine	-89	+99
acetylcholine +hexamethonium	-40	± 0
acetylcholine +atropine	-72	+80

[d]Each additive was present at 100 µmol/L in the presence of the radio-isotope. The incubation period with [2-^{3}H]glycerol was 30 min ("short-term") or 180 min ("long-term").

The specificity of the "short-term" and "long-term" effects of cholinergic stimulation was studied by the addition of hexamethonium and atropine, respectively. The "short-term" inhibition of PC biosynthesis was not affected by atropine and could be slightly reduced by hexamethonium if compared with CaCh. In comparison with ACh plus Es, the two blockers increased the inhibitory effect. In contrast, the "long-term" stimulation of PC biosynthesis as induced either by ACh plus Es or by CaCh was specifically abolished by hexamethonium (Table 2). Hence it seems that the "short-term" effect is less specifically associated with receptor activity.

The "long-term" effect on [2-^{3}H]glycerol incorporation into cellular PC was also to be seen in some other glycerolipids. At 10^{-9} mol/L of the stimulus radioactivity, PA was significantly enhanced whereas the labeling of the zwitterionic lipids was less changed (Fig. 5). Incubation with higher de novo concentrations of CaCh resulted in a stimulation of the formation of various glycerolipids de novo as follows: phosphatidic acid (a 30-fold increase)>phosphatidylinositol>phosphatidylcholine> diacylglycerol>phosphatidylethanolamine. Only phosphatidylserine (PS) and a chromatographic spot that was tentatively identified as cytidine 5'-diphosphate diacylglycerol (CDP-DG) showed reduced radioactivity. These results were obtained after a 30 min preincubation with the cholinergic stimulus. It is worth noting that the pattern of the introduction of radiolabeled glycerol into individual glycerolipids was changed with respect to PC when the incubation conditions were altered. Hence it is possible that the de novo biosynthesis of other glycerophospholipids might be affected by cholinergic stimuli. This consideration prompted us to search for evidence that might indicate the specificity of the neuronal PC-effect.

At first we focussed primarily on subcellular activities and "chase" experiments with labelled glycerol. Synaptosomes and microsomes were prepared from phase I,b explants of CC that were stimulated with ACh plus Es (100 µmol/L each) for a 3 h period, i.e. "long-term" condition. The fractions showed specific changes in the de novo biosynthesis of glycerolipids (Table 3). The results obtained with the microsomes confirmed in part the data obtained from total tissue namely enhanced formation of PA followed by PC>PE>PI. Microsomal DG and PS were reduced in radioactivity. Synaptosomal lipids incorporated the label to a much lesser extent in spite of a much longer incubation period. Practically

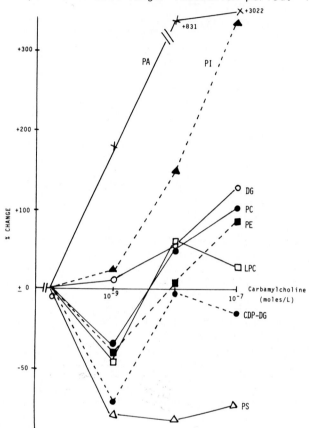

FIG. 5. Regulation of cellular glycerolipids by carbamylcholine under "long-term" conditions. Results are averages from four individual determinations.

TABLE 3. De novo biosynthesis of subcellular glycerolipids[a]

SUBCELLULAR LIPIDS	dpm x mg protein[-1]					
MICROSOMES	PA	DG	PC	PE	PS	PI
no prestimulation	107	531	1880	544	533	2325
with prestimulation	400	139	3981	827	83	2977
SYNAPTOSOMES						
no prestimulation	188	1773	433	1178	194	422
with prestimulation	22	8268	228	152	89	67

[a]Subcellular fractions were prepared from phase I,b cultures of cerebral cortex previously stimulated with acetylcholine plus eserine (each compound 100 μmol/L) for a 3 h period. The fractions were incubated with [^{14}C]glycerol-3-phosphate as described in the methods section. Microsomes were incubated for 10 min, synaptosomes for a 30 min period.

all lipid bound radioactivity (89%) was accumulated in DG. Whether this
finding is the expression of a cholinergically induced activation of
phosphatidate phosphohydrolase as suggested earlier by Schacht and
Agranoff (33) and Abdel-Latif et al. (1) remains obscure at present.
    The most significant findings from chase experiments with [2-^{3}H]-
glycerol introduced into cellular lipids from viable cells are
summarized in Fig. 6. Among the degradation products of PI and PC that
were measured, the label was accumulated specifically and exclusively in
lyso-PC with respect to time (Fig. 6,a). ACh plus Es was more effective
than CaCh. The degradation of PC occurred in the microsomes but was
absent in synaptosomes (Fig. 6,b). According to the time required for
the degradation of microsomal PC (10 min) this event can be attributed
to the "short-term" effects of cholinergic stimulation. Because of the
heterogeneous composition of membrane fragments in the 100000xg pellet
and the cell surface localization of the cholinergic receptor it is
concluded that the stimulation of phospholipase A is based on the
structural proximity of the enzyme and the receptor. If that is the
case lyso-PC should play a key role in regulation of the synthesis of
the endoplasmic reticulum as suggested from glycerol-3-phosphate
incorporation (Table 3).

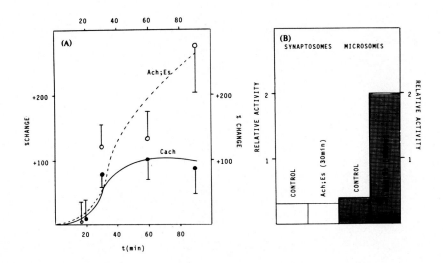

FIG. 6. Phospholipase A activity in CC explants. Fig. 6,a shows the
percentage increase of [2-^{3}H]glycerol accumulation in lyso-PC as a
function of time measured in total tissue fragments. The results
represent averages from triplicate experiments obtained after 2.5 h
prelabeling of the cultures. The label was chased with unlabelled
glycerol (10 µmol/L). Fig. 6,b shows the subcellular localization of
the enzyme activity. Synaptosomes and microsomes were obtained from
prelabelled cultures. The label was chased as above in the presence of
cholinergic agonists and NaF (10 mmol/L) to inhibit phosphatidate
phosphohydrolase activity. The results are expressed as averages from
triplicate determinations in the form of relative activity as calculated
from the ratio lyso-PC/PC. ACh, Es and CaCh were added to all
incubations at a final concentration of 100 µmol/L each.

Phospholipid Methylation

The use of tritiated S-adenosyl-L-methionine has an advantage over glycerol since only some of the zwitterionic lipids and no acidic phospholipids are labelled.   Phosphatidyl-N-monomethylethanolamine (PME), phosphatidyl-N-dimethylethanolamine (PDE) and PC labelled from SAM have been reported to be localized in the cell surface membrane with an asymmetric distribution across the membrane (5).   We have chosen a 10 min incubation period of the label in order to evaluate the "short-term" effect of cholinergic stimulation.   Furthermore, incubation of SAM for 3 h produced a random distribution of tritium among the lipids.   Fig. 7 shows the results in terms of phospholipid methylation as a function of CaCh concentration.   The stimulus induced a several-fold increase in the methylation of PME whereas all other methylation products including lyso-PC were reduced.   The stimulation of PDE formation required a concentration of the stimulus two magnitudes higher than that for the inhibition of the other lipids.   The CaCh induced inhibition of PC formation with "short-term" conditions required a lower concentration of the stimulus as measured by the methylation pathway whereas the

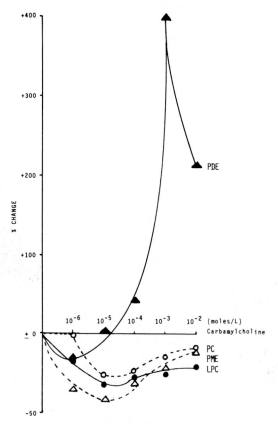

Fig. 7.   Phospholipid methylation in CC explants.   Cholinergic stimulation was achieved by preincubation under "short-term" conditions. The label (SAM) was present for 10 min at 200 µmol/L.   Averages from quadruplicate determinations are given.   Abbreviations are explained in the text.

inhibitory effect of CaCh was more potent as measured by glycerol incorporation.

Because of the enzyme-mediated asymmetric distribution of PE and PME (cytoplasmic side) on the one hand and of PDE and PC (external side) on the other as suggested by Axelrod and collaborators (5,15), the CaCh-effect on the methylation pathway was measured under "cytoplasmic" and "external" conditions. According to the findings of these authors, a low concentration of SAM (1 μmol/L) leads to the formation of PME, and a high concentration of the precursor (200 μmol/L) leads to PDE and PC. As can be seen in Table 4 cholinergic stimulation led to a specific increase in PDE formation with either experimental condition. We observed only a small difference, namely a two fold stimulation, with "cytoplasmic" conditions and a fourfold increase with "external" conditions. Also, reduced utilisation of SAM for PC formation could not be observed with "cytoplasmic" conditions.

These data suggest that the "short-term" effect of CaCh is associated with events occurring on the external surface of a given cellular plasma membrane. However, it also seems possible that the difference in exogenous SAM concentration is inappropriate for the identification of an enzyme-mediated translocation of membrane PL in living neurons. That this experimental arrangement is appropriate for nerve ending preparations (5) and for reticulocyte ghosts (16) may be explained by the topology of membrane lipids that may be stationary in centrifuged pellets whereas the lipids in living neurons could be undergoing a fast transmembrane movement. Even applications of phospholipase C in order to discriminate between cytoplasmic and external surface would not necessarily give the correct answer unless an enzymatically introduced transbilayer movement could be excluded. Problems associated with the topology and the dynamics of membrane lipids have been comprehensively discussed by van Deenen (34).

TABLE 4. Phospholipid methylation with "cytoplasmic" and "external" conditions[d]

Methyl-incorporation	1 μmol/L		200 μmol/L	
	femtomoles	%	picomoles	%
PME				
without stimulus	143.5±42.1	25.0	3.00±0.38	22.0
with stimulus	105.9±24.7	10.4	1.68±0.52	4.7
PDE				
without stimulus	368.4±24.6	64.1	6.33±2.20	46.7
with stimulus	814.9±102	80.0	31.19±8.99	88.7
PC				
without stimulus	25.5±3.8	4.4	1.76±0.17	13.0
with stimulus	48.7±12	4.8	1.22±0.13	3.4
lyso-PC				
without stimulus	37.4±13	6.5	2.47±0.48	18.3
with stimulus	49.5±16	4.9	1.18±0.49	3.3

[a]Cholinergic stimulation was achieved by preincubation of the cultures with CaCh (1 mmol/L) for 30 min. SAM was provided for 10 min thereafter (concentration as indicated). The spec. radioactivity of SAM was 29.7 dpm/fmol under "cytoplasmic" conditions and 368 dpm/pmol under "external" conditions. The results are expressed as the averages of four determinations ± SD in the form of moles labelled methyl groups incorporated/mg protein.

Enzymes Involved in Phasphatidylcholine Biosynthesis

     CTP:cholinephosphate cytidylyltransferase (EC 2.7.7.15) and CDPcholine:1,2-diacylglycerol cholinephosphotransferase (EC 2.7.8.2) were measured in subcellular fractions obtained from phase I,b cultures that were previously stimulated with CaCh or ACh plus Es under "long-term" conditions.

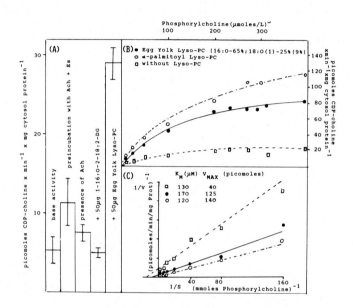

Fig. 8. Regulation of CTP:cholinephosphate cytidylyltransferase (EC 2.7.7.15) activity in phase I,b cultures of cerebral cortex. Experimental conditions are indicated. Lyso-PC was present at 40 µg per assay in saturation experiments (8b,c). Lineweaver-Burk plots derive from data in 8,b.

     The findings for CDPcholine formation, catalyzed by the most likely pacemaker enzyme (19), are summarized in Fig. 8. Prestimulation of the cultures with ACh plus Es (100 µmol/L each) for 2.5 h resulted in doubling the baseline activity. This effect cannot be explained by the physical contact of the enzyme with the neurotransmitter (Fig. 8,a). Hence other natural components arising from cholinergic stimulation should serve as mediators. Two lipids could play that role. The first is diacylglycerol stemming from PI-hydrolysis in brain (14) and other tissues (21). The second is lyso-PC as indicated by our own observations (see Fig. 6) and recent observations of Woelk et al. (36). Both compounds have detergent activities but only lyso-PC stimulated the formation of CDPcholine (Fig. 8,a) in a concentration dependent and fatty acid-specific manner (Fig. 8,b). It is known that the activity of the enzyme in rat liver and intestinal musosa does depend on the lipid environment (8,29). Lyso-PC has a similar effect to that obtained in brain cultures. Stimulation of the enzyme activity can also be achieved by sodium dodecyl sulphate in a way that the high molecular weight forms (4). Under physiological conditions this effect might be caused by lyso-PC as expressed by a three fold increase in V_{max} at a relative constancy of the K_m value (Fig. 8,c). It is tempting to speculate that upon cholinergic stimulation receptor-associated phospholipase A_2 is activated and as a consequence of the lyso-PC operates in a kind of feed-back mechanism regulating two conformational states of cytidylyltransferase, namely the dissociated form when the receptor is activated and the aggregated form composed of at least three monomers, when no cholinergic stimulation occurs. The intracellular amount of CDPcholinewill determine the amount of PC that is to be synthesized in the nerve cells.

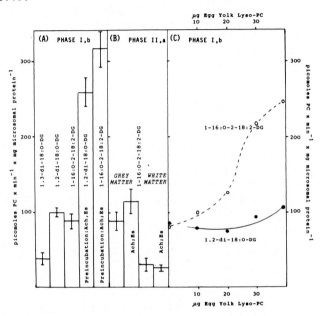

FIG. 9. Regulation of CDPcholine:1,2-diacylglycerol cholinephosphotransferase (EC 2.7.8.2) in grey matter (phase I,b and II,a) and white matter explants (phase II,a).

The formation of PC from CDPcholine and DG was also enhanced by a factor of three after "long-term" stimulation of phase I,b explants with ACh plus Es (Fig. 9,a). A most interesting finding was made with respect to the fatty acid composition of DG. Without stimulation the enzyme recognized primary hydroxyl groups but did not show any specificity towards the acyl groups in the 1- and 2-positions. After cholinergic stimulation a significant preference for unsaturated acyl residues in the 2-position was observed. This event occurs in nerve cells since cholinergic stimulation did not affect the enzyme activity in phase II,a cultures of grey matter and white matter (Fig. 9,b).

Since the intracellular level of CDPcholine determines the activity of the microsomal enzyme (19), the effects of cholinergic stimulation of the cytosolic enzyme may be expressed in the form of increased utilization of cellular DG. This consideration, however, would not explain the positional specificity for diacylglycerol fatty acids with respect to double bonds that is exhibited by the enzyme after treatment with the neurotransmitter. As can be seen in Fig. 9,c the discriminatory potency of the enzyme can be mimicked by lyso-PC, in assays in vitro. Lyso-PC had no effect on the utilization of saturated DG whereas PC formation from unsaturated DG was significantly enhanced in a concentration-dependent way.

One has certainly to ask whether the amount of lyso-PC stemming from cholinergic stimulation of CC explants can cause the effects on both enzymes. The phospholipase A assay we have used indicates that during "short-term" treatment with ACh approximately 20 picomoles of lyso-PC would be generated. This amount, however, would be insufficient. Nevertheless, this calculation does not exclude a mediator role of lyso-PC. One reason is that our assay might be inappropriate. This view is supported by the findings of others who studied the enzyme by using exogenous PC instead of endogenous substrate (36). These authors found in nerve cell preparations a norepinephrine-sensitive phospholipase A_2 activity in the nanomolar range. If that is the case in explants, the calculation will tip the balance in favour of the mediator role of lyso-PC.

Phospholipids and GABA-Binding to Receptors and Carriers

With the explant culture system available, a most challenging problem was to localize on a cellular basis the cholinergically induced formation of PDE ("short-term" effect) and of PC ("long-term" effect). The organotypic structure of the tissue fragments, i.e. the functional relationship between different types of neurons, was used to approach that aim. The experiments were designed on the assumption of the presence of synaptic contacts between inhibitory and excitatory neurons that were established in phase I,b.

Although the final concept of the balance between inhibition and excitation is not yet understood it seems that cellular PL may play an important role. Membrane PL are known to regulate a number of functional proteins. In connection with a possible role for PL in the binding of GABA to receptors, Lloyd and Beaumont (23) have provided evidence that a possible dysfunction of GABAergic neurons in epilepsy, schizophrenia, Parkinson's disease and Huntington's chorea is accompanied at least in part by changes in the PL composition of synaptic membranes. It has also been shown that antipsychotics increase the turnover of GABA in the globus pallidus suggesting that the release of the amino acid is facilitated and that perhaps these GABA containing neurons may impinge on cholinergic nerve cells producing their inhibition (24). Zsilla et al. (38) have reported that GABA receptor stimulants, diazepam and muscimol, reduce the turnover of acetylcholine in cerebral cortex.

Since GABA is a major inhibitory neurotransmitter in cerebral cortex (for review see ref. 28) on one hand and acetylcholine is the excitatory equivalent on the other, a simplified model depicting the functional relationship between inhibition and excitation in the explants is suggested (Fig. 10). The neuronal circuit is composed of a GABAergic nerve cell transmitting its inhibitory input on to a cholinergic neuron via an axosomatic synapse whereas the cholinergic cell provides stimulation of the GABAergic cell via an axodendritic synapse. Both forms of synapses are established in phase I,b cultures of CC (10).

Cholinergically induced stimulation of PDE and PC would possibly affect lipid-dependent membrane proteins in a GABAergic neuron if the postsynaptic acetylcholine receptor is activated. If receptors on the plasma membrane of the cholinergic neuron are activated the lipid effect could be associated with functional proteins in this cell type. GABA binding to carriers or GABA transport were chosen as parameters in the

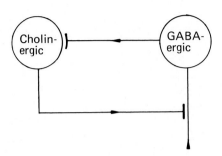

Fig. 10. Model of the functional relation between a GABAergic and a cholinergic nerve cell in cerebral cortex.

first case and GABA binding to receptors in the second. Previous studies in our laboratory have clearly shown that the kinetics of the carrier molecules binding the amino acid are specifically regulated by the polar head group as well as by the acyl groups of glycerophospholipids that are components of the microenvironment of the protein (11). Fiszer de Plazas and De Robertis (9) have earlier demonstrated the lipoprotein nature of the GABA receptor.

Results obtained from cholinergic stimulation of the cultures under "short-term" and "long-term" conditions are listed in Table 5. The stimulus enhanced selectively and specifically the affinity of the receptor for GABA. "Long-term" conditions were more potent than "short-term" application of the stimulus although the concentration of CaCh was three magnitudes lower in the first case. The increase in affinity for the ligand could be mimicked in membranes from cultures that were previously enriched with PL. PDE turned out to be more effective than PC. This finding strongly indicates that the CaCh-induced lipid effects occur in cholinergic neurons. This view is supported by the GABA-carrier assays. In contrast to the GABA-receptor-binding, cholinergic stimulation of the cultures did not affect the carrier system either with "short-term" or with "long-term" conditions although the activity of the protein is regulated by PL as measured from GABA-transport in viable cells.

Because of the "multiplicity" of GABA receptive sites we added in another series of experiments with bicuculline which is considered to be a highly selective inhibitor of the postsynaptic GABA-receptor (6,27). The drug was effective in displacing the ligand from the receptor in the control and after cholinergic stimulation (Table 6). Removal of FA from PL on the external side of the plasma membrane by incubation of viable cells with phospholipase A_2 resulted in a 40% reduction of GABA binding. Moreover, the displacement capacity of bicuculline was abolished.

TABLE 5. GABA-receptor, -carrier and -transport kinetics[a]

Isothermal GABA-binding	Na+-independent		Na+-dependent	
	$\overline{B}_{max}$ (pmol)	K_D (μmol/L)	B_{max} (pmol)	K_D (μmol/L)
control	21	0.9	750	13
carbamylcholine ("long-term")	21	0.2	800	17
carbamylcholine ("short-term")	24	0.3	700	14
			GABA-transport	
control			3500	40
PC-di-18:2	57	0.6	5500	120
PDE-di-16:0	47	0.3	3500	50

[a]Pretreatment of phase I,b cultures was carried out by addition of CaCh under "long-term" conditions (10^{-7} mol/L for 30 min followed by a 3 h incubation in Medium M-199) and "short-term" conditions (10^{-4} mol/L for 30 min). Introduction of exogenous PL into cell membranes was achieved by incubation of viable cells with PC or PDE as indicated. The lipids were solubilized in Medium M-199 (50 μg/ml) by ultrasonication. The kinetic data were obtained from Scatchard analysis. B_{max} is given in pmol/mg protein.

TABLE 6. Regulation of the postsynaptic GABA-receptor[a]

GABA-binding (Na+-independent)	(pmol/mg protein)		% change
	-bicuculline	+bicuculline	
control	2.43 ± 0.19	1.00 ± 0.28	-59
CaCh (10^{-4} mol/L)	10.30 ± 1.87	7.58 ± 0.61	-26
phospholipase A_2	1.37 ± 0.11	1.31 ± 0.74	± 0

[a]The displacement of GABA (120 nmol/L) from the postsynaptic receptor was achieved with bicuculline (50 nmol/L) present in the incubation mixture. The association experiment was carried out in postnuclear homogenates obtained from phase I,b cultures of cerebral cortex that were pretreated with carbamylcholine for 30 min or with phospholipase A_2 for 10 min. The enzyme was given to each coverslip in a concentration of 21 units in 0.2 ml Medium M-199. Results are given as averages ± SD from four independent determinations.

These findings confirm our suggestion that cholinergic stimulation of CC explants induces the formation of PDE ("short-term" effect) and of PC ("long-term" effect) in cholinergic nerve cells.

The experiments also show that membrane PL may play an important role in the concept of excitation and inhibition in the central nervous system. The dynamics of PL-mediated receptor functioning were previously demonstrated in our laboratory even without application of a neurotransmitter (10,12,13). In growing active synapses CaCh induced the formation of polyunsaturated fatty acids in target cells, affected the formation of various phospholipids and reduced the binding of inhibitory amino acid neurotransmitters.

ACKNOWLEDGEMENT

We are endebted to Zeiss (Köln, Germany) for giving us the opportunity to use a scanning photometer microscope.

REFERENCES

1. Abdel-Latif, A.A., Yau, S.-J. and Smith, J.P. (1974): J. Neurochem., 22:383-393.
2. Bartlett, G.R. (1959): J. Biol. Chem., 234:466-468.
3. Borkenhagen, L.F. and Kennedy, E.P. (1957): J. Biol. Chem., 227:951-962.
4. Choy, P.C., Lim, P.H. and Vance, D.E. (1977): J. Biol. Chem., 252:7673-7677.
5. Crews, F.T., Hirata, F. and Axelrod, J. (1980): Neurochem. Res., 5:983-991.
6. Curtis, D.R. and Felix, D. (1971): Brain Res., 34:302-321.
7. Durell, J. and Sodd, M.A. (1966): J. Neurochem., 13:487-491.
8. Fiscus, W.G. and Schneider, W.C. (1966): J. Biol. Chem., 241:3324-3330.
9. Fiszer de Plazas, S. and De Robertis, E. (1975): J. Neurochem., 25:547-552.
10. Giesing, M. (1978): Habilitationsschrift, University of Bonn.
11. Giesing, M., Schmitz, B., Kempfle, M., Egge, H. and Zilliken, F. (1981): In: New Trends in Nutrition, Lipid Research and Cardiovascular Diseases, edited by N.G. Bazán, J.M. Iacono, and R. Paoletti, (in press). Alan R. Liss, New York.
12. Giesing, M. and Zilliken, F. (1977): In: Cell Culture and its Application, edited by R. Acton, and J.D. Lynn, pp. 417-432. Academic Press, New York.
13. Giesing, M. and Zilliken, F. (1980): Neurochem. Res., 5:257-269.
14. Hawthorne, J.N. and Pickard, M.R. (1979): J. Neurochem., 32:5-14.
15. Hirata, F. and Axelrod, J. (1978): Proc. Natl. Acad. Sci. USA, 75:2348-2352.
16. Hirata, F., Strittmatter, W.J. and Axelrod, J. (1979): Proc. Natl. Acad. Sci. USA, 76:368-372.
17. Hokin, L.E. and Hokin, M.R. (1959): J. Biol. Chem., 234:1387-1390.
18. Horwitz, A.F., Hatten, M.E. and Burger, M.M. (1974): Proc. Natl. Acad. Sci. USA, 71:3115-3119.
19. Infante, J.P. (1977): Biochem. J., 167:847-849.
20. Kurokawa, M., Sakamoto, T. and Kato, M. (1965): Biochem. J., 97:833-844.
21. Lapetina, E.G. and Michell, R.H. (1973): FEBS Letters, 31:1-10.
22. Lester, B.R. and Peck, Jr., E.J. (1979): Brain Res., 161:79-97.
23. Lloyd, K.G. and Beaumont, K. (1980): Brain Res. Bull., 5:285-290.
24. Mao, C.C., Marco, G., Revuelta, A., Bertilsson, L. and Costa, E. (1977): Biol. Psychiat., 12:359-371.
25. Martin, D.L. (1973): J. Neurochem., 21:345-356.
26. McIlwain, H. (1959): Biochemistry and the Central Nervous System. Boston, Mass., Little Brown.
27. Möhler, H. and Okada, T. (1977): Nature (Lond.), 267:65-67.
28. Nistri, A. and Constanti, A. (1979): Prog. Neurobiol., 13:117-235.
29. O'Doherty, P.J.A., Smith, N.B. and Kuksis, A. (1977): Arch. Biochem. Biophys., 180:10-18.

30. Possmayer, F. and Mudd, J.B. (1971): Biochim. Biophys. Acta, 239:217-233.
31. Rickli, E.E., Ghazanfar, S.A.S., Gibbons, B.H. and Edsall, J.T. (1964): J. Biol. Chem., 239:1065-1078.
32. Roussel, G., Delaunoy, J.P., Nussbaum, J. and Mandel, P. (1979): Brain Res., 160:47-55.
33. Schacht, J. and Agranoff, B.W. (1974): J. Biol. Chem., 249:1551-1557.
34. Van Deenen, L.L.M. (1981): FEBS Letters, 123:3-15.
35. Whiting, P.H., Bowley, M., Sturton, R.G., Pritchard, P.H., Brindley, D.N. and Hawthorne, J.N. (1977): Biochem. J., 168:147-153.
36. Woelk, H., Arienti, G., Gaiti, A., Kanig, K. and Porcellati, G. (1981): Neurochem. Res., 6:23-32.
37. Yavin, E. and Menkes, J.H. (1973): J. Neurochem., 21:901-912.
38. Zsilla, G. Cheney, D.L., Racagni, G., and Costa, E. (1976): J. Pharmac. Exp. Ther., 199:662-668.

Phospholipids in the Nervous System, Vol. 1: Metabolism, edited by L. Horrocks, et al. Raven Press, New York © 1982.

Effects of Phosphatidylserine on Brain Cholinergic Mechanisms

P. Mantovani, *F. Aporti, *A. C. Bonetti, and G. Pepeu

*Department of Pharmacology, Florence University, 50134 Florence; *Department of Biochemistry, Fidia Research Laboratories, Via Ponte della Fabbrica 3/A, 35031 Abano Terme, Italy*

Phospholipids may affect brain cholinergic mechanisms in at least two ways. First, by increasing the supply of choline, which in turn may stimulate ACh synthesis (22) or act directly on muscarinic receptors (10). This is the case of phosphatidylcholine, whose administration increases the serum levels of free choline (8). Phosphatidylethanolamine may also be considered to some extent a precursor for phosphatidylcholine synthesis (2).

Second, phospholipids may have intrinsic pharmacological properties. One example is phosphatidylserine (PS), which according to Casamenti et al. (4), stimulates the release of ACh from the cerebral cortex in urethane anaesthetized rats. The stimulation is prevented by dopaminergic antagonists and by septal lesions. These findings suggest that 1) PS acts indirectly by stimulating a dopaminergic system which in turn enhances ACh output from the cholinergic nerve endings, and that 2) the cholinergic fibres stimulated by PS originate from or, what is more likely, pass through the septum (5).

It has also been shown that PS prevents the scopolamine-induced disruption of spontaneous alternation in naive rats (15).

This paper presents further work demonstrating pharmacological effects of PS on brain cholinergic mechanisms and its functions.

The following investigations have been carried out:

1) The interactions between PS and scopolamine on electrocorticogram (ECoG) have been studied in unanaesthetized freely moving New Zealand adult male rabbits and adult male rats of Sprague-Dawley strain. Epidural screw electrodes were implanted in the skull on each hemisphere. The animals were connected through long leads to a Galileo electroencephalograph. Recording was carried out in the morning by placing the animal in a sound-proof box with dim light. The electrocorticogram was qualitatively examined through a monitor (x - y Monitor O.T.E. R.35). The quantitative analysis of the electrocortical recording was carried out using a Berg-Fourier frequency analyzer (O.T.E.) supplemented by period and power spectrum analysis using a digital computer program for a 6060 Olivetti computer.

2) The effect of single and repeated administrations of PS on ACh content in

the cerebral cortex and striatum was studied in the rat. Adult male Sprague-Dawley rats were killed by microwave radiation. ACh content was extracted either by the method of Beani and Bianchi (1) and quantified by bioassay or by a radioenzymatic method (11). Striatal ACh contents measured by the two methods showed no statistical differences.

3) The effect of PS on ACh output was studied in striatal slices incubated in eserinized Ringer solution (3) and ACh was quantified by bioassay on the guinea-pig ileum.

Immediately before the use, PS was sonicated in 0.05 M Tris buffer under a nitrogen stream in order to obtain liposomes as described by Casamenti et al. (4). PS produced by Fidia Research Laboratories was used throughout the experiments.

Interactions between scopolamine and PS on the ECoG

Scopolamine, a powerful muscarinic antagonist, is an useful tool for impairing the central cholinergic mechanism (see references in 14).

Since it has been shown (15) that PS antagonizes the disruption of spontaneous alternation induced by scopolamine in naive rats, in the present study we investigated whether PS also antagonizes the effects of scopolamine on the ECoG. The administration of antimuscarinic drugs is followed by changes in the ECoG pattern characterized by the appearance of bursts of high voltage slow waves (13). Fig. 1 illustrates the effect of scopolamine and PS on the electrocortical activity in the 0 - 4 Hz wave-frequency range. The activity is expressed as per cent change over the controls. It can be seen that at this frequency range scopolamine (2 mg/kg i.p.) caused an increase in electrical activity, which was then prevented by the administration of PS (30 mg/kg i.p.). On the other hand PS alone had no significant effects on the ECoG.

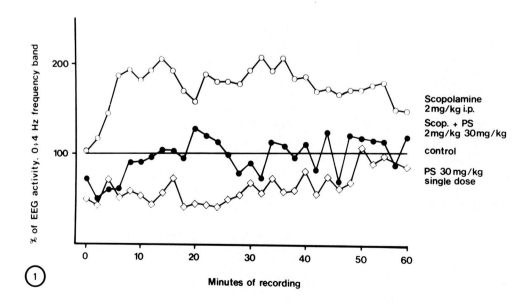

Fig. 2 shows that also repeated administrations of PS (30 mg/kg i.p.) for 10 days had no effect on the normal ECoG but antagonized the increase in electrical activity induced by scopolamine.

PS also antagonized the electrocorticographic effect of scopolamine in the rabbit as shown in Fig. 3.

In order to explain these findings we might assume that the increase in ACh output from the cerebral cortex elicited by PS (4) displaces scopolamine from the muscarinic receptors in the cerebral cortex, thus antagonizing its effects.

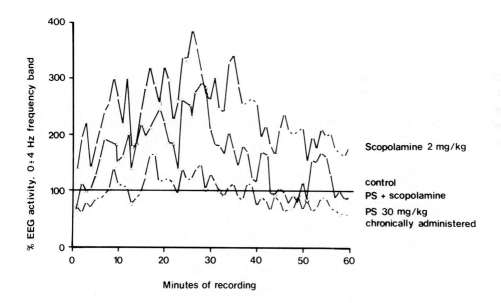

FIG. 2. Effect of a daily administration of PS for 10 days on the ECoG in the rat. Tracings as in Fig. 1.

FIG. 1. Effect of a single administration of PS on the ECoG in the rat. Each point of the tracings represents the mean of the percent changes in total electrical activity from the controls of any given time. For each treatment at least 8 rats were used. Note the antagonism between PS and scopolamine.

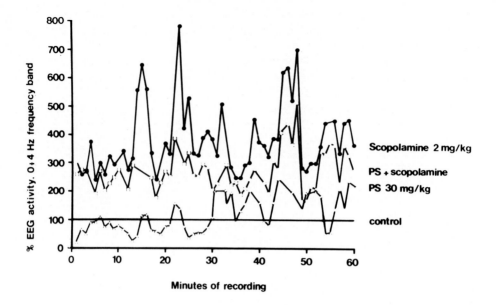

FIG. 3. Effects of a single administration of PS on the ECoG in the rabbit. Each point of the tracings as in Fig. 1. For each treatment at least 6 rabbits were used.

Effect of PS on ACh level in the rat cerebral cortex

Giarman and Pepeu (7) demonstrated that all centrally-acting anticholinergic drugs bring about a decrease in brain ACh. This effect is not uniform since it particularly involves the cerebral cortex and does not occur in the brain stem. The decrease is paralleled by an increase in ACh release (19), caused by the anticholinergic agents' blockade of the presynaptic muscarinic receptors which inhibit ACh output from the cholinergic nerve endings (20).

Fig. 4 shows the dose-dependent decrease in ACh content following scopol-ami ne administration. The repeated administration of PS (30 mg/kg i.p. for 10 days) enhanced the effect of scopolamine. A single administration of PS (30 mg/kg i.p.), however, neither affected the basal ACh level nor modified the decrease in ACh content induced by scopolamine.

A sommation of the releasing effect of PS and scopolamine could explain these findings but it is still difficult to understand why ACh released by PS seems unable to displace scopolamine from the presynaptic receptors.

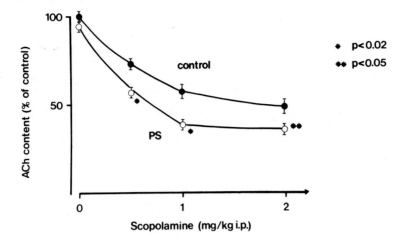

FIG. 4. Effect of increasing doses of scopolamine on ACh content in the cerebral cortex of control rats (upper tracing) and of rats treated daily for 10 days with PS, 30 mg/kg i.p. (lower tracing). ACh content in the cerebral cortex of control rats: 20.5 ± 0.5 nmol/g ± S.E. (n= 9).

Effect of PS on ACh levels in the rat caudate nucleus

Since PS seems to enhance ACh output from the cerebral cortex through the stimulation of a subcortical dopaminergic system (4), an attempt was made to ascertain whether PS exerted dopaminergic effects on the striatal cholinergic neurons as well.

It has been shown repeatedly that dopaminergic agonists increase ACh content in the striatum (11, 16) by decreasing ACh output from the cholinergic intrinsic neurons (17).

Table 1 shows that bromocriptine, a direct dopaminergic agonist (9), brought about the expected significant increase in striatal ACh level. It also shows that while a single administration of 50 mg/kg i.p. of PS had no effect on ACh content, repeated administration of the same dose for 10 days brought about a significant increase in ACh level. Larger doses of PS were needed in order to cause a dose-dependent increase in ACh content with a single administration. The increase was effectively prevented by pretreating the rats with haloperidol. On the other hand haloperidol administration was followed by the expected marked decrease in ACh level (6).

In rats treated with the largest doses of PS we observed an increase in spontaneous mobility which was prevented by haloperidol.

TABLE 1. Effect of phosphatidylserine (PS) on ACh content in the caudate nucleus of the rat

Drug	Dose mg/kg i.p.	N° rats	ACh nmol/g ± S.E.	% change	P
Saline	-	33	48.92 ± 4.6	-	
Bromocriptine	10	12	70.45 ± 5.0	+44.0	<0.01
PS	50	8	49.07 ± 5.2	-	
PS	50 x 10 days	8	60.43 ± 9.8	+23.5	<0.05
PS	150	15	57.30 ± 7.2	+17.1	<0.05
PS	300	10	61.78 ± 8.3	+26.2	<0.01
Haloperidol	1	5	26.33 ± 1.4	-46.2	<0.01
Haloperidol + PS	1 300	5	23.87 ± 0.6	-51.2	<0.01

Effect of PS on ACh output from striatal slices

A further confirmation that PS acts through the dopaminergic system was sought by investigating PS effect on spontaneous ACh output from striatal slices. It has been shown (18) that dopaminergic agonists decrease ACh output from the striatum also "in vitro". Table 2 demonstrates that sonicated PS added to the incubation medium also brought about a decrease in the spontaneous ACh output.

TABLE 2. Effect of phosphatidylserine (PS) on ACh output from striatal slices incubated in Krebs solution

Drug	Concentration nmol/ml	N° expts.	ACh output ng/g/min	% change	P
none	-	10	26.55 ± 2.3	-	-
PS	175	5	24.62 ± 3.1	-7.3	n.s.
PS	350	5	18.93 ± 2.6	-28.7	<0.05

It is pertinent to mention here that PS at similar concentrations has no effect on spontaneous and K$^+$ stimulated ACh output from cortical slices (4).

CONCLUSIONS

The antagonism exerted by PS on the electrocorticographic effects of scopolamine in rats and rabbits confirms that PS influences the cortical cholinergic mechanisms as indicated by the previously reported (4) increase in ACh output from the cerebral cortex.

The findings that haloperidol antagonizes the increase in striatal ACh level induced by PS in a dose-dependent manner, and that PS decreases the spontaneous ACh output from striatal slices, together demonstrate that PS is able to activate dopamine receptors in the caudate nucleus. This supports the hypothesis that the stimulation of ACh output from the cerebral cortex might also be mediated through the activation of subcortical dopaminergic mechanisms.

From our experiments no information can be obtained as to whether PS acts directly or indirectly on the dopaminergic receptors. As indirect mechanism is however supported by two observations (21): that PS increases the turnover of noradrenaline and dopamine in several brain areas in rats and mice, and that the increase in turnover is accompanied by adenylate cyclase activation.

It should also be noted that PS can exert cumulative effects since doses apparently ineffective after a single administration affected the electrocortical actions of scopolamine and increased striatal ACh levels after repeated administrations. A long-lasting progressive modification of some biochemical mechanism could explain this finding.

REFERENCES

1. Beani, L., and Bianchi, C. (1963): J. Pharm. Pharmac., 15:281-282.
2. Blusztajn, J.K., Zeisel, S.H., and Wurtman, R. (1979): Brain Res., 179:319-327.
3. Casamenti, F., Mantovani, P., and Pepeu, G. (1978): Br. J. Pharmac., 63:259-265.
4. Casamenti, F., Mantovani, P., Amaducci, L., and Pepeu, G. (1979): J. Neurochem., 32:529-533.
5. Casamenti, F., Pedata, F., Sorbi, S., Lo Conte, G., and Pepeu, G. (1981): In: Cholinergic Mechanisms: Phylogenetic Aspects, Central and Peripheral Synapses, Clinical Significance, edited by G. Pepeu, and H. Ladinsky, pp. 685-694. Plenum Publishing Co., New York.
6. Consolo, S., Ladinsky, H., and Bianchi, S. (1975): Eur. J. Pharmacol., 33:345-351.
7. Giarman, N.J., and Pepeu, G. (1964): Br. J. Pharmac., 23:123-130.
8. Hirsch, M.J., Growdon, J.H., and Wurtman, R.J. (1978): Metabolism, 27:953-960.
9. Johnson, A.M., Loew, D.M., and Vigoret, J.M. (1976): Br. J. Pharmac., 56:59-68.
10. Krnjevic, K., and Reinhard, W. (1979): Science, 206:1321-1323.
11. Ladinsky, H., Consolo, S., Bianchi, S., Samanin, R., and Ghezzi, D. (1975): Brain

Res., 87:221-226.

12. Ladinsky, H., Consolo, S., Bianchi, S., and Gori, A. (1976): Brain Res., 108:351-361.

13. Longo, V.G. (1966): Pharmacol. Rev., 18:965-996.

14. Pepeu, G., and Corradetti, R. (1980): In: Advances in Neurotoxicology, edited by L. Manzo, pp. 329-333. Pergamon Press, Oxford.

15. Pepeu, G., Gori, G., and Bartolini, L. (1980): In: Aging of the Brain and Dementia, edited by L. Amaducci, A.N. Davidson, and P.A. Antuono, pp. 271-275. Raven Press, New York.

16. Sethy, V.H., and Van Woert, M.H. (1974): Res. Commun. Chem. Pathol. Pharmacol., 8:13-28.

17. Stadler, H., Lloyd, K.G., Gadea-Ciria, M., and Bartholini, G. (1973): Brain Res., 55:476-480.

18. Stoof, J.C., Thieme, R.E., Vrijmoedde-Vries, M.C., and Mulder, A.H. (1979): Naunyn-Schmied. Arch. Pharmacol., 309:119-124.

19. Szerb, J.C., Malik, H., and Hunter, E.G. (1970): Canad. J. Physiol. Pharmacol., 48:180-186.

20. Szerb, J.C., and Somogyi, G.T. (1973): Nature New Biology, 241:121-122.

21. Toffano, G., and Bruni, A. (1980): Pharmacol. Res. Commun., 12:829-845.

22. Wecker, L., and Schmidt, D.E. (1980): Brain Res., 184:234-238.

Phospholipids in the Nervous System, Vol. 1: Metabolism, edited by L. Horrocks, et al. Raven Press, New York © 1982.

Fate of Phosphatidyl-L-(U-^{14}C)Serine in Mice

G. Toffano, A. Battistella, S. Mazzari, *P. Orlando, *P. Massari, and *C. Giordano

*Department of Biochemistry, Fidia Research Laboratories, 35031 Abano Terme; *Università Cattolica del Sacro Cuore, Centro Radioisotopi, 00135 Roma, Italy*

Phosphatidylserine (PS), the major acidic phospholipid of mammalian membranes is involved in several membrane linked events such as fusion (21), excitability (5), enzyme activation (14, 21, 29) and histamine release (8, 17). Sonicated preparations of PS, purified from ox brain and injected in vivo, modify cerebral and peripheral parameters in rats and mice (for a review see 26). Significant for their pharmacological implications are the effects of PS on cerebral catecholaminergic (13, 25) and cholinergic (4, 16) functions.

The intimate mechanism of these effects in vivo is only partially understood. Since conversion of PS into its monoacylderivative, namely lysoPS, enhances pharmacological potency of PS, it has been suggested that the deacylation-reacylation process is involved in the PS effect (2, 3). In addition, the requirement for the carboxylate and unsubstituted ammonium group of the serine polar head (Bigon et al., submitted) shows that specific conformation of the phospholipid head group is responsible for the pharmacological effect. Whether the effects induced by PS on the central nervous system reflect the penetration of phospholipids in this area or are consequent to peripheral interactions in an unsolved question. A direct central effect is supported by the finding that intracerebroventricularly and intravenously injected PS shows the same stimulatory effect on the impaired learning capability of aged rats (6). However, this is not sufficient to decide whether PS is active per se or after its metabolic conversion in districts other than the brain. A main difficulty in the investigation of this point has been the lack of radioactive PS of adequate specific activity. Recently Orlando et al. (19) reported a method to obtain phosphatidyl-L-(U-^{14}C)serine from ox brain phosphatidylcholine with high specific activity and with the same fatty acid composition of the native molecule. In this work the distribution and metabolism of intravenously injected radioactive PS in mice has been investigated.

PREPARATION OF ^{14}C-LABELED PS FROM OX CEREBRAL PS

Highly labeled phsophatidyl-L-(U[14]C)serine was prepared by the procedure previously reported (18), the only exception being the source of phosphatidic acid (Table 1).

Table 1. Synthesis of Phosphatidyl-L-(U-^{14}C)-Serine

1)

PHOSPHATIDYL-SERINE (PS)   PHOSPHOLIPASE D   PHOSPHATIDIC ACID (PA)   +   SERINE

2)

PA   +   CYTIDINE-5-MONOPHOSPHATE (CMP) ⇌ CYTIDINE-DIPHOSPHATE-DIGLYCERIDE (CDP-DG)   + H$_2$O

3)

CDP-DG   L-(U-^{14}C)SERINE   PHOSPHATIDYL-TRANSFERASE   PHOSPHATIDYL-L-(U-^{14}C)SERINE   CMP

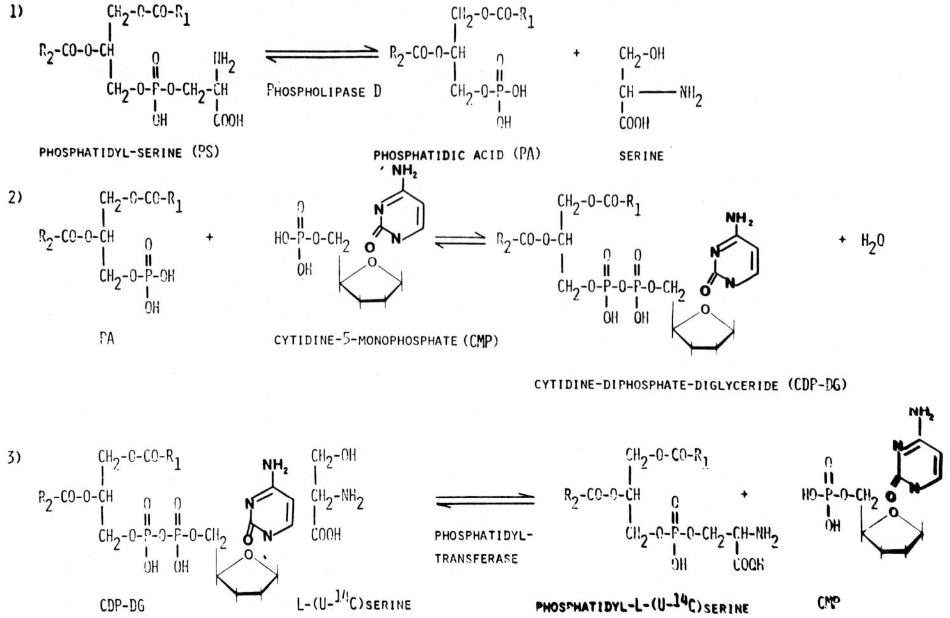

Pure phosphatidic acid (PA) was prepared by incubating ox brain PS, purified according to Bigon et al. (1), with phospholipase D (EC 3.1.4.4.) following the Wurster and Copenhaver procedure (30). Then PA and cytidine-5-monophosphate-morpholidate (CMP) were allowed to react in pyridine for 65 hours at room temperature. The resulting product, cytidine-di-phosphate-diglyceride (CDP-DG), was extracted in methanol-chloroform (1:1, v/v), washed with 10^{-4} M HCl and extracted again with methanol-2M NH$_4$OH (2:1, v/v). The synthesis of PS uniformly labeled with ^{14}C into the serine group was performed by a modification of Kanfer and Kennedy (12) procedure. CDP-DG was incubated with (^{14}C)-serine (170 μCi) in an appropriate medium containing a crude preparation of CDP-diglyceride: L-serine phosphatidyltransferase prepared from E. Coli. The incubation was performed at 37° C for 1 hour in the presence of 10^{-6} M hydroxylamine in order to inhibit, almost completely, the PS$_4$ decarboxylase activity present in the E. Coli crude extracts. Phosphatidyl-L-(U^{14}C)serine was purified by TLC on silica gel-G plates by using chloroform-methanol-1M NH OH (65:25:4, v/v/v). The purity of the product lipid was over 99%, the specific activity was 170 Ci/mol, and the molecular species composition similar to that of natively occurring PS (Table 2).

Table 2. Fatty acid composition of reagent and product lipids

Main fatty acid	Phosphatidylserine	
	Native	Final product
16:0	6.05 ± 0.2	5.85 ± 0.2
16:1	2.24 ± 0.2	2.22 ± 0.2
18:0	20.70 ± 0.9	20.10 ± 1.2
18:1	18.55 ± 1.1	27.32 ± 1.2
18:2	1.59 ± 0.3	1.62 ± 0.3
18:3	5.21 ± 0.8	5.62 ± 0.5
20:0	1.27 ± 0.3	1.25 ± 0.2
20:2	1.52 ± 0.2	1.50 ± 0.2
20:4	9.40 ± 0.5	9.36 ± 0.4
22.6	9.20 ± 0.6	9.00 ± 0.6

Values are percent ± S.D. GLC was carried out on a PYE UNICAM GDC chromatograph.

FATE OF PHOSPHATIDYL-L-(U-^{14}C)SERINE

Mice were injected intravenously with a sonicated preparation of (^{14}C)PS in 50 mM Tris-HCl buffer, pH 7.4 (20 mg/kg, 1.6 mCi/kg), corresponding to approximately 533 nmoles per mouse, and sacrified 5, 10, 20 and 30 minutes later by decapitation. Organs were rapidly dissected out and extracted according to Folch et al. (7). Phospholipids were separated by TLC (23). Spots were visualized by iodine spraying and plates divided in 0.5 cm sections, each being then scraped off and measured for radioactivity. The amount of radioactivity was determined in blood, liver and brain. Blood contamination in the tissues, as determined by injecting the mice with (^{14}C) inuline, was subtracted from the total counts. The distribution of total radiocativity after various time intervals from the injection of (^{14}C)PS is reported in Fig. 1.

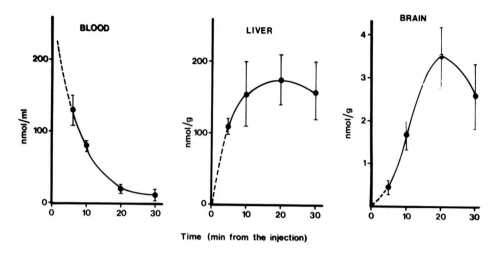

Mice were injected with 20 mg/kg (1.6 mCi/kg) of [U-14C] PS. Values are means ± S.D. of three experimental data. Blood contamination in the liver and brain, as determined by injecting mice with 14C-inuline, was substracted from the total counts.

Fig. 1. Distribution of radioactivity in the blood, liver, and brain after intravenous injection of (14C)PS.

There was a rapid decline of radioactivity in the blood although the kinetics were clearly biphasic. The initial fast rate was completed in about 10 minutes and led to the disappearance of approximately 90% of the injected amount. The rapid phase was then followed by a slow decline. As expected, the radioactivity increased rapidly in the liver and, at a lower extent, in the brain. These findings agree with previous studies on the distribution of phospholipid liposomes *in vivo* (23).

The amount of radioactive material recovered in the liver was 36% of the injected dose with a peak (180 nmol/g) at 20 minutes. The amount recovered in the brain was 0.25% of the injected dose with a peak also at 20 minutes. Considering that the brain weight is about 1.5% of the total body weight, the amount of radioactivity detected in the brain is significant.

Thin layer chromatographic analysis of blood, liver and brain lipidic extracts revealed that, at any time, about 90-95% of radioactivity was recovered as PS (Table 3).

Table 3. Percentage of different labeled phospholipids in blood, brain and liver extracts.

Samples	LysoPS	PS	PE
Blood			
5'	2.7 ± 0.5	93 ± 4	2.6 ± 0.5
10'	2.3 ± 0.2	94 ± 3	3.2 ± 0.6
20'	3.8 ± 0.8	92 ± 6	4.4 ± 2.0
30'	4.4 ± 0.7	90 ± 5	5.8 ± 0.8
Liver			
5'	4.6 ± 1.0	87 ± 8	6.0 ± 0.5
10'	3.0 ± 0.5	94 ± 2	4.0 ± 1.0
20'	1.8 ± 1.0	92 ± 4	5.0 ± 1.0
30'	1.2 ± 1.0	92 ± 5	6.0 ± 1.0
Brain			
5'	6.3 ± 2.0	86 ± 5	5.3 ± 1.0
10'	3.7 ± 1.0	85 ± 4	5.1 ± 2.0
20'	1.4 ± 0.5	91 ± 5	5.0 ± 0.5
30'	1.3 ± 0.5	90 ± 6	4.7 ± 2.0

Animals were injected intravenously with 20 mg/kg (1.6 mCi/kg) phosphatidyl-L-(U¹⁴C)serine.

A small but significant amount of labeled phosphatidylethanolamine (PE), indicative of the extent of PS decarboxylation, was found. This amount increased with time in the blood and remained constant in the liver and brain. Radioactive lysophosphatidylserine (lysoPS) was also found. The concentration of this phospholipid gradually increased in the blood and decreased in the liver and brain. Probably this reflected the rate of reacylation of lysoPS occurring in the liver and brain (9). As suggested (2) a site for the formation of lysoPS may be the blood stream where the conversion can be mediated by a phospholipase A_2 (20).

The amount of radioactivity in the hydrosoluble extract was also determined (Table 4).

Table 4. <u>Distribution of radioactivity in hydrosoluble extracts (Folch's washings).</u>

Time	Blood	Brain	Liver
5'	4.0 ± 0.5	0.1 ± 0.01	9.4 ± 1
10'	1.4 ± 0.3	0.14 ± 0.02	8.8 ± 1
20'	1.4 ± 0.3	0.35 ± 0.07	13.6 ± 2
30'	1.0 ± 0.2	0.81 ± 0.05	14.4 ± 1

Values are expressed as nmoles/g of wet weight.

In the brain and in the liver this amount increased gradually from 0.1 to 0.8 nmol/g and from 9 to 14 nmol/g after 5 and 30 minutes, respectively. In contrast, the radioactivity present in the hydrosoluble extract from blood tended to decrease from 4 to 1 nmol/ml after 5 and 30 minutes from injection.

DISCUSSION

The view that liposomes reach the brain and affect directly the cerebral metabolism is supported only by circumstantial evidence. Jonah et al. (1975) following the fate of EDTA entrapped in liposomes composed of phosphatidylcholine, cholesterol and PS, has shown a limited (0.4%) uptake by the brain. Furthermore, GABA encapsulated in PS liposomes is capable to counteract the penicillin induced epileptic seizures (15) and the isoniazide-induced convulsions (18). Since EDTA and GABA are polar compounds, they do not cross the blood brain barrier without appropriate vehicle. This vehicle seems to be the PS liposome. The presence of the negative charge seems a specific requirement in view of the fact that GABA entrapped in neutral phosphatidylcholine liposomes, fails to show anticonvulsant effect (18, 27). In agreement with these indications, this paper shows that a small amount of PS enters the brain. When this phospholipid is injected intravenously, in form of sonicated oligolamellar vesicles, 0.25% of the injected radioactivity enters the brain and most of it is recovered as PS (90-95%). The amount of PS found in the brain is suitable to elicit pharmacological activity. In fact, it has been observed (6) that 10 μg of PS injected intraventricularly in aged rats has been as effective as 20 mg/kg injected intravenously in stimulating acquisition of active avoidance. In both cases the amount of PS found in the brain is about 4-5 nmoles per g.

Although the concept that PS liposomes enter the brain as intact structures is not generally accepted (11), the present data and other reported in this meeting (18, 28) suggest that a limited penetration does occur. Alternatively, PS liposomes could be fragmented in the blood stream and distributed in the body fluids as small lipoprotein complexes. The binding of liposomes to high density lipoproteins has been shown to facilitate the interaction with cell membranes (23). An additional finding of pharmacological interest is that the injected PS is poorly metabolized by the liver. The simplest interpretation of this result is that the phospholipid is incorporated more into the cell membrane than distributed in the cell cytosol. This implies that the injected liposomes undergo mostly fusion with the phospholipid bilayer of the liver cell plasma membrane, rather than being extensively taken up through phagocytotic processes. However, further studies are required to corroborate this interesting but preliminary suggestion.

REFERENCES

1. Bigon, E., Boarato, E, Bruni, A., Leon, A. and Toffano, G. (1979): Br. J. Pharmacol., 66:167-174.
2. Bigon, E., Boarato, E., Bruni, A., Leon, A. and Toffano, G. (1979): Br. J. Pharmacol., 67:611-616.
3. Calderini, G., Teolato, S., Bonetti, A.C., Battistella, A. and Toffano, G. (1981): Life Sci., 28:2367-2375.
4. Casamenti, F., Mantovani, P., Amaducci, L. and Pepeu, G. (1979): J. Neurochem., 32:529-533.
5. Cook, A.M., Low, E. and Ishijmi, M. (1972): Nature New Biol., 239:150.
6. Drago, F., Ippolito, G., Binaglia, L., Giordano, C. and Porcellati, G. (1980): J. Lipid Res., 21:1053-1057.
7. Folch, J., Lees, M. and Sloane-Stanley, G.H. (1957): J. Biol. Chem., 226:497-503.
8. Hirata, F., Axelrod, J. and Crews, F.T. (1979): Proc. Natl. Acad. Sci. USA, 76:4813-4816.
9. James, O.A., Mc Donald, G. and Thompson, W. (1979): J. Neurochem., 33:1061-1066.
10. Jonah, M.M., Cerney, E.A. and Rahman, Y.E. (1975): Biochem. Biophys. Acta, 401:336-348.
11. Juliano, R.L. (1981): TIPS, 2:39-42.
12. Kanfer, J. and Kennedy, E.P. (1964): J. Biol. Chem., 239:1720-1726.
13. Leon, A., Benvegnù, D., Toffano, G., Orlando, P. and Mazzari, S. (1978): J. Neurochem., 30:23-26.
14. Lloyd, T. and Kaufman, S. (1974): Biochem. Res. Commun., 59:1262-1269.
15. Loeb, C., Benassi, E., Tanganelli, P. and Besio, G. (1978): IRCS Med. Sci., 6:488.
16. Mantovani, P., Pepeu, G. and Amaducci, L. (1976): Adv. Experim. Med. Biol.,72:285-292.
17. Martin, T.W. and Lagumoff, D. (1978): Proc. Natl. Acad. Sci. USA, 75:4997-5000.
18. Mazzari, S., Zanotti, A., Orlando, P. and Toffano, G. (1981): this meeting.
19. Orlando, P., Ippolito, G., Binaglia, C., Giordano, C. and Porcellati, G. (1980): J. Lipid Res., 21:1053-1057.
20. Paysant, M., Bitran, M., Etienne, J. and Polorovski, J. (1969): Bull. Soc. Chem. Biol., 51:863-873.
21. Portis, A., Newton, C., Pangborn, W. and Papahadjopoulos, D. (1979): Biochemistry, 18:780-790.
22. Raese, J., Patrick, R.L. and Barchas, J.D. (1976): Biochem. Pharmacol., 25:2245-2250.
23. Scherphof, G., Roerdink, F., Hoekstra, D., Zborowski, J. and Wisse, E.

(1980): In: Liposomes in Biological Systems, edited by G. Gregoriadis and A.C. Allison, pp. 179-205. John Wiley, Chichester.

24. Skipski, V.P. and Barclay, M. (1969): Meth. Enzymol., 14:530-587.

25. Toffano, G., Leon, A., Mazzari, S., Savoini, G., Teolato, S. and Orlando, P. (1978): Life Sci., 23:1093-1102.

26. Toffano, G. and Bruni, A. (1980): Pharmacol. Res. Commun., in press.

27. Tökes, Z.A., Kulcsar St. Peter, A. and Todd, J.A. (1980): Brain Res., 188:282-286.

28. Vecchini, A., Orlando, P., Binaglia, L., Mazzari, S., Giordano, C. and Porcellati, G. (1981): this meeting.

29. Wheeler, K.P. and Whittam, R. (1970): Nature, 225:449-450.

30. Wurster, C.F.Jr. and Copenhaver, J.H.Jr. (1966): Lipids, 1:422-424.

Phospholipids in the Nervous System, Vol. 1:
Metabolism, edited by L. Horrocks, et al. Raven
Press, New York © 1982.

Studies on Sphingomyelinase

S. Gatt

Laboratory of Neurochemistry, Hebrew University–Hadassah Medical School, Jerusalem, Israel

Sphingomyelinase (sphingomyelin choline phosphohydrolase, EC 3.1.4.12) **is** an enzyme which degrades the phospho-sphingolipid, sphingomyelin (SPM) to choline-phosphate and ceramide (N-acylsphingosine; Scheme 1). Further hydrolysis of ceramide to sphingosine and fatty acid (6,7,25) completes the degradation of SPM to its constituents. Studies on this enzyme began in the author's laboratory in 1962 and interest in it persisted to date. Thus, the first report was published in 1963 (22) and the last in 1980 (24). This manuscript summarizes, briefly, the various aspects of this research. It is not a general review of the subject, therefore studies done in other laboratories are referred to only when directly related to those done in the laboratory of the author.

$$
\begin{array}{c}
\textsf{Ceramide-phosphorylcholine} \\
\downarrow \textsf{Sphingomyelinase} \\
\textsf{Ceramide+Phosphorylcholine}
\end{array}
$$

Scheme 1

1. ISOLATION OF AND PURIFICATION OF THE LYSOSOMAL SPHINGOMYELINASE

The initial investigations described the properties of the enzyme of rat brain particles (1). Radioactively-labelled SPM, prepared by catalytic hydrogenation with tritium gas, was dispersed in detergent (Triton X-100 and sodium cholate) and used as substrate. The greatest specific activity was located in a 25,000 x g particulate fraction, from which the enzyme could be extracted by treatment with sodium cholate. The enzyme could be further purified and separated from other enzymatic activities by precipitation at pH 5.5. Further solubilization in buffered sucrose provided an enzyme which was about 20-fold purified. This preparation hydrolyzed SPM to ceramide and choline phosphate. Optimal rates were obtained at about pH 5 and a detergent, such as Triton X-100, cholate or taurocholate was needed. The kinetics conformed with the Michaelis and Menten theory. The direct product, ceramide as well as the end products (sphingosine or fatty acids) were inhibitory and the natural stereoisomer (D-erythro-SPM) as well as the non-natural L-erythro or DL-threo isomers were degraded. Subsequent studies showed that extracts of rat brain particles also contain a phospholipase which hydrolyzes the ester linkage in the 1-position of glycerophospholipid ("phospholipase A1", ref.8). The latter enzyme did not sediment at pH 5.5 and could thus be separated from the sphingo-myelinase.

Further investigation showed that the enzyme of rat brain particles could be extracted with water, buffer or an isotonic solution of sucrose (12), thus providing a rapid and easy procedure for solubilizing the enzyme. The preparation which had been extracted with isotonic sucrose was about 100-fold purified, did not sediment at 100,000 x g and on gel filtration had a molecular weight of about 300,000 daltons. This suggested that sphingomyelinase is not an intrinsic component of the membranes of the brain particles from which it can be detached easily. Also, the high molecular weight suggested that the solubilized prepar-ation probably was a multi-protein aggregate. Addition of Triton X-100 decreased the molecular weight to about 200,000 daltons. The enzyme could be further purified (Gatt, unpublished) by binding to concanavalin A and eluting with methyl mannoside or methyl glucoside. Already at this stage sphingomyelinase was free of most other sphingo-lipid hydrolases. It was then subjected to chromatography on a column of Sepharose-bound sphingosylphosphorylcholine. The enzyme adsorbed onto this column and could not be eluted by extensive washing with buffer or Triton X-100, although this detergent seemed to remove other protein contaminants. This suggested that the above column indeed constituted a true "affinity" rather than a hydrophobic chromatographic procedure. Sphingomyelinase was eluted with a mixed-micelle of SPM and Triton X-100 in buffer, at pH 5.0; namely by a dispersion which simulated the incubation mixture used for enzymatic hydrolysis, again suggesting that the sphingosylphosphorylcholine-Sepharose was indeed an affinity-label. The resulting enzyme contained no other detectable sphingolipid hydrolases, but because of the small quantities of enzyme obtained from rat brain, the specific activity could not be assessed accurately. These purification studies have not been pursued but the potential use of Sepharose-bound sphingolipids as affinity-labels for the various enzymes has been recently assessed, using glucosylcere-broside or sphingosylglucoside (glucosyl psychosine) bound to Sepharose for the purification of glucocerebrosidase (Grabowski, Devine, Dagan, Gatt and Desnick, unpublished) and galactosylpsychosine or cerebroside bound to Sepharose for the purification of cerebroside sulftotransferase (Siegrist, Herschkowitz and Gatt, unpublished).

2. LIPOSOMAL DISPERSIONS OF SPHINGOMYELIN

Sphingomyelinase activity is most commonly estimated using a mixed-micelle of SPM and detergent(s). This procedure makes it impossible to distinguish between the role of the detergent in dispersing the substrate and its possible direct effect on the enzymatic protein. To permit a separate analysis of these two effects we developed a procedure in which sphingomyelinase activity was measured using a liposomal dispersion of SPM, without any detergent (11). For this purpose, sphingomyelin was dried onto the wall of a test tube and dispersed, as multilamellar liposomes or, as sonically irradiated, unilamellar vesicles. The effect of several lipids when included in the liposomes is shown in Table I. The data of this table show that, depending on the lipid additive, up to 55% of the rates obtained with mixed micelles of SPM and Triton X100 could be achieved. There was no correlation between the rate of SPM hydrolysis and the surface charge of the liposome measured in a microelectrophoresis apparatus. This study showed that liposomal dispersions of SPM, without detergent, could be used as substrates for the solubilized lysosomal sphingomyelinase. It is anticipated that, using more advanced techniques for preparing sphingomyelin-vesicles, even greater rates of SPM hydrolysis might be attained.

TABLE I

Effect of lipid additives on the rates of hydrolysis of liposomal sphingomyelin.

Additive	Molar ratio additive: sphingomyelin	Relative reaction rate (%)
A) Sonicated liposome		
–	–	100*
Phosphatidylcholine (egg)	0.15	102
Lysophosphatidylcholine (egg)	0.10	50
Phosphatidic acid (egg)	0.15	230
Phosphatic acid (dipalmitoyl)	0.15	220
Phosphatic acid (dilauroyl)	0.15	210
Phosphatic acid (mixed)	0.15	226
Dicetylphosphate	0.15	223
Octadecylamine	0.10	137
Methyl oleate	0.25	242
Methyl palmitate	0.25	250
Cholesterol	0.15	151
Glycerol monooleate	0.15	86
Triton X-100	0.20	152
Triton X-100	2.70	415
B) Non-sonicated liposome		
–	–	30
Phosphatidic acid (mixed)	0.15	96
Methyl oleate	0.15	35
Triton X-100	0.20	150
Triton X-100	2.70	415

In a more recent investigation (17), liposomal dispersions were used to transport sphingomyelin into cultured skin fibroblasts. [3H]-Choline-labelled SPM was mixed with a long-chain amine, such as hexadecyl or octadecylamine; about 15 mole% of the amine was used. Sonically irradiated dispersions of this mixture were added to the growth medium of cultured skin fibroblasts. Uptake of SPM into the cells was practically linear for at least 24 hours when about 5% of the total radioactivity became cell-associated. Some radioactivity migrated with cellular phosphatidylcholine, probably because of reutilization of choline which was released as a consequence of the metabolic degradation of SPM. As a consequence of the internalization of SPM, there was a very marked reduction of the binding, internalization and degradation of low density lipoproteins. Concomitantly, incorporation of $[^{14}C]$ acetate into cholesterol increased 4-10 fold. The presence of the SPM-octadecylamine liposomes did not affect cell growth, and the reduction of LDL-uptake, as well as the increased utilization of acetate reversed when the cells were transferred to a medium to which SPM had not been added. These experiments suggested that intake of SPM affects cholesterol metabolism, perhaps by forming an association of the internalized SPM with the intracellular cholesterol. Other, more recent studies of uptake of SPM into cultured cells and their metabolic utilization are discussed under the heading of Colored and Fluorescent Derivatives of Sphingomyelin.

3. NON-LYSOSOMAL, MAGNESIUM-DEPENDENT SPHINGOMYELINASE

Sphingomyelinase is a component of the lysosomes of all animal cells. This enzyme, which shows optimal activity at pH 5, does not require any confactor. In 1967, Schenider and Kennedy (23) mentioned the presence of a second sphingomyelinase, with a neutral or alkaline pH optimum. In 1967 we described the properties of a sphingomyelinase which requires a divalent metal and whose optimal pH is between 7 and 8 (10,13). Similar, independent investigations on this enzyme were published by Rao and Spence (20). This enzyme differed from the lysosomal sphingomyelinase in the following properties. 1: An absolute requirement for divalent ions. Magnesium and manganese could be used, while calcium was less effective. 2: EDTA abolished enzymatic activity. Thus, assaying with and without EDTA was used to assess the relative contents of the lysosomal and magnesium-dependent enzymes in crude preparations. 3: Optimal hydrolysis was obtained at pH 7-8. 4: The enzyme was present in several cellular membrane fractions, but showed no enrichment in lysosomes. 5: Brain showed the greatest total and specific activities; extraneural tissues had only 1-4% of the enzymatic activity of brain. 6: The enzyme showed a pronounced developmental pattern, having considerably greater activity in the brain of young humans or rats. 7: Dissimilar to the lysosomal enzyme which is absent in Niemann-Pick disease, Type A, the magnesium-dependent enzyme showed close to normal activity in the brain of these patients (15, Fig.1).

The enzyme required detergents for optimal activity. Bile salts (Fig.2) or Triton X-100 could be used. Dissimilar to the lysosomal enzyme, hydrolysis of SPM by the magnesium-dependent enzyme in the presence of Triton X-100 exhibited complex kinetics. The dependence of hydrolysis on enzyme concentration yielded non-linear, parabola-like curves with the magnesium-dependent enzyme (Fig.3). The extent of deviation from linearity was a function of the concentration of Triton X-100 (Fig.4). In parallel, the curves which described the activity as a function of increasing concentrations of this detergent were biphasic, each having ascending and descending portions and an optimum. The detergent concentration yielding this optimal rate depended on the concentration of the enzyme (Fig.5). Superimposed on this was the observation that enzymatic preparations contain a "heat-stable" factor composed of protein and lipids which, when added to the reaction mixtures considerably increased the reaction rates and changed the parabolic v versus S curves to straight lines (Fig.6)

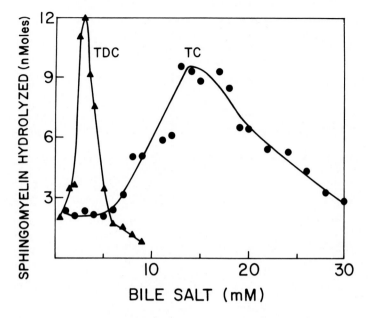

FIG 1: Hydrolysis of SPM by the magnesium-dependent enzyme of normal
and Niemann-Pick brain.

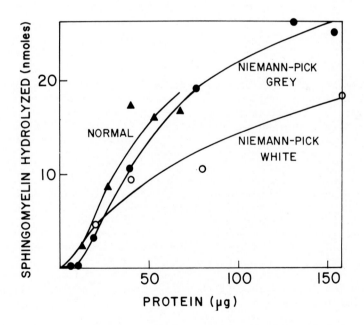

FIG 2: Hydrolysis of SPM by the magnesium-dependent enzyme as a
function of increasing concentrations of taurodeoxycholate
taurocholate.

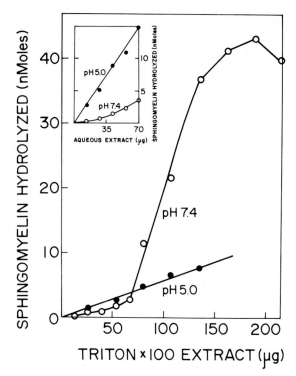

FIG 3:   Effect of increasing concentration of brain extract on the
         hydrolysis of SPM by the lysosomal enzyme at pH 5 and the
         magnesium-dependent enzyme at pH 7.4.

These observations could be explained by the hypothesis that the
magnesium-dependent enzyme requires lipids for optimal activity. Triton
X-100, which is needed to disperse the substrate (SPM) has a secondary
effect of displacing the lipid from the active site of the enzyme.   The
"heat-stable factor" counteracts this, displaces the Triton X-100 and
again supplies the lipid to the active sites.

     It is interesting to speculate on the role of the alkaline,
magnesium-dependent enzyme. Since its activity in young brain greatly
exceeds that of the lysosomal sphingomyelinase (10,9), it might provide
an alternative, non-lysosomal pathway of SPM degradation. The ceramide
produced could be further degraded by the lysosomal or alkaline
ceramidases (7,25). Also, the presence of the very active, magnesium-
dependent sphingomyelinase in brain tissue of Niemann-Pick, Type A
patients provides a metabolic pathway for SPM-degradation and might be
the reason that these patients show no excessive accumulation of this
lipid in brain tissue (15).

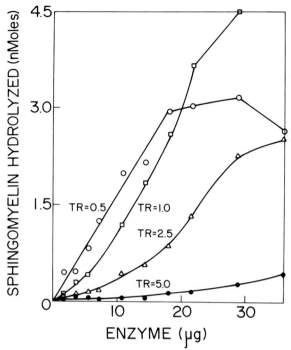

FIG 4: Effect of increasing concentration of the magnesium-dependent enzyme on the hydrolysis of SPM at several concentrations of Triton X100.

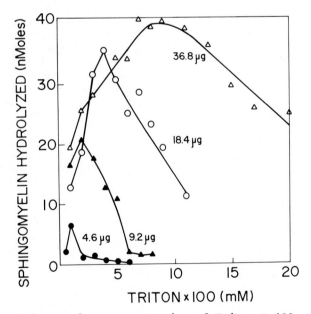

FIG 5: Effect of increasing concentration of Triton X-100 on the hydrolysis of SPM at several concentrations of the magnesium-dependent enzyme.

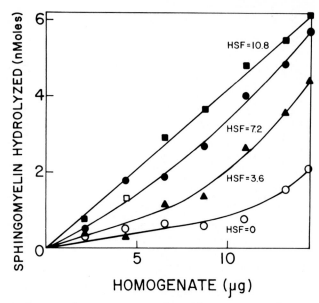

Fig6: Effect of increasing concentration of the magnesium-dependent
enzyme on the hydrolysis of SPM at several concentrations of
"heat-stable" factor

4. LATENT SPHINGOMYELINASE OF CHICKEN ERYTHROCYTE MEMBRANES

Hirschfeld and Loyter observed that hypotonic lysis of chicken
erythrocytes was followed by hydrolysis of the SPM of the RBC membrane
(18). A follow-up study (19) showed that treatment for as little as
5 to 10 min with a hypotonic medium activated a "latent" sphingomyelinase which could degrade practically all the SPM in the membrane of
the "ghost". This hydrolysis occurred, even when the medium was
adjusted to iso-or hypertonicity. Furthermore, once evoked, the RBC
enzyme could hydrolyze SPM, not only in its own membranes (intramembrane hydrolysis), but also that residing in an external membrane,
such as in lyzed, human erythrocyte "ghosts" (intermembrane hydrolysis)
(Fig.7). Further experiments showed that, while intermembrane hydrolysis
followed Michaelis-Menten kinetics, yielding hyperbolic v versus S
curves using SPM-containing human RBC "ghosts" or liposomal dispersions
of this lipid (Fig. 8), intramembrane hydrolysis was characterized
by parabola-like dependence of reaction rates on substrate concentration (see inset in Fig. 9).

Although the mechanism of activation of the membranous sphingomyelinase is not yet entirely clear, it provides an example of a latent
enzyme whose activity is probably not expressed during the entire life-
cycle of the intact avian erythrocyte. This implies that the enzyme
does not degrade the SPM for many weeks in the circulation, but that a
brief lysis in a hypotonic medium makes the enzyme accessible to the
substrate. Then, because of its considerable catalytic potential, it
hydrolyzes the entire SPM of the membrane in about 1 hour. It is
possible that latency and activation of membranous enzymes might
represent an important mechanism which has not yet been explored.

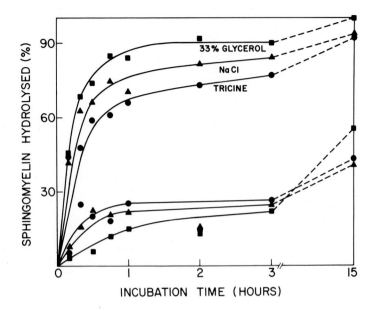

FIG 7: Time course of hydrolysis by the enzyme in chicken erythrocyte "ghosts" of SPM in the same membranes (intramembrane hydrolysis, upper 3 curves) and in membranes of human erythrocyte "ghosts" (intramembrane hydrolysis, lower 3 curves).

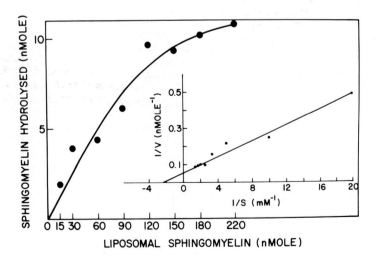

FIG 8: Effect of increasing concentration of SPM in liposomal dispersion on its hydrolysis by the chicken erythrocyte enzyme.

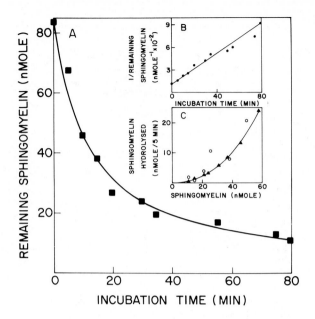

FIG 9:   Time course of hydrolysis of SPM in chicken erythrocyte
         "ghosts" by the enzyme following hypotonic treatment. The
         lower inset shows the effect on increasing SPM, in these
         membranes, on its rate of hydrolysis by the intramembrane
         route.

5:   COLORED AND FLUORESCENT DERIVATIVES OF SPHINGOMYELIN

    The most common substrate used for estimating sphingomyelinase
activity is sphingomyelin labelled with a radioactive tracer in the
ceramide or phosphorylcholine moieties (1,19,24). A chromogenic
substrate, which is not related to SPM, was introduced by Gal et al.
(5) and bis(4-methylumbelliferyl) phosphate was also used as substrate
(2,4). To circumvent the use of hazardous radioactivity and, nevertheless permit spectrophotometric or fluorometric analysis using the
natural substrate, we introduced two groups of SPM-derivatives. The
first is SPM in which the natural fatty acid was replaced by trinitro-
phenylaminolauric acid (TNPAL) (14). This compound (TNPAL-SPM), is a
yellow derivative of the natural lipid, which, when hydrolyzed by the
enzyme yields the yellow trinitrophenylaminolauroyl-sphingosine
(TNPAL-ceramide) as product. This can be isolated by a single solvent-
extraction step and its color intensity estimated in a spectrophoto-
meter. The rate of hydrolysis of TNPAL-SPM was very close to that
observed with radioactively-labelled SPM. Extracts of Niemann-Pick,
Type A cells did not hydrolyze this compound (Fig. 10).

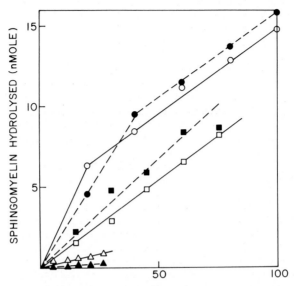

FIG 10: Hydrolysis of trinitrophenylaminolauroyl-SPM and radioactively-
labelled SPM by extracts of fibroblasts (circles), amniotic
cells (squares) and fibroblasts, cultured from skin of a
patient with Niemann-Pick disease (triangles).

    The TNPAL derivative provides a simple spectrometric procedure
while being, essentially, an analog of natural SPM. It can be prepared
in large quantities, is stable and provides the molar concentrations of
the product within minutes after termination of the reaction. Its
only disadvantage is its somewhat low color yield. Its molar extinction
was about 14,000 absorbance units when estimated at 330 nm and 23,000
absorbance units when estimated in an alkaline pH range. Therefore,
when using cells with low enzymatic activity, long incubations may be
required to attain sufficient product for a reliable spectrophotometric
estimation. The second group of SPM-derivatives which we synthesized
overcomes this difficulty by having a fluorescent probe attached to the
fatty acyl residue of SPM (16). SPMs were prepared having the following
fluorescent probes attached to the fatty acyl moiety: anthracene,
anthracene carboxylic acid ester, pyrene, carbazole, NBD [(N-methyl-N-
7-nitrobenz-2-oxa-1,3-diazole-4-yl)] , DANSYL [(11-(5-dimethylaminon-
aphthalene-1-sulfonyl)] and more recently, also fluorescein, rhodamine
and tetramethylrhodamine (Dagan, Barenholz and Gatt, unpublished). The
excitation and emission spectra of the respective compounds ranged from
the ultraviolet to the upper, red region of the visible spectrum.
Because of the great sensitivity of the fluorescent probe, the
fluorescent-SPM was diluted 10-20 fold with natural SPM and this
mixture used as substrate for sphingomyelinase. The hydrolysis of
anthroyloxyundecanoyl-SPM was followed by extracting the reaction

product (anthroyloxy-ceramide) into a heptane-rich phase and estimating the fluorescence intensity in a spectrofluorometer. Its rates of hydrolysis equalled those of radioactively labelled SPM and were about zero using cells of Niemann-Pick Type A patients (25).

The fluorescent derivatives of sphingomyelin provide analogs of the natural lipid whose rates of hydrolysis can be estimated fluorometrically. Furthermore they can be utilized for cell biological studies to follow dynamic aspects, such as transport through cell membranes, exchange of lipids between organelles and membranes, and fusion process. We dissolved fluorescent-SPM in dimethylsulfoxide and introduced this solution into the growth medium of cultured skin fibroblasts. Uptake of the fluorescent lipid could be followed by viewing in a fluorescence microscope. Extraction of the cells, followed by separation on thin layer plates of silica gel showed that a considerable portion of the ingested SPM was degraded to ceramide. Some fluorescence was also observed in other phospholipids (e.g., phosphatidylcholine and phosphatidylethanolamine), perhaps as a consequence of reutilization of the fluorescent fatty acid relased by metabolic degradation of the SPM. To date, it was impossible to differentiate between normal and Niemann-Pick cells when fluorescent SPM was introduced into these respective cells and accumulation of either SPM or ceramide was measured.

6. MIXED DISPERSIONS OF SPHINGOMYELIN AND DETERGENT:
    CORRELATING PHYSICO-CHEMICAL PROPERTIES OF ENZYMATIC HYDROLYSIS

In the vast majority of experiments studying the hydrolysis of SPM to sphingomyelinase, this lipid is "solubilized" in a detergent. The two most common detergents used for this purpose are the nonionic detergent Triton X-100 or an anionic bile salt, such as sodium taurocholate or taurodeoxycholate. In the early 70s, we began a series of investigations whose purpose was to analyze the mixed dispersion of detergent and lipid and correlate its physico-chemical characteristics to enzymatic utilization. In the first study (26), attention was paid to the mode of solubilization of SPM by Triton X-100 and the nature of the dispersions. Turbidity, sedimentation and electron microscopy were used for this purpose. Dispersion of sphingomyelin in water or buffer yields a multilamellar liposome. When mixed with an aqueous solution of Triton X-100, below its critical micellar concentration (when the detergent is present as a monomolecular solution), the detergent molecules did not affect the liposomal structure of the lipid and probably did not penetrate the bilayer to any significant extent. When the concentration of the detergent was increased above its critical micellar concentration (when micelles are present) the bilayered, liposomal structure disintegrated and mixed micelles of SPM and Triton X-100 formed. These experiments were then repeated, but the two components were premixed as solutions in an organic solvent. The solvent was subsequently evaporated and the dry residue dispersed in an aqueous medium. At concentrations greater than the critical micellar concentration of the detergent, the mixed micelles of detergent and Triton X-100 were similar to those obtained using the previous procedure. But, even below this concentration , mixed disperions of SPM and Triton X-100 were present which under the electron microscope seemed to be small uni- or oli-golamellar bilayered vesicles.

Subsequent studies (3,27) characterized the physical parameters of
the mixed micelles of SPM and Triton X-100. Light scattering was used
to measure the diffusion coefficient at increasing ratios of Triton X-100
to SPM (3). Later (27), sedimentation coefficients were also measured
and these two parameters used to calculate molecular weights of the
mixed micelles. This permitted calculating the aggregation numbers
(namely, the number of molecules of Triton X-100 or SPM in each micelle).
Table II shows the results of these experiments.

TABLE II

AGGREGATION NUMBERS OF MIXED MICELLES
OF TRITON X100 AND SPHINGOMYELIN

RATIO TR/SM	SM MOLAR FRACTION	MOLECULAR WEIGHT	AGGREGATION NUMBERS		
			N_{TR}	N_{SM}	N_{Total}
—		86,000	134	—	134
3.80	0.21	163,000	192	50	242
3.16	0.24	187,000	210	66	276
1.90	0.34	220,000	209	110	319
1.58	0.39	238,000	209	133	342
0.95	0.51	272,000	186	196	382
0.79	0.56	293,000	180	228	408
0.63	1.61	334,000	179	282	461
0.47	0.68	479,000	210	442	652

It is of interest that in spite of the increasing ratios of SPM to
Triton X-100 the aggregation number of the detergent was constant, but
the molecular weight of the mixed micelle increased because of a greater
number of SPM molecules in each micelle. The solubilizing effect of the
detergent was evident from the observation that when the molar fraction
of Triton X-100 increased from 0.32 to 0.79, the aggregation number of
SPM decreased from 442 to 50; that of Triton X-100 remained constant at
about 196. These studies also permitted calculating the radii, numbers
and surface areas of these micelles (Table III) and led to a hypothesis
on the structure of the micelles at various ratios of detergent to lipid
(see Fig. 11). This model suggests that, when the mole fraction of Triton
X-100 is 0.79, the mixed micelle is spherical. But when it decreases to
0.38 (namely SPM constitutes 62 mole%), the mixed micelle is eliposidal
with an uneven distribution of molecules of Triton X-100 and
sphingomyelin (27).

TABLE III

RADII, SURFACE AREAS AND CONCENTRATIONS OF MIXED

MICELLES OF TRITON X100 AND SPHINGOMYELIN

RATIO TR/SM	TRITON MOLAR FRACTION	STOKES RADIUS (A)	SURFACE AREA of MICELLE ($A^2 \times 10^{-3}$)	NUMBER of MICELLES* $\times 10^{-14}$	TOTAL SURFACE AREA (m^2)
0.47	0.32	78.8	78.0	1.35	0.10
0.63	0.39	74.1	69.0	2.12	0.15
0.79	0.44	70.9	63.1	2.62	0.16
0.95	0.49	68.2	58.4	3.05	0.18
1.58	0.61	61.9	48.1	4.51	0.22
1.90	0.66	60.0	45.2	5.43	0.24
3.16	0.76	55.8	39.1	9.00	0.35
3.80	0.79	54.5	37.3	11.85	0.44

*Number of micellar units in 1 ml at 0.1 mM SM

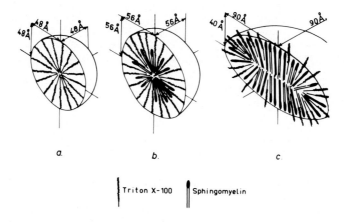

FIG 11:   Cutaway models for the structures of micelles of pure Triton
X-100 and of mixed micelles of this detergent and SPM, at two
ratios of detergent to lipid. The respective mole fractions
of Triton X-100 are a. 1.0;   b. 0.79;   c. 0.32.

Subsequent studies measured the rates of hydrolysis by rat
brain sphingomyelinase of mixed dispersions of SPM and Triton X-100 (28)
or bile salts (29). Rates of hydrolysis of SPM were measured at several
fixed ratios or alternatively, fixed concentrations of the two components of the mixed micelle. The type of complex kinetics observed is
exemplified in Fig. 12, which shows v versus S curves at several fixed
ratios of Triton X-100 to sphingomyelin. It was rewarding, that utilizing the physico-chemical parameters measured for the mixed micelles,

these curves were considerably simplified and interpreted (Fig. 13).The last study (29) utilized mixed dispersions of SPM with the dihydroxy bile salt taurodeoxycholate or the trihydroxy bile salt, taurocholate. The rate of hydrolysis is a function of increasing concentrations of bile salt followed by a multiphasic pattern. Turbidity studies suggested that hydrolysis of SPM begins at that bile salt concentration which solubilizes the lipid and incorporates it into a mixed micelle of detergent and lipid. Ultracentrifugation studies suggested that the effects of the two respective bile salts on the size of the mixed micelles was dissimilar. Thus in the case of taurodeoxycholate, it was the ratio of bile salt to lipid, while with taurocholate, it was the absolute concentration of the bile salt which determined the micellar size.

7. CONCLUSIONS

These studies used the sphingomyelinase-sphingomyelin system as a model for probing several,varied aspects of the enzymology of complex lipid substrates. These included studies on the properties, solubilization and purification by affinity chromatography of this lysosomal enzyme, as well as the problematics of enzyme multiplicity (i.e lysosomal extra lysosomal and plasma membrane sphingomyelinases) and the effect of the physical state of the lipid substrate, which is present in an aqueous dispersion, on its interaction with the enzyme. More recently, this system was used for two other approaches. In the first, the sphingomyelinase of the plasma membrane of the chicken erythrocytes was studied as a model for the activation of a latent, membranous enzyme and for intra- and intermembrane interaction between membranous enzymes and for membrane-embedded lipid substrates. In the second approach, sphingomyelin was introduced into cells, cultured from normal persons and from patients with Niemann-Pick disease. The effects of SPM intake on cellular metabolism (e.g, the receptor-mediated LDL intake and cholesterol biosynthesis) and on the intracellular hydrolysis of internalized, fluorescent SPM were investigated.

A projection on the future course of research on sphingomyelinase suggests two main parallel approaches. One will use purified enzyme to determine the active site and the nature of the molecular mutation in Niemann-Pick disease. Attempts will be made to prepare a template DNA for the enzyme and subsequently introduce this into the genome of the cells to produce large quantities of the enzyme. Production of monoclonal antibody should facilitate studies of enzyme polymorphism.

In parallel, a regression from the pure enzyme level to that of the biological membrane and the cell is most warranted. Relatively little is known to date on the mechanism involving the interaction of sphingomyelinase and sphingomyelin in the leaflets of the bilayered, biological membrane. Similarly, the exact nature of the cellular biosynthetic and degradative reactions is still rather obscure. In spite of the difficulty of working with these multi-enzyme systems, the time might be ripe to attempt a study of the exact mechanism of cellular turnover of sphingomyelin.

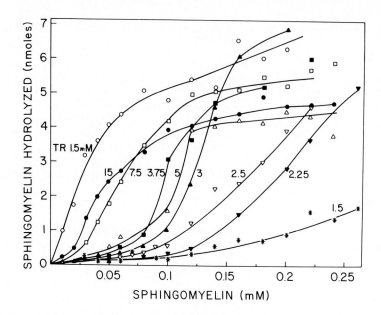

FIG 12: Effect of increasing concentration of SPM on its hydrolysis
by the lysosomal enzyme of rat brain at several fixed molar
ratios of Triton X100 to SPM.

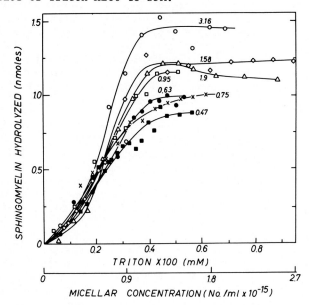

FIG 13: Effect of increasing concentration of Triton X100 on hydrolysis of SPM by the lysosomal enzyme of rat brain at
several fixed molar ratios of Triton X100 to SPM. The second
abcissa describes the concentrations of the mixed micelles of
detergent and lipid.

8. ACKNOWLEDGEMENTS

The following colleagues participated in these studies.
Y. Barenholz, G.V. Cooper, T. Dinur, A. Herzl, Z. Leibowitz-BenGershon,
A. Loyter, A. Roitman, and S. Yedgar.

The experimental part of this work was generously supported for
2½ years by NIH Grant NS-02967.

REFERENCES

1. Barenholz, Y., Roitman, A. Gatt, S. (1966): J. Biol. Chem. 241: 3731-3737.
2. Beasley, G.T.N. (1977): FEBS Letters 80:71-74.
3. Cooper, V.G., Yedgar, S., Barenholz, Y. (1974): Biochim. Biophys. Acta 363:86-97.
4. Fensom, A.H., Benson, P.F., Babrik, A.W., Grant, A.R., Jacobs, L. (1977): Biochem. Biophys. Res. Comm. 74:877-883.
5. Gal, A.E., Brady, R.O., Hibbert, S.R., Pentchev, P.G. (1975): New Engl. J. Med. 293:632-636.
6. Gatt, S. (1963): J. Biol. Chem. 238:3131-3133.
7. Gatt, S. (1966): J. Biol. Chem. 241:3724-3730.
8. Gatt, S. (1968): Biochem. Biophys. Acta 159:304-316.
9. Gatt, S. (1970): Chem. Phys. Lipids 5:235-249.
10. Gatt, S. (]976): Biochem. Biophys. Res. Comm. 68:235-241.
11. Gatt, S., Herzl A., Barenholz, Y. (1973): FEBS Letters 30:281-285.
12. Gatt, S., Gottesdiner, T. (1976): J. Neurochem. 26:421-422.
13. Gatt, S., Dinur, T., Leibowitz-BenGershon, Z. (1978): Biochem. Biophys. Acta 531:206-214.
14. Gatt, S., Dinur, T. Barenholz, Y. (1978): Biochim. Biophys. Acta 530:503-507.
15. Gatt, S., Dinur, T., Kopolovic, J. (1978): J. Neurochem. 31:547-550.
16. Gatt, S., Dinur, T., Barenholz, Y. (1980): Clin. Chem. 26:93-96.
17. Gatt, S., Bierman, E.L. (1980): J. Biol. Chem. 255:3371-3376.
18. Hirschfeld, D., Loyter, A. (1975): Arch. Biochem. Biophys. 67:186-192.
19. Kanfer, J.N., Young, O.M., Shapiro, D., Brady, R.O. (1966): J. Biol. Chem. 241:1081-1084.
20. Rao, B.G., Spence, M.W. (1976): J. Lipid Res. 17:506-515.
21. Record, M., Loyter, A., Gatt, S. (1980): Biochem. J. 187:115-121.
22. Roitman, A., Gatt, S. (1963): Israel J. Chem. 1:190.
23. Schneider, P.B., Kennedy, E.P. (1976): J. Lipid Res. 8:202-209.
24. Stoffel, W. (1975): Methods Enzymol. 35:533-548.
25. Yavin, Y., Gatt, S. (1969): Biochemistry 8:1692-1698.
26. Yedgar, Y., Hertz, R., Gatt, S. (1974): Chem. Phys. Lipids 13:404-414.
27. Yedgar, S., Barenholz, Y., Cooper, V.G. (1974): Biochim. Biophys. Acta 363:98-111.
28. Yedgar, S., Gatt, S. (1976): Biochemistry 15:2570-2573.
29. Yedgar, S., Gatt, S. (1980): Biochem. J. 185:749-754.

Phospholipids in the Nervous System, Vol. 1:
Metabolism, edited by L. Horrocks, et al. Raven
Press, New York © 1982.

On the Metabolism of Etherphospholipids in Glial Cell Cultures

H. Debuch, B. Witter, H. K. Illig, and J. Gunawan

*Institut für Physiologische Chemie, Lehrstuhl II, Universität zu Köln,
D-5000 Köln 41 (Lindenthal), Federal Republic of Germany*

Glial cells are of more and more biochemical interest, since we know that they differ not only in morphology (Fig. 1) but also in function.

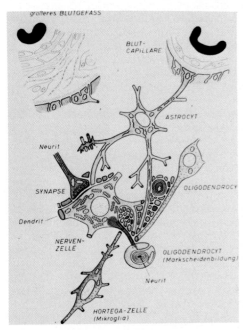

Fig. 1. Morphology of brain cells. Figure courtesy of Dr. A. Oksche, from A. Oksche and L. Vollrath (1980): Handbuch der mikroskopischen Anatomie des Menschen, Vol. IV, 10. Teil Neuroglia I, p. 53. Springer Verlag Heidelberg.

Only about 20 years ago, oligodendrocytes were considered to play a role comparable to that of Schwann cells for the peripheral nerves, namely to form the myelin sheath within the central nervous system (10,14). Although myelin is a unique membrane, electron microscopical studies (9) seem to show that the ensheathment of the axons is a much more complicated process than can be explained by the simple wrapping hypothesis (9). Be that as it may, myelin can be regarded as an enormous extension of the plasma membrane of oligodendrocytes. These cells therefore have to produce the constituents of myelin such as proteins and lipids. The latter comprise up to 75% of the dry weight and consist of about equal parts of cholesterol, glycolipids and phospholipids. Since myelin is one of the richest sources of plasmalogens in mammalian tissues we wanted to study its biosynthesis within these cells.

We decided to work with dissociated cells from newborn rats for different reasons, mainly to be sure of obtaining living cells, although we had to take into account the fact that our primary cell cultures were mixed populations of astrocytes and oligodendrocytes.

Cell culturing was performed according to the method by Booher and Sensenbrenner (1); brain extract from newborn rats (17) was added on and after the fifth day. At the 16th or 17th day in culture, the cells were characterized by histological as well as by immunohistochemical methods. They consisted mainly of astrocytes (both types: protoplasmic and fibrillary) and oligodendrocytes (Fig. 2). The latter showed positive reactions to the monoclonal antibodies to galactocerebrosides (16) and furthermore to monoclonal antibodies "04" (19), which are regarded as specific for some immature oligodendrocytes. No neurons could be detected, whereas some fibroblasts grew under the cell layers. Analysis revealed a protein content of 1.26 mg ± 0.26 (n=406) and an average phospholipid content of 0.26 mg per dish (result of 4 individual cultures). Phospholipid analysis (Table 1) at the 16th day showed that phosphatidylcholine is the main phospholipid, the phosphatidylethanolamine fraction (including plasmalogens) accounting for about 1/4 of the total phospholipids. This fact is of special interest since fetal calf serum contains only trace amounts of phosphatidylethanolamine, about 1% of total phospholipids (22). Therefore it seemed to be reasonable to study the metabolism of ethanolamine phospholipids.

At this stage these cells were incubated with 1-[^{3}H]monoradyl-GPE. As recently published (7,21), 1-[^{3}H]alkyl-GPE (1-alkyl-sn-glycerophosphoethanolamine; substrate A) and 1-[^{3}]alkenyl-GPE (1-alkenyl-sn-glycerophosphoethanolamine; substrate B) were prepared from the ethanolamine phospholipid fraction from rat brain, obtained after intracerebral injection of [^{3}H]hexadecanol. All incubations were performed with similar quantities of radioactivity but varying quantities of substrate. This was achieved by dilution of the radioactive labeled material with unlabeled material, prepared in the same way. We chose the monoradyl compounds because i) it could be assumed that these lipids were better internalized by the cells compared to the diradyl lipids and ii) because we showed by in vivo experiments that alkyl-GPE is the best precursor for plasmalogen biosynthesis in the 14 day old rat brain (6,20).

As far as we are aware, plasmalogen biosynthesis has never been studied in primary glial cell cultures. Yavin and Kanfer (24,25) investigated ethanolamine phospholipid metabolism in mixed neuron-glial cell cultures derived from embryonic rat brain, whereas Poduslo et al. (13) used bulk isolated oligodendroglia from calf and lamb. Eichberg et al. (3) described some important features of phospholipid composition and metabolism in so-called astroglial cultures from newborn hamster brain using radioactive labeled glucose, acetate and inorganic phosphate as precursors. They found some incorporation of ^{32}P into plasmalogens, mainly in the choline type with trace amounts in the ethanolamine plasmalogens.

TABLE 1. Phospholipids (% of total) of Brain or Glial Cells from Rat

Age	Cell Suspension	Whole Brain	Primary Culture		Astrocytes (bulk isolated)	
			Glial Cells	Astrocytes[c]		
	new born[a] (n=2)	14 days[b] (n=6)	16th day[a] (n=9)	14th day[d]	14 days[a] (n=4)	10 days[e] (n=2)
Phosphatidyl -Choline Fract.	56.1	44.8	52.4	50.4	50.0	53.7
-Ethanolamine Fraction	22.7	32.8	22.9	20.7	29.4	26.0
(including Plasmalogens)	(6.3)	(12.5)	(7.5)	(11.5)	(3.3)	(9.4)
-Inositol	4.2	4.8	5.8	4.8	4.6	5.5
-Serine	9.0	9.3	6.2	2.4	8.0	7.2
Sphingomyelin	1.8	3.8	7.0	11.1	2.4	4.6
Cardiolipin	1.1	4.3	2.5	-	2.5	-
Unidentified	5.1	-	3.2	-	3.1	3.3

a) see Ref. 22; b) Etzrodt, A., Diss. Köln (1972), Robbers, G., Diss. Köln (1975); c) hamster; d) see Ref. 3; e) see Ref. 12.

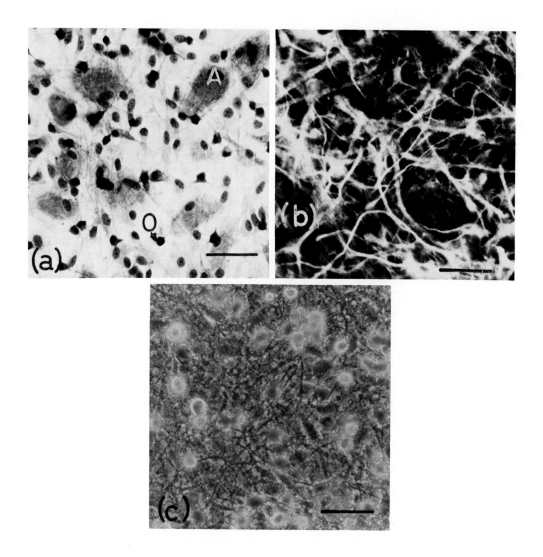

Fig. 2 a-c Photomicrographs of glial cells from rat brain primary culture (16th day).

a) Staining with Haidenhain's iron haematoxylin (15) A: Astrocyte, O: Oligodendrocyte. Scale bar = 50 μm.
b) GFA positive astrocytes. A 17 day old cell culture was fixed with 3.5% paraformaldehyde in buffer and labeled with rabbit anti-GFA serum, followed by fluorescein labeled goat anti-rabbit IgG. Fluorescence optic.
c) Phase contrast optic, same field as b), Scale bar (for b and c) = 40 μm.

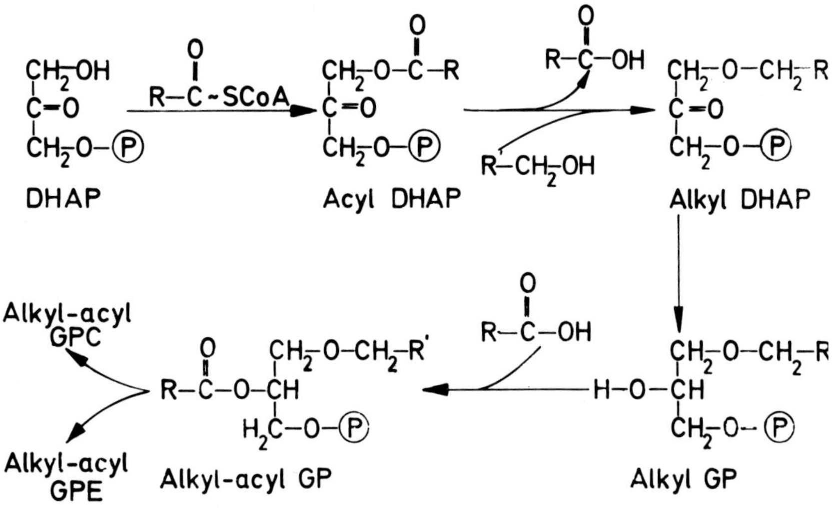

Fig. 3. Biosynthetic pathway for formation of alkylacyl phospholipids (18). DHAP: Dihydroxyacetonephosphate; GP:Glycerophosphate.

Although the main steps toward biosynthesis of plasmalogen (Fig. 3) seem to be well established (18), the mode of introduction of the alkenyl double bond is still unclear. As mentioned above we found some evidence for desaturation of the monoradyl compound, whereas other authors (23,8) working with Ehrlich ascites cells or with brain subcellular fractions who only used 1-alkyl-2-acyl-GPE (1-alkyl-2-acyl-sn-glycerophosphoethano-lamine) for plasmalogen formation concluded from their results that de-saturation takes place only with the acylated compound.

The results we present here were obtained after incubating the glial cell culture described above with both substrates (A and B) for different times (1-20 h) as well as with different quantities (30-300 nmol/mg cell protein). After incubation, the cells were rinsed with saline buffer three times and pelleted after scraping off the surface of the dish. Protein content was estimated, the lipids of the cells extracted according to Folch et al. (4) and the radioactivity was measured. The total lipid extracts were separated on tlc (22) and the radioactivity of the indivi-dual spots (identified by standards) was measured in the presence of silica gel.

All results reported here were evaluated by computing, using the statistical package for the social sciences (SPSS, Version 8,0) (Lit. 11), for details see (22). As shown in Fig. 4 after 3 h incubation both sub-strates were internalized by the cells. Although the rate of uptake is quite different for A or B, we found near linearity with the substrate supply within some ranges. 1-Alkyl-2-acyl-GPE and 1-alkenyl-2-acyl-GPE (1-alkenyl-2-acyl-sn-glycerophosphoethanolamine = plasmalogen), respec-tively, were found to be the main products after the first three hours of incubation. The acylation reactions follow hyperbolic curves (Fig. 5). Some radioactivity could also be detected in choline-containing phos-pholipid fractions at that time (Fig. 6). After incubation with 1-alkyl-GPE, a hydrolysis product, 1-alkyl-G (1-alkyl-sn-glycerol), was observed in small amounts as well as some 1-alkenyl-2-acyl-GPE (Fig. 6).

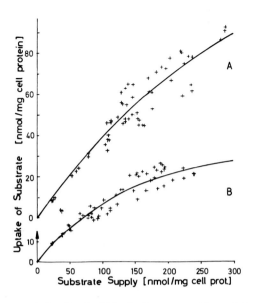

Fig. 4. Internalization of 1-alkyl-GPE (substrate A) and 1-alkenyl-GPE
         (substrate B) by glial primary cultures after 3 h incubation.

The experimental data showed not only that the quantity of the substrate supply influenced the intensity of substrate uptake by the cells,
but also the time of incubation. Therefore experiments had to be performed with increasing substrate concentrations for 1, 2, 3, 6, 12 and 20
h. From all these results we show here only those, observed at internalization of 50 nmol substrate per mg cell protein, obtained under analogous conditions (Fig. 7).

Thus, we found that although the concentration of substrate B
(alkenyl-GPE) in the cell is very low, its acylation rate is much higher
than that of substrate A. The acylated compounds are mostly accumulated
in the cells between 2 and 6 h incubation time. In contrast, the alkenylacyl-GPE derived from alkyl-GPE increased up to 12 h and showed under the
conditions used no precursor-product relationship to substrate A. With
regard to the results demonstrated in Fig. 7 one has to ask the question: which compound is the direct precursor of alkenylacyl-GPE (plasmalogen). During the incubation no alkenyl-GPE was found from alkyl-GPE.
If one, however, compares the affinity of the acylating enzyme system
(Fig. 8) for 1-alkyl-GPE (substrate A) with that for 1-alkenyl-GPE (substrate B) one realizes that the K_m for the latter is 1.7 nmol/mg cell
protein, whereas that of 1-alkyl-GPE is 5.0 nmol/mg cell protein.
Furthermore, the Lineweaver-Burk plot reveals that both substrates compete
for the active center of the enzyme.

On the other hand the desaturation enzyme system is very slow-
reacting. Because these experiments were made with living cells, supplied with phospholipids, the results of shorttime experiments were un-
satisfactory. However, the following observations on Fig. 7 can be made.
After 3 h incubation with alkenyl-GPE the substrate concentration in the
cells is only 3.5 nmol/mg cell protein. Its acylated product amounts to
28.5 nmol/mg cell protein. The real concentration of alkyl-GPE under the
same conditions is 9.5 nmol/mg cell protein and the acylated product

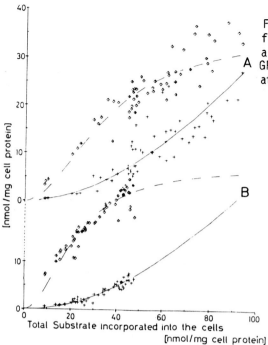

Fig. 5. Formation of alkylacyl-GPE (◇) from 1-alkyl-GPE (substrate A, +) and alkenylacyl-GPE (◇) from 1-alkenyl-GPE (substrate B; +) by glial cells after 3 h incubation.

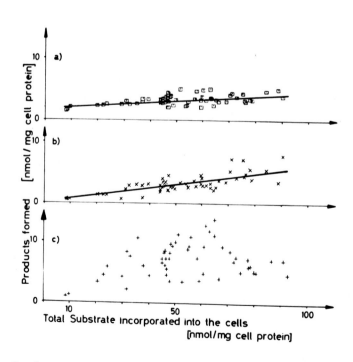

Fig. 6. Products from the substrate 1-[^{3}H]alkyl-GPE by glial cells after 3 h incubation. a) 1-alkenyl-2-acyl-GPE (plasmalogen); b) 1-alkyl-glycerol; c) 1-alkyl-2-acyl-GPC.

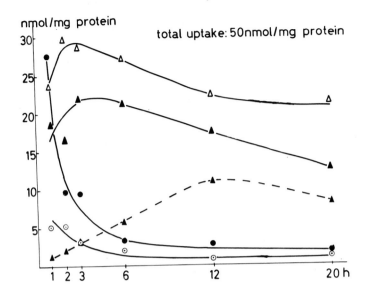

Fig. 7. Time course of product formation from alkyl-GPE (●) and alkenyl-GPE (ⵔ). ▲ solid line: alkylacyl-GPE; ▲ dashed line: alkenylacyl-GPE, derived from alkyl-GPE (●); Δ alkenylacyl-GPE, derived from alkenyl-GPE (ⵔ).

3h Incubation

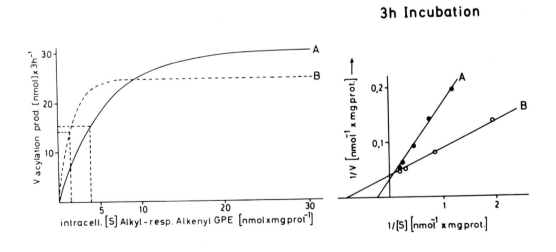

Fig. 8. Acylation rates of substrate A (1-alkyl-GPE) and substrate B (1-alkenyl-GPE). Lineweaver-Burk plot (right) indicating that A and B react as competitive inhibitors.

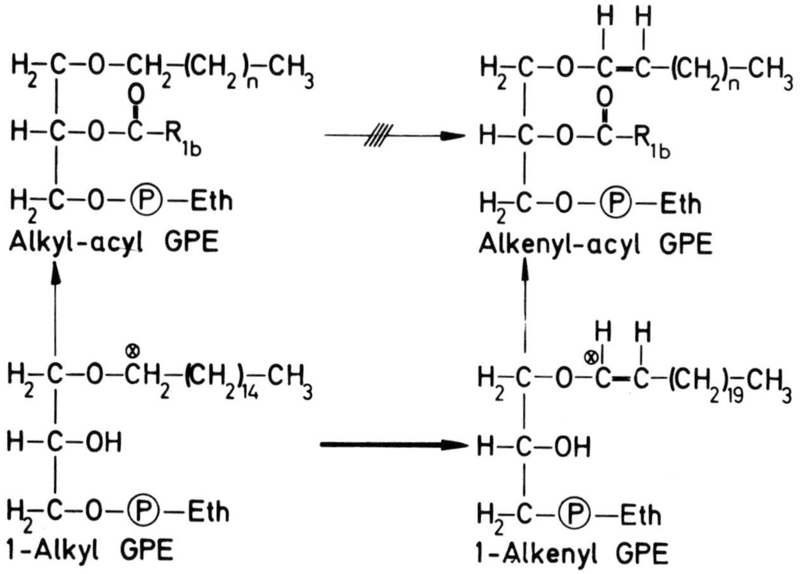

Fig. 9.   Pathway of plasmalogen formation proved by experiments.

22.0 nmol/mg cell protein.   Again, at the same time and under the same conditions, the desaturated product derived from alkyl-GPE is only 3.0 nmol/mg cell protein.   Of course, the product formation is dependent on the substrate concentration within the cells.   If one assumes that the concentration of alkyl-GPE would be the same as that of alkenyl-GPE, that is 3.5 nmol/mg cell protein, the respective acylated product - 1-alkyl-2-acyl-GPE - would account for 8.1 nmol/mg protein and the desaturated compound would be 1.1 nmol/mg protein.   The conclusion can then be drawn that if the substrate concentration of alkyl-GPE is 3.5 nmol/mg cell protein, the desaturation of alkyl-GPE then would be 1 nmol/mg protein but the acylation of the alkenyl-GPE is 25 nmol/mg protein.   That is the explanation for the fact that, although alkenyl-GPE originates from alkyl-GPE, it cannot be observed since the velocity of its acylation is much higher.

Therefore one has to assume that the introduction of the alk-1-enyl double bond into plasmalogen takes place with the monoradyl compound (Fig. 9).

Finally, with longer incubation times we found increasing radioactivity in the PC-fraction (phosphatidylcholine) (Fig. 10).   We cannot decide yet whether this conversion is due to base-exchange reactions (5) or is due to stepwise methylation (2) of 1-alkyl-2-acyl-GPE.   Here again 1-alkenyl-2-acyl-GPE seems to be the better substrate.   1-Alkylglycerol - a hydrolysis product - was found in a nearly constant but low concentration.

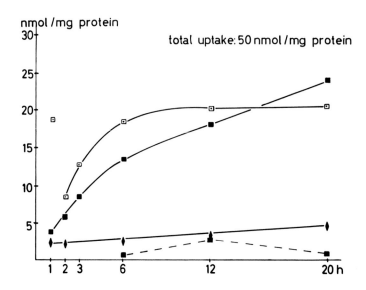

Fig. 10. Time course of product formation after incubation of glial cells with monoradyl-GPE as substrate. ■ solid line: 1-alkyl-2-acyl-sn-glycero-phosphocholine; ■ dashed line: 1-alkenyl-2-acyl-sn-glycerophosphocholine; ◆ alkylglycerol (derived from 1-alkyl-GPE); ⊡ 1-alkenyl-2-acyl-sn-glycerophosphocholine (derived from 1-alkenyl-GPE).

CONCLUSION

Mixed populations of glial cells derived from dissociated newborn rat hemispheres can be used for studies of phospholipid metabolism. They internalize monoradyl-glycerophosphoethanolamines. Except for a small degradation rate, these are mainly acylated and base-exchanged. It could be shown that the acylating enzyme system possesses a higher affinity for 1-alkenyl-GPE compared to 1-alkyl-GPE. Desaturation of the latter, however, is a very slow reaction, probably 25 times slower than the acylating one. Therefore, one has to conclude that the monoradyl compound is desaturated prior to acylation - the last step in plasmalogen biosynthesis.

REFERENCES

1. Booher, J. and Sensenbrenner, M. (1972): Neurobiology, 2:97-105.

2. Crews, F.T., Hirata, F., and Axelrod, J. (1980): J. Neurochem., 34:1491-1498.

3. Eichberg, J., Shein, H.M., and Hauser, G. (1976): J. Neurochem., 27:679-685.

4. Folch, J., Lees, M., and Sloane-Stanley, G.H. (1957): J. Biol. Chem., 126:497-509.

5. Goracci, G., Blomstrand, C., Arienti, G., Hamberger, A., and Porcellati, G. (1973): J. Neurochem., 20:1167-1180.

6. Gunawan, J. and Debuch, H. (1977): Hoppe-Seyler's Z. Physiol. Chem., 358:537-542.

7. Gunawan, J., Vierbuchen, M., and Debuch, H. (1979): Hoppe-Seyler's Z. Physiol. Chem., 360:971-978.

8. Horrocks, L.A. and Radominska-Pyrek, A. (1972): FEBS Letters, 22:190-192.

9. Knobler, R.L., Stempak, J.G., and Laurencin, M. (1976): J. Ultrastructure Res., 55:417-432.

10. Krey, S. (1960): Arch. Neurol., 2:140-145.

11. Nie, N.H., Hull, C.H., Jenkins, J.G., Steinbrenner, K., and Bent, D.H. (1975): Statistical Package for the Social Sciences. McGraw-Hill, Inc., New York.

12. Norton, W.T. and Poduslo, S.E. (1971): J. Lipid Res., 9:129-136.

13. Poduslo, S.E., Miller, K., and McKhann, G.M. (1978): J. Biol. Chem. 253:1592-1597.

14. de Robertis, E., Gerschenfeld, H., and Wald, F. (1958): J. Biophys. Biochem. Cytol., 4:651-658.

15. Romeis, B. (1948): Mikroskopische Technik. Leibniz Verlag, München.

16. Schachner, M., Kim, S.K., and Zehnle, R. (1981): Developmental Biology, 83:328-338.

17. Sensenbrenner, M., Springer, N., Booher, J., and Mandel, P. (1972): Neurobiology, 2:49-60.

18. Snyder, F. (1972): In: Ether Lipids-Chemistry and Biology, edited by F. Snyder, pp. 152-156. Academic Press, New York.

19. Sommer, J. and Schachner, M. (1981): Developmental Biology, 83:311-327.

20. Tjiong, H.B., Gunawan, J., and Debuch, H. (1976): Hoppe-Seyler's Z. Physiol. Chem., 357:707-712.

21. Vierbuchen, M., Gunawan, J., and Debuch, H. (1979): Hoppe-Seyler's Z. Physiol. Chem., 360:1091-1097.

22. Witter, B. and Debuch, H. (1981): submitted for publication.

23. Wykle, R.L., Blank, M.L., Malone, B., and Snyder, F. (1972): J. Biol. Chem., 247:5442-5447.

24. Yavin, E. and Kanfer, J.N. (1975): <u>J. Biol. Chem.</u>, 250:2885-2890.

25. Yavin, E. and Kanfer, J.N. (1975): <u>J. Biol. Chem.</u>, 250:2891-2895.

Phospholipids in the Nervous System, Vol. 1: Metabolism, edited by L. Horrocks, et al. Raven Press, New York © 1982.

Plasmalogenase Activity in Isolated Oligodendroglia— Subcellular Location and Regulation in the Metabolism of Myelin Plasmalogen

Eric M. Carey, Angela Carruthers, and Neil Freeman

Department of Biochemistry, University of Sheffield, Sheffield S10 2TN, United Kingdom

Plasmalogens (1-alk-1'-enyl-glycerophospholipids) account for a substantial proportion of the phospholipids of the mammalian brain and are present in highest amounts in myelin (9). Around 70% of the ethanolamine glycerophospholipid fraction of bovine myelin consists of 1-alkenyl-2-acyl-GPE.

The accumulation of 1-alkenyl-2-acyl-GPE during brain development parallels the appearance of myelin which is a specialised plasma membrane of the oligodendroglial cell (13). During the myelination phase of brain development, oligodendroglia synthesise myelin membrane components which are incorporated into the extending plasma membrane. The cytoplasmic faces of the plasma membrane condense together and further membrane extension results in the formation of the multi-lamellar structure of the myelin sheath which surrounds the nerve axon (29).

1-Alkenyl-2-acyl-glycerophospholipids are synthesised from 1-alkyl-2-acyl-glycerophospholipids by a desaturase which has highest activity at the time of myelination (21). In a competing reaction, the ether bond of 1-alkyl-2-acyl-phospholipids is cleaved by a mixed function oxidase but in brain tissue the enzyme has a low activity. In the developing brain, the formation of the precursor alkyl-DHAP from acyl-DHAP is favoured when the tissue concentration and synthesis of long chain alcohols from fatty acids increases.

Although the pathway for the synthesis of plasmalogens is well understood, their function in myelin and other plasma membranes is uncertain. There are physico-chemical differences between 1-alkenyl-2-acyl and diacyl-glycerophospholipids. The surface potential exerted by 1-alkenyl-2-acyl-glycerophospholipids is lower than that of diacyl-glycerophospholipids (15), and the absence of a carbonyl group may affect lipid-protein interactions. With the exception of the double bond between carbons 1 and 2, the alkenyl groups of plasmalogens are highly saturated and the proportion of alkenyl groups with a 9,10 double bond increases only slightly during brain development. Because of the alkenyl group, plasmalogens are more saturated than diacyl-glycerophospholipids.

The alkenyl group of 1-alkenyl-2-acyl-glycerophospholipids is hydrolytically cleaved in a reaction catalysed by a specific hydrolase, 'plasmalogenase'. The enzyme was first shown by Warner and Lands (16) to be present in liver and later Ansell and Spanner (1) found that brain tissue rapidly hydrolyses the alkenyl ether bond of plasmalogens. However, the alkenyl ether double bond can also be oxidatively cleaved by ascorbate (22).

In their study of plasmalogenase activity in brain, D'Amato et al (4) found that the enzyme was competitively inhibited by diacyl-GPE. Woelk and Porcellati (19) showed that the membrane bound phospholipase A_1 of nervous tissue is inhibited by 1-alkenyl-2-acyl-glycerophospholipids. This competitive inhibition may serve an important regulatory function in reducing both the turnover of all diradyl glycerophospholipids in the plasma membrane and the formation of monoradyl glycerophospholipids. Plasmalogens may therefore contribute to membrane stability in two ways - by enhancing hydrophobic interactions of membrane lipids and by modulating the catabolism of diacyl-glycerophospholipids. Plasmalogenase may hydrolyse the alkenyl group from 1-alkenyl-2-acyl-glycerophospholipids (5) and from 1-alkenyl glycerophospholipids after removal of the acyl group from the 2 position by phospholipase A_2 (8).

Plasmalogenase has a higher activity in brain white matter compared with grey matter (1). The ontogenic development of plasmalogenase activity coincides with the period of myelination and it is likely that enzyme activity is expressed during the differentiation of the myelinating oligodendroglial cell. This paper describes some of the properties of plasmalogenase from isolated oligodendroglia and the relationship between enzyme activity and the concentration of 1-alkenyl-2-acyl-glycerophospholipids in brain tissue during the course of experimentally induced demyelination and subsequent remyelination.

RESULTS AND CONCLUSIONS

Distribution and subcellular location of plasmalogenase

Oligodendroglia, neuronal perikarya and astrocytes were prepared from white matter dissected from adult bovine brain and myelinating rat brain. Oligodendroglial cell preparations were characterized by light and electron microscopy, by indirect immunofluorescence using galactocerebroside antiserum and by the presence of 2'3'-cyclic nucleotide 3'-phosphohydrolase and UDP-galactose:ceramide galactosyl transferase (3). The degree of contamination in each type of cell preparation was not more than 10%. Plasmalogenase activity was assayed in tissue homogenates and disrupted cell preparations by the procedure of Williams et al. (19) which involves the specific iodination of the alkenyl ether double bond in plasmalogen remaining after incubation. In membrane fractions obtained from isolated oligodendroglia, plasmalogenase was assayed by the conversion of released aldehydes to the corresponding alcohols in the presence of NADH and liver alcohol dehydrogenase (6). Details of the assay are given in the legend to Table 3. Purified ethanolamine plasmalogen (12) was used as a substrate for all incubations.

Oligodendroglia had the highest specific activity of plasmalogenase (Table 1). The activity in astroglia and neuronal perikarya could be due to contamination by oligodendroglia. The ratio of plasmalogenase

TABLE 1. Plasmalogenase activity in neuronal perikarya, astroglia and oligodendroglia[d]

Cell Type	Rat Brain	Bovine white matter
	(nmol/mg protein/min)	
Neuronal perikarya	0.4 ± 0.2	1.2 ± 0.3
Astroglia	0.7 ± 0.3	2.1 ± 0.4
Oligodenroglia	4.8 ± 1.2	11.2 ± 3.1
		(umol/g tissue/h)
White matter (corpus callosum)		12 ± 2
Grey matter (cerebral cortex)		1.5 ± 0.6

[d]Activity ± S.E.M. (n = 5)

activity in oligodendroglia to that in neuronal perikarya was in the order of 10:1 which is similar to the ratio of activity in white and grey matter (1). Our results with isolated brain cell preparations are similar to earlier results of Dorman et al. (5), confirming that plasmalogenase is predominantly localised in oligodendroglia. Oligodendroglia isolated from adult bovine brain had a higher plasmalogenase activity than oligodendroglia isolated from myelinating rat brain (Table 1), suggesting that plasmalogenase activity is expressed as part of oligodendroglial differentiation. This would also support the earlier observation that the increase in plasmalogenase activity in whole brain parallels myelin accumulation (1). The content of 1-alkenyl-2-acyl glycerophospholipids is also higher in isolated oligodendroglia compared with neuronal perikarya. In contrast to the almost exclusively oligodendroglial location of plasmalogenase, phospholipase A_1 and A_2 activities are 2-fold higher in neuronal perikarya compared with oligodendroglia (18).

Membrane fractions from isolated oligodendroglia were prepared by the method of Poduslo (14) and characterised by the distribution of various 'marker' enzymes (Table 2). Plasmalogenase had the highest specific activity in the plasma membrane fraction, with some activity in other fractions. A heavy myelin fraction derived from the oligodendroglial cell preparations had some activity, although myelin isolated from bovine brain white matter and subjected to osmotic shocking and purification by density gradient centrifugation had no measurable plasmalogenase activity (results not presented). Phospholipase A_1 and A_2 are also absent from light myelin fractions. The plasmalogenase localised in the plasma membrane could function in the catabolism of myelin ethanolamine plasmalogen without the necessity of transfer to intracellular membranes by phospholipid exchange proteins.

Ansell and Spanner (2) studied the distribution of plasmalogenase in subcellular fractions derived from whole brain and found the highest specific activity in a mitochondrial fraction which would also contain lysosomal particles, with some activity in a microsomal membrane fraction containing plasma membrane. The distribution of plasmalogenase was similar to that of phospholipases A_1 and A_2, which are present in membrane-bound and soluble lysosomal forms with different pH optima (19). This would suggest a dual location of plasmalogenase. Isolated oligodendroglial cell bodies have few subcellular particles which are mainly concentrated in cell processes, lost during the isolation

TABLE 2. Distribution of plasmalogenase and 'marker' enzymes
          in membrane fractions derived from isolated
                      oligodendroglia.

Fraction (sucrose conc)	Relative specific activity				
	CNP'ase	5'NT ase	NADPH-cyt.c reductase	CGal transferase	Plasmalo-gemase
Oligodendroglia	1.0	1.0	1.0	1.0	1.0
Myelin (0.85 M)	5.1	1.7	0.1	0.6	3.0
Plasma membrane (1.0 M)	5.3	4.6	0.1	2.8	5.5
Endoplasmic reticulum (1.5 M)	3.7	1.5	4.3	4.4	3.7

CNP'ase; 2'3'-cyclic nucleotide 3'-phosphohydrolase (myelin)
5'-NT'ase; 5'-nucleotidase (plasma membrane)
NADPH-cytochrome c reductase (E.r.)
CGal Transferase; UDP-galactose:ceramide galactosyl transferase
(oligodendroglia)
Membrane fractions were prepared by the method of Poduslo.

procedure. The properties of the plasmalogenase described in the next
section are those of a membrane-bound form of the enzyme.

Properties of plasmalogenase from isolated bovine oligodendroglia

     The cleavage of the alkenyl group of 1-alk-1'-enyl-GPE, prepared by
mild alkaline hydrolysis of 1-alkenyl-2-acyl-GPE, was lower than that
obtained with 1-alkenyl-2-acyl-GPE as substrate (Table 3). With both
substrates, the concentration of Triton X-100 in the assay (0.025%) was
the same. Gunawan et al. (9) showed that brain microsomes from 14 day
old rats possess a plasmalogenase activity which is considerably more
active towards 1-alkenyl-GPE than towards 1-alkenyl-2-acyl-GPE. This
lysoplasmalogenase activity, with a neutral pH optimum, has a requirement for divalent cations unlike the plasmalogenase from bovine oligodendroglia. The precise cellular location of the lysoplasmalogenase was
not determined. In brain tissue therefore there appears to be at least
two enzyme activities able to hydrolyse the alkenyl group of plasmalogens.
     The activity of plasmalogenase from oligodendroglia, with
alkenyl-acyl-GPE as substrate, was influenced by the concentration of
the non-ionic detergent Triton X-100 (Table 3). The highest activity
was obtained at a concentration of 0.025%, and higher concentrations
were inhibitory. Plasmalogenase activity was lower when deoxycholate
(an anionic detergent) was used instead of Triton X-100 (Table 3). Presumably the surface charge on the lipid-detergent micelles influences
enzyme activity. Differences between 1-alkenyl-2-acyl-GPE and alkenyl-
GPE as substrates could be due to different physico-chemical properties, with alkenyl-GPE acting as a detergent.
     The addition of magnesium ions or EDTA was found to have no effect
on plasmalogenase activity and dialysis of disrupted oligodendroglia
preparations did not significantly affect enzyme activity. Ansell and
Spanner (1) found that the cleavage of alkenyl groups from plasmalogen

TABLE 3. Factors affecting the activity of plasmalogenase in isolated oligodendroglia from bovine brain white matter

Modified conditions from standard assay	Enzyme Activity (nmol aldehyde released) /mg protein/min).
None	11.1 ± 1.4
Substrate 0.24 mM 1-alk-1'-enyl-GPE	4.0 ± 0.3
Detergent solubilisation	
Triton X-100 0.01% (final concn)	8.7
0.025	13.2
0.1	7.7
0.5	3.0
Sodium deoxycholate 0.05%	6.9
Stability	
Assayed 1 day after glial preparation	13.2
2 days	10.3
3 days	5.7
after freeze/thawing	6.7

Incubations (in 1.0 ml); disrupted glial cell suspension (50-250 μg protein), 0.24 mM 1-alk-1'-enyl-2-acyl-GPE (isolated from bovine white matter), 0.025% (w/v) Triton X-100, 1 mM dithiothreitol, 100 mM Tris-HCl, pH 7.4, 0.3 mM NADH and 0.1 mg liver alcohol dehydrogenase (0.3 units nominal activity with ethanol as substrate).

by acetone extracted powders from rat brain had an absolute requirement for Mg^{++}. The deoxycholate concentrations used to solubilise the acetone extracted brain tissue could have been inhibitory. The addition of magnesium ions causes the precipitation of insoluble magnesium deoxycholate.

When kept at 0°C the plasmalogenase activity of oligodendroglial preparations progressively lost activity (Table 3). Disruption of membranes by freezing and thawing resulted in loss of activity, suggesting that the membrane-bound plasmalogenase is sensitive to alteration in membrane structure.

The activity of plasmalogenase was determined over a range of pH from 6.6 to 7.9 and the pH optimum was between 7.0 and 7.4. A pH optimum of 7.4 was found for the enzyme in acetone-extracts of whole rat brain, over a range of pH between 6.0 and 11.5 (1). The reported pH optima for phospholipase A_1 and A_2 in glia are 5.4 and 8.0 respectively (19). There is no information on whether there is any significant plasmalogenase activity at a pH below 6.0.

The metabolism of the alkenyl group of ethanolamine plasmalogen

1-[9,10-^{3}H]alkenyl-2-acyl-GPE was used as a substrate to determine directly the release of ^{3}H-aldehyde by disrupted oligodendroglia (Fig. 1). In the absence of NADH, radioactive aldehydes could not be detected. The radioactivity in the alkenyl group of the phospholipid substrate (determined by GLC as the aldehyde-dimethylacetal) declined as the radioactivity in esterified fatty acid increased. The appearance of radioactivity in lysophosphatidylethanolamine and in aldehyde only occurred in the presence of NADH. The further addition of a liver alcohol dehydrogenase preparation resulted in the conversion of long-chain aldehydes to the corresponding alcohols. One possible explanation is that oligodendroglia oxidised the released aldehyde to fatty acid which was reincorporated into diacyl phospholipid without the accumulation of lysophospholipid. In support of this conclusion we found an active aldehyde dehydrogenase in oligodendroglia which was specific for long-chain fatty aldehydes and inhibited by NADH.

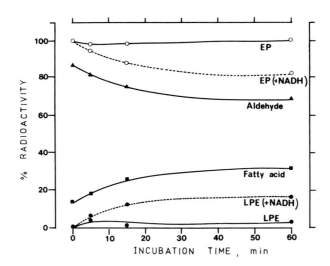

Fig. 1. The metabolism of 1-[9,10-^{3}H]alk-1'-enyl-2-acyl-glycerophosphoethanolamine by bovine oligodendroglia. Incubations (in 0.5 ml) contained: 100 mM Tris-HCl, pH 7.4, 1 mM dithiothreitol, disrupted oligodendroglia (250 μg protein), 0.24 mM [^{3}H]plasmalogen (45,000 dpm added as a 2.4 mM solution containing 0.5% Triton X-100 and solubilised by sonication) and (where shown with broken lines) 0.3 mM NADH. The specific activity of the [^{3}H]plasmalogen was 0.169 Ci/mol based on phospholipid-P, and the specific activity of the alkenyl group, determined as the hydrazone, was 0.187 Ci/mol. From the analyses of the fatty acid methyl esters and aldehyde dimethyl acetals produced by BF$_3$ methanolysis, the ratio of radioactivity in the alkenyl and acyl groups was 5:1. After incubation lipids were extracted and analysed by TLC. Radioactivity in ethanolamine phospholipid (EP) and lysophosphatidylethanolamine (LPE) was determined after scraping the appropriate areas of silica gel into liquid scintillant. Fatty acids and aldehydes were analysed by radio GLC.

The activity of plasmalogenase in relation to demyelination

In brain regions undergoing active demyelination there is a loss of ethanolamine plasmalogen and other myelin sheath components. The activities of plasmalogenase (2) and phospholipases A$_1$ and A$_2$ (20) have been found to be higher in apparently normal white matter adjacent to demyelinating regions in the human brain during the course of multiple sclerosis. Plasmalogenase has also been reported to show increased activity in virus-induced CNS demyelination in the dog (7). It has not been established whether the increased activity of plasmalogenase or phospholipases is an early event in myelin loss or whether such changes in catabolic activity are secondary to myelin breakdown.

Cuprizone (biscyclohexanone oxaldihydrazone), a copper chelating agent, causes extensive demyelination of myelinated tracts in different brain regions of the mouse (10), while neurons and their axons are mostly unaffected. Demyelination and loss of oligodendroglia is accompanied by the proliferation of reactive astrocytes, and macrophages are also evident (10). The sensitivity of oligodendroglia to cuprizone may be due to its effects on mitochondrial respiration and oxidative phosphorylation. Cuprizone-induced demyelination is reversible although the reformed myelin sheaths are thinner and the internodal lengths shorter. The cells functioning in the remyelination process are probably oligodendroglia, formed by differentiation of glioblasts, although this has not been definitely established.

In our experiments, Cuprizone was administered in the diet (0.4% by weight) to weanling male mice (at 3 weeks of age) for periods of up to 3 weeks, followed by a return to a normal laboratory diet. The brain weight was permanently reduced by 7-10%, while body weight returned to that of controls.

The brain was sectioned vertically into 5 sections. The amount of myelin was estimated from activity of the activity of 2',3'-cyclic nucleotide-3'-phosphohydrolase (CNP'ase) an enzyme present in myelin and also in oligodendroglia. The increase in CNP'ase activity occurs primarily between weeks 2 and 4, the myelination phase of brain development. Cuprizone treatment, commenced at 3 weeks of age, resulted in a decrease of CNP'ase activity between weeks 4 and 6 followed by partial recovery on a return to normal diet (Fig. 2). Section 1 contains the white matter of the frontal region of the cerebral cortex and section 2, the mid-cortical region and corpus callosum. The least affected areas were the mid-brain region and cerebellum (sections 4 and 5). Brain sections which had been fixed and stained to reveal myelinated fibres showed extensive loss of myelin in sub-cortical white matter of the cerebral cortex and corpus callosum. Based on the activity of CNP'ase, around 80% of myelin in cerebral cortical white matter was lost over the 3 week period of Cuprizone administration. In the recovery phase, CNP'ase activity increased to about 35% of that of control animals. There was a permanent deficit of myelin in the cerebral cortex, but not in the cerebellum, and following recovery animals showed no apparent neurological signs.

The increase in plasmalogenase ctivity during mouse brain development paralleled that of CNP'ase, suggesting that both enzymes are expressed during oligodendroglial differentiation. During the period of Cuprizone-induced demyelination, plasmalogenase activity was elevated above controls. The highest activity (after 2 weeks on the Cuprizone diet) was reached while the CN'ase activity was still declining. The increase in plasmalogenase activity (on a gram wet weight basis) cannot be accounted for by the decrease in brain weight. McKeown and Allen (11) found an increase in the activity of a number of lysosomal enzymes in apparently normal white matter surrounding actively demyelinating plaque regions in multiple sclerosis. The source of the enzymes was considered to be reactive astrocytes rather than macrophages because of the noticeable astrocytosis. The increase in plasmalogenase activity in response to Cuprizone (and phospholipase A_1 and A_2 activities in

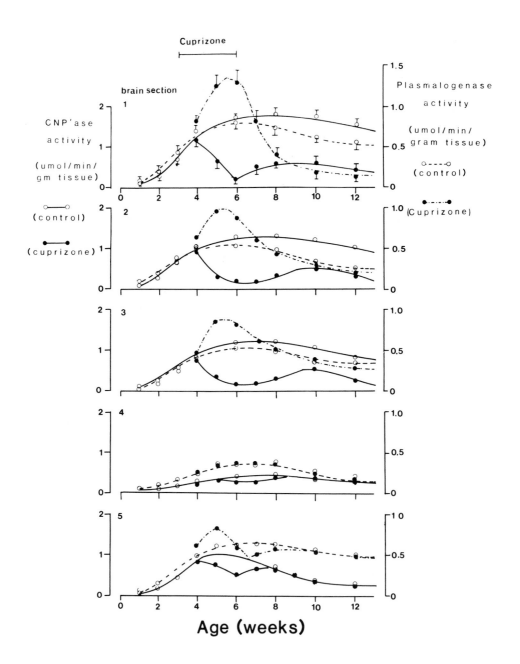

Figure 2. Activity of CNP'ase and plasmalogenase in different brain regions in response to cuprizone.

multiple sclerosis) could be astrocytic in origin. In reactive astrocytes there may be increased hydrolytic activity compared with normal astrocytes (Table 1). It is unlikely that the increased activity is due to activation of the plasmalogenase in the oligodendroglial plasma membrane.

Following recovery from Cuprizone administration, plasmalogenase activity in sections 1 and 2 was about 30% of control values. Sections 4 and 5 were least affected as for CNP'ase, with no deficit in plasmalogenase activity. In the cerebellum it therefore appears that any effect of Cuprizone on oligodendroglia and myelin is transitory and reversible.

The plasmalogen content on a gram wet weight basis of the different brain regions was determined three weeks after returning animals to a normal diet (Figure 3). Significant differences between control and Cuprizone-treated animals were found for sections 1 and 2. The reduced plasmalogenase activity was accompanied by an elevated plasmalogen content. In normal development and in brain sections from control animals at 9 weeks of age there was a good correlation between plasmalogenase activity and plasmalogen content. This might be expected because both parameters reflect oligodendroglial differentiation. However following recovery from Cuprizone-administration, plasmalogenase activity in sections 1 and 2 was lower than controls. This could be a consequence of a reduction in oligodendroglial cell numbers by as much as 70%. In the recovery phase there may also be an imbalance between myelin synthesis and catabolism producing an altered myelin composition.

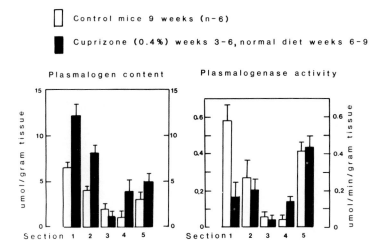

Figure 3. Plasmalogen content and plasmalogenase activity in different brain regions following recovery from cuprizone-induced spongiform encephalopathy.

Acknowledgement

The work was supported by a grant from the Multiple Sclerosis Society of Great Britian. A.C. was a recipient of an M.R.C. studentship.

References

1. Ansell, G.B. and Spanner, S. (1965): Biochem. J., 88:56-64.
2. Ansell, G.B. and Spanner, S. (1968): Biochem. J., 108:207-209.
3. Carruthers, A. and Carey, E.M. (1979): Biochem. Soc. Trans., 7:718-719.
4. D'Amato, R.A., Horrocks, L.A. and Richardson, K.E. (1975): J. Neurochem., 24:1251-1255.
5. Dorman, R.V., Toews, A.D. and Horrocks, L.A. (1977): J. Lipid Res., 18:115-117.
6. Freeman, N.M. and Carey, E.M. (1980): Biochem. Soc. Trans., 8:612-613.
7. Fu, S.C., Mozzi, R., Krakowka, S., Higgins, R.J. and Horrocks, L.A. (1980): Acta Neuropathol., 49:13-18.
8. Gunawan, J., Vierbuchen, M. and Debuch, H. (1979): Hoppe-Seyler's Z. Physiol. Chem., 360:971-978.
9. Horrocks, L.A. (1968): J. Lipid Res., 9:469-472.
10. Kesterton, J.W. and Carlton, W.W. (1971): Exp. Mol. Pathol., 15:82-96.
11. McKeown, S.R. and Allen, I.V. (1978): Neuropathol. Appl. Neurobiol., 4:471-481.
12. Paltauf, F. (1978): Lipids, 18:165-166.
13. Peters, A. and Vaughn, J.E. (1970): Myelination, C.C Thomas, Springfield, Illinois.
14. Poduslo, S. (1975): J. Neurochem., 24:647-654.
15. Shah, D.O. and Schulmann, J.H. (1965): J. Lipid Res., 6:341-349.
16. Warner, H.R. and Lands, W.E.M. (1961): J. Biol. Chem., 236:2404-2409.
17. Williams, J.N., Anderson, C.O.E. and Jasik, A.D. (1962): J. Lipid Res., 3:378-381.
18. Woelk, H., Goracci, G., Gaiti, A. and Porcellati, G. (1973): Hoppe-Seyler's Z. Physiol. Chem., 354:729-736.
19. Woelk, H. and Porcellati, G. (1973): Hoppe-Seyler's Z. Physiol. Chem., 354:729-736.
20. Woelk, H. and Peiler-Ichikawa, K. (1974): J. Neurol., 207:319-326.
21. Wykle, R.L. and Schremmer Lockmiller, J.M. (1975): Biochim. Biophys. Acta 380:291-298.
22. Yavin, E. and Gatt, S. (1972): Eur. J. Biochem., 25:431-437.

Phospholipids in the Nervous System, Vol. 1: Metabolism, edited by L. Horrocks, et al. Raven Press, New York © 1982.

Studies of Phospholipid Synthesis in Mammalian and Invertebrate Axons and Terminals

*R. M. Gould, **H. Pant, †H. Gainer, and ‡M. Tytell

*Marine Biology Laboratory, Woods Hole, Massachusetts 02543; *Institute for Basic Research in Developmental Disabilities, Staten Island, New York 10314; **National Institute on Alcohol Abuse and Alcoholism, Rockville, Maryland 20852; †National Institute of Child Health and Human Development, National Institutes of Health, Bethesda, Maryland 20205; ‡Department of Anatomy, Bowman Gray School of Medicine, Wake Forest University, Winston-Salem, North Carolina 27103*

Neurons have extensive processes containing membranous and cytoplasmic elements. With its single nucleus, the neuron's transcriptional and translational activities are restricted to the soma and proximal dendrites. A sophisticated system of axonal transport (8) functions to continually supply the axon and terminals with needed proteins, nucleic acids, and other macromolecules. Membrane proteins and their associated phospholipids are axonally transported at very rapid rates, presumably because of their roles in the functional properties of the axon (e.g. impulse propagation) and terminals (e.g. chemical transmission). In addition, there is evidence that phospholipid synthesis occurs in axons (5,6,9,12) and terminals (1,2,14).

Using an autoradiographic approach, we found that the myelinated and unmyelinated axons of mouse sciatic nerve actively form phosphatidyl-inositol from [2-^{3}H]myo-inositol (Fig 1A,5), while axonal synthesis of phosphatidylcholine from [methyl-^{3}H] choline was not observed (Fig 1B,7). Like myo-inositol, tritiated glycerol incorporation is localized to unmyelinated fibers (Fig 1C). Possibly the small caliber axons selectively take up and synthesize phospholipid from this precursor. Furthermore, in crush injured nerves, choline labels many myelinated axons (Fig 1D). This finding suggests a latent choline lipid synthesis in axons, which is expressed in injured axons because of a greater accessibility of labeled substrate and/or an activation of (a) latent enzyme(s). These autoradiographic results have been strengthened by biochemical studies (11, Gould and Cohen, unpublished observations), which have shown that CDP diglyceride-inositol transferase (EC 2.7.8.11), and possibly CDPcholine:1,2-diacyl-glycerol choline phosphotransferase (EC 2.7.8.2) and ATP:diacylglycerol phosphotransferase (EC 2.7.1.-) are axonally transported. Their transport would support an axonal localization of these synthetic enzymes.

The squid giant axon is a unique tissue, ideally suited for investigations to elucidate axonal lipid synthesis. Larrabee and Brinley (12) used this preparation to show that axoplasm synthesized phosphatidylethanolamine, phosphatidylinositol, and phosphatidic acid from precursor ^{32}P-phosphate. Recently, Brunetti et al. (4) reported that squid giant

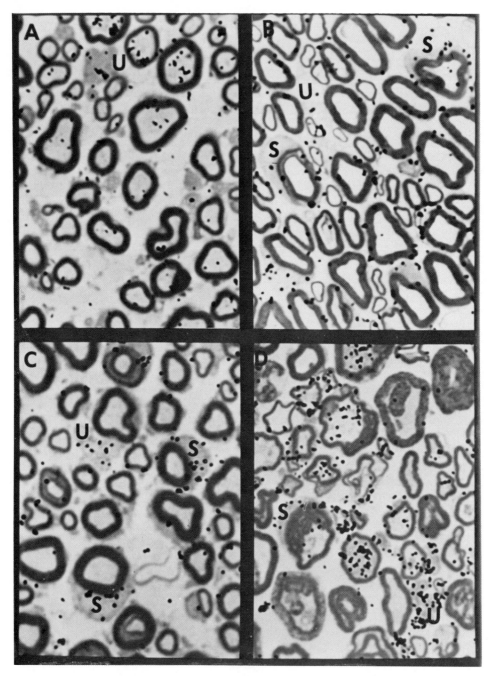

Legend: Light microscopic autoradiographs of transverse sections of mouse sciatic nerve labeled in vivo with (A) [2-^{3}H]myo-inositol, (B&D) [methyl^{3}H]choline and (C) [2-^{3}H]glycerol for 2 h. One of the nerves (D) was crushed 6 h before injection of the precursor. The fixation, embedment and preparation of the autoradiographs are as previously described (7). Symbols: U - unmyelinated fibers   S - Schwann cell cytoplasm axons incubated with tritiated choline synthesized phosphatidylcholine, some of which was found in extruded axoplasm.

TABLE I. Incubation with intact giant axons

Precursor (# of axons)	Extruded Axoplasm Lipid	L/A^{X}100	Sheath Lipid	L/A^{X}100	A/S^{X}100
Choline (3)	0.68	0.81	13.2	5.2	5.2
myo-Inositol (3)	0.68	0.65	2.8	9.3	24.3
Glycerol (3)	1.56	0.79	34.2	77.2	4.6
Phosphate (4)	7.73	0.11	51.6	10.7	15.0

Dissected giant axons were cleaned of attached small fibers and incubated (4-5 hrs at 19-20°C) in troughs containing 0.2 ml of artificial seawater (430 mM NaCl, 10 mM KCl, 10 mM CaCl$_2$, 50 mM MgCl$_2$, and 20 mM Tris-HCl, pH 7.6) and labeled precursor (200 μCi). Following the incubations the nerves were rinsed in seawater and the axoplasm was separated from the sheaths by extrusion. Lipid was extracted from axoplasm and homogenized sheaths in chloroform:methanol (2:1 v:v, for choline and glycerol) or chloroform:methanol:conc. HCl (2:1:0.075 v:v:v for myo-inositol and glycerol). Following extractions (15-30 min) the lipids were partitioned with 0.9% KCl or 1N HCl. Portions (0.3 ml) of the upper phase were used to determine aqueous radioactivity, while portions (0.3 ml) of a three time washed lower phase were used to determine lipid extractable radioactivity. Lipid values are presented as incorporated cpm (x10^{-3}) per hr of incubation. L/A (lipid/aqueous) ratios are calculated from cpm in the original samples. The A/S (axoplasm/sheath) ratios are computed from the lipid values.

We have expanded these studies to further elucidate axonal lipid synthesis in the squid giant axon. Specifically we examined a number of potential precursors to determine the extent of phospholipid metabolism in intact giant axons and in axoplasm separated from the axon by extrusion.

All of the precursors tested were incorporated into phospholipids by the giant axon (Table I). [^{32}P]phosphate and [2-^{3}H]glycerol were more effective precursors than tritiated choline and myo-inositol. Most of the radioactive lipids were recovered from the sheath which was comprised of Schwann cells, axolemma and cortical axoplasm. The sheath synthesized all the major phospholipids, choline and ethanolamine phosphoglycerides, phosphatidylserine, phosphatidylinositol, sphingomyelin and polyphosphoinositides from ^{32}P phosphate (Table III). Tritiated choline and myo-inositol were incorporated largely into phosphatidylcholine and phosphatidylinositol, respectively.

Table II. Incubations with extruded axoplasm

Precursor	# of incubations	Incorporation	Major lipid product(s)
Choline	2	750 + 140	PC
myo-Inositol	6	7200 + 3930	PI
Glycerol	2	680 + 80	TG,PI,PA
Serine	4	6060 + 3800	PS
ATP	5	4370 + 1370	PI-P
Phosphate	5	4680 + 4970	PI-P

Axoplasm was extruded from giant axons and suspended in artificial axoplasm (300 mM potassium methylsulfate, 150 mM taurine, 100 mM potassium glutamate, 12.9 mM magnesium chloride, 3 mM calcium chloride, 10 mM EGTA (ethylene bis (oxyethylene-nitrilo) tetraacetic acid), 20 mM imidazole, pH 7.3, modified from Rubinson and Baker (17)). Incubations were with 5-20 μCi of radioactive precursors [methyl-^{3}H] choline chloride, myo(2-^{3}H)inositol, (2-^{3}H)glycerol, L-[^{3}H-(G)]serine, [γ-^{32}P]-adenosine triphosphate, [^{32}P]inorganic phosphate) for 1-4 hrs at 19°-22°C in 50 μl of axoplasm. Lipid was extracted with chloroform:methanol (choline or glycerol) or acidified chloroform:methanol (other precursors) and water-soluble precursors removed by washing (see Table I). Values are expressed as cpm·μCi^{-1}·mg protein^{-1} + standard deviation. The major lipid products were determined following separation on TLC sheets (Silica gel 60, EM reagent, Curtin Matheson Scientific). Solvent systems were (1) chloroform:methanol:acetic acid:water 65:40:1:4 v:v:v:v,10); (2) chloroform:methanol:28% ammonium hydroxide:water 90:90:7:22 v:v:v:v,18) and (3) hexane:ether:acetic acid 70:30:1.5 v:v:v,16) for separation of phospholipids, polyphosphoinositides and neutral lipids, respectively. Abbreviations: PC, phosphatidylcholine; PI, phosphatidylinositol; PA, phosphatidic acid; TG, triglyceride; PS, phosphatidylserine and PI-P, phosphatidylinositol phosphate.

To determine if axoplasm synthesizes phospholipids, we incubated extruded axoplasm with different phospholipid precursors, and measured rates of incorporation into lipid product (Table II). All of the precursors tested were incorporated into lipid in a time dependent fashion. Extruded axoplasm showed a different preference for precursors than the intact giant axon. Radioactive myo-inositol, serine, ATP and phosphate were incorporated into lipid more rapidly than tritiated choline and glycerol. The main products formed by axoplasm were the acidic lipids: phosphatidylinositol from myo-inositol and glycerol, phosphatidylserine from serine, and phosphatidylinositol phosphate from ATP and phosphate.

The autoradiographic pattern of [^{32}P]lipid recovered from extruded axoplasm following incubations of the giant axon with [^{32}P]phosphate was similar to that of the sheath, and different from that of extruded axoplasm incubated separately with this precursor (Table III). Larrabee and Brinley (12) also found differences in the phospholipid labeling by extruded axoplasm incubated alone or as part of the intact axon. Because they used neutral chloroform:methanol extractions, they failed to detect labeled polyphosphoinositides. However, in both studies labeled phosphatidylethanolamine was a dominant lipid in axoplasm extruded after incubation, while extruded axoplasm formed little of this precursor from [^{32}P]phosphate.

Table III. Distribution of labeled lipids formed in axon and axoplasm

Precursor	Phospholipid (%)					
Phosphate	PPI	PC	PE	PI	PS	PA
E-AX	80-90	3-4	0-1	2-4	1-2	1-4
AX	10-20	20-26	24-32	2-4	8-16	3-8
SH	13-18	23-30	22-35	3-5	8-15	5-12
Glycerol						
E-AX	8-1	0-1	42-46	23-30	0-1	3-5
AX	1-2	3-4	45-66	6-8	7-8	10-11
SH	0-1	2-4	70-80	4-5	3-4	10-15

Portions of the radioactive lipid formed during incubations of giant axons (sheath (SH) and axoplasm (AX) were separated after the incubations) or extruded axoplasm (E-AX) were chromatographed on thin layer sheets (Table II) with total lipids prepared from squid brain as standards. After visualization of the lipids with iodine vapor, the sheets were cut up and radioactivity migrating with the individual phospholipids counted. The range of percentages of label in individual lipids (2-3 samples) is shown for experiments with [^{32}P]phosphate (upper) and [2-^{3}H]glycerol (lower) as precursors. Symbols: PPI, for polyphosphoinositides (mainly PI-P with extruded axoplasm incubations), PC for phosphatidylcholine, PE for phosphatidylethanolamine, PI for phosphatidylinositol, PS for phosphatidylserine, and PA for phosphatidic acid.

Using acid extractions, we found that phosphatidylinositol phosphate was the primary lipid formed by extruded axoplasm incubated with [^{32}P]-phosphate (Tables II,III). Far higher levels of labeled PC, PE and PS are found in axoplasm extruded after incubation of the giant axons with [^{32}P]phosphate (Table III). Levels of radioactivity associated with polyphosphoinositides are reduced.

Tritiated glycerol was a poor substrate for extruded axoplasm. Phosphatidylethanolamine and phosphatidylinositol were the main phospholipids formed. Some neutral lipid, mainly triglyceride, was also formed. Giant axons synthesized phosphatidylethanolamine and phosphatidic acid from glycerol. Some labeled lipid comigrated with phosphatidylcholine, phosphatidylinositol and phosphatidylserine. As with [^{32}P]phosphate, axoplasm extruded after incubation contained different proportions of the labeled lipid from that incubated alone with precursor. The distributions of label among the different phospholipids were similar for axoplasm and sheath separated after incubation. These studies suggest that most of the labeled phospholipids present in axoplasm following incubation of the giant axons with [^{32}P]phosphate are transferred to the axoplasm following synthesis in the sheath. Most likely the synthetic machinery is in the Schwann cells, although it is possible that some of the phospholipids are made in the axolemma or cortical axoplasm. This suggested glial-axon transfer of phospholipid may be coupled to the

glial-axon transfer of protein demonstrated in squid (13) and, furthermore, suggest a mechanism of transfer involving membrane vesicles (9).
The findings that the phospholipids synthesized by axoplasm do not re-
semble those present in axoplasm after incubation of the giant axon indicate that the sheath cells act as a barrier preventing the utilization
of the precursors by enzymes of lipid synthesis in the axon. In addition, the differences may be a reflection that many of the axoplasmic
reactions require an organization which is destroyed during the extrusion or suspension in medium.

Having characterized lipid synthesis in axoplasm, we decided to compare the synthesis with that present in cell bodies and terminals. Homogenates of stellate ganglia and synaptosomes prepared from squid brain
optic lobes (15) were incubated with the radioactive precursors, and
rates of lipid synthesis measured (Table IV).

TABLE IV. Comparison of homogenized ganglia and synaptosomes with
           axoplasm

Precursor	Ganglia(G/A)	Synaptosomes(S/A)	G/S
Choline	8.7	4.7	1.8
myo-Inositol	67.4	10.2	6.6
Glycerol	13.1	62.8	0.2
Serine	4.1	2.1	2.0
ATP	3.1	1.7	1.8
Phosphate	0.6	1.5	0.4

Stellate ganglia and optic lobe synaptosomes were homogenized in
artificial axoplasm (Table II) and incubated for 90 min at 19-22°C with
precursor (5-10 µCi). Radioactive lipid was extracted and washed to
remove precursor (Table I) and the rates of incorporation (cpm·µCi^{-1}·h
$^{-1}$·mg protein^{-1}) were calculated and averaged from two-three experiments.
Rates were divided by the rates calculated for axoplasm (Table II) and
expressed as ganglia/axoplasm (G/A) and synaptosome/axoplasm (S/A)
ratios. A ganglia/synaptosome (G/S) ratio was also calculated.

Like axoplasm, these preparations synthesized lipid from every precursor. The rates of incorporation were generally highest for the stellate ganglia homogenates when calculated on a protein basis. Synaptosomal homogenates synthesized lipid more actively than axoplasm, especially with tritiated glycerol, myo-inositol and choline precursors. Surprisingly, the rates of lipid synthesis from tritiated glycerol were
higher in synaptosomes than ganglia '(five-fold)' and axoplasm (sixty-
fold). This result may be a reflection of active acylation reactions
localized in nerve terminals (1). The major lipid products were phosphatidylinositol (26%), neutral lipid (21%), and phosphatidic acid (11%).
A significant proportion of the radioactivity (13%) remained at the
origin of the TLC plates, possibly reflecting an active synthesis of
polyphosphoinositides. These results demonstrate that acidic phospholipids are actively synthesized by all parts of the neuron, while glia
(sheath cells) actively synthesize abundant amphipathic choline and
ethanolamine phosphoglycerides.

Finally, we compared lipid biosynthesis in ganglion cell bodies and
synaptosomes with homogenates of these tissues. The integrity of the
preparations was found to profoundly influence the rates of lipid

synthesis (Table V). With every precursor, except myo-inositol, the intact ganglia synthesized phospholipid far better than the homogenized preparation. Tritiated choline and [^{32}P]phosphate incorporation rates were compromized the most. Similar trends were observed for intact vs homogenized synaptosomes, i.e. the intact synaptosomes more actively synthesized phospholipid than the homogenized preparations. The differences between intact and homogenized synaptosomes were less pronounced than those observed with the ganglia. Myo-inositol and glycerol were more effective lipid precursors with homogenized vs intact synaptosomes.

TABLE V. Comparison of lipid synthesis in intact and homogenized preparations

Precursor	Ganglia Intact/Homogenized	Synaptosome Intact/Homogenized
Choline	78.8	1.6
myo-Inositol	0.26	0.10
Glycerol	4.1	0.76
Serine	7.7	2.6
ATP	12.7	2.3
Phosphate	31.9	2.8

Precursors were incubated with intact synaptosomes or ganglia suspended in artificial seawater (composition in Table I) or with homogenates of synaptosomes or ganglia in artificial axoplasm (composition in Table II). The rates of incorporation (cpm·μCi^{-1}·h^{-1}·mg protein^{-1}) were calculated from 2 to 3 experiments and intact/homogenized ratios were calculated from these values.

The preferential incorporation of myo-inositol into lipid in homogenized systems suggests that this precursor is poorly transported across the intact plasma membranes of ganglion cells and synaptosomes. Homogenization apparently exposes the transferase to exogenous substrates which enhance the rate of phosphatidylinositol synthesis. With the other precursors, the facilitation observed with intact systems might result from the required integrity of the multi-step reactions involved in the incorporation of other precursors into the complex lipids.

Besides affecting the rates of synthesis, the intactness also altered distribution of label among the phospholipids. With [^{32}P]phosphate and [γ-^{32}P]ATP, the percentage of label associated with phosphatidylinositol phosphate decreased dramatically. The radioactivity in all the other phospholipids, including phosphatidylinositol diphosphate, increased in intact vs homogenized preparations.

In summary, these studies demonstrate similarities in axonal lipid synthesis between squid and mammalian nerves. Both preparations preferentially synthesize acidic phospholipids in the axons. In contrast, the supportive glial cells more actively synthesize choline and ethanolamine phosphoglycerides. In squid and mammals it is apparent that lipid synthesis, unlike that of proteins, occurs in all parts of the neuron, i.e., cell bodies, axons and terminals. Enzymes of acidic phospholipid biosynthesis are dominantly expressed throughout the neuronal cytoplasm.

One factor which was found to have profound influence on lipid synthesis was the integrity of the preparation. Axoplasm extruded after the incubation of intact giant axons with precursors, [^{32}P]phosphate and [2-³H]glycerol, contained different distributions of phospholipids from those formed during incubations of extruded axoplasm with precursor. One explanation for this difference is that in an intact giant axon, the axoplasm obtains its lipids from the sheath (glial-axon transfer mechanism) and does not synthesize lipids from precursors in the incubation medium. This explanation would also mean that the sheath can influence axonal lipid metabolism by controlling precursor availability. Another possible explanation for this difference is that extruded axoplasm incubated without its surrounding axolemma is less able to perform multi-step enzyme reactions. For example, [³²P]phosphate or [γ-³²P]ATP are readily used by homogenized preparations (synaptosomes and ganglia) for phosphorylation of phosphatidylinositol (formation of phosphatidylinositol phosphate). In intact preparations of ganglia and synaptosomes, the complex sequence of reactions leading to the incorporation of phosphate into the backbone of glycerolipids more readily occurs. Further experimentation is required to explain how the different labeling patterns arise when axoplasm is incubated alone or within the intact axon.

ACKNOWLEDGMENTS

This research was supported by grant NS-13980 from the National Institutes of Health. We are grateful to Drs. I. Tasaki and R.J. Lasek in whose laboratories this work was performed, to George Pappas and Rochelle Cohen for preparation of the synaptosomes and to Fred Connell, Gary Mattingly and Edna Troiano for their help in the preparation of this manuscript.

REFERENCES

1. Baker, R.R., Dowdall, M.J., and Whittaker, V.P. (1976): Biochem. J. 154:65-75.

2. Bleasdale, J.E. and Hawthorne, J.N. (1975): J. Neurochem. 24:373-379.

3. Broekhuyse, R.M. (1969): Clin. Chim. Acta 23:457-461.

4. Brunetti, M., Guiditta, A., and Porcellati, G. (1979): J. Neurochem. 32:319-324.

5. Gould, R.M. (1976): Brain Research 117:169-174.

6. Gould, R.M. (1980): Biol. Bull. 159:484.

7. Gould, R.M., and Dawson, R.M.C. (1976): J. Cell. Biol. 68:480-496.

8. Grafstein, B. and Forman, D.S. (1980): Physiol. Rev. 60:1167-1283.

9. Holtzman, E. and Mercurio, A.M. (1980): Int. Rev. Cytol. 67:1-67.

10. Hughes, B.P. and Frais, F.F. (1965): Biochem. J. 96, 6P.

11. Kumara-Siri, M.H., and Gould, R.M. (1980): Brain Res. 186:315-330.

12. Larrabee, M.G., and Brinley, Jr., F.J. (1968): J. Neurochem. 15:

533-545.

13. Lasek, R.J., Gainer, H., and Barker, J.L. (1977): J. Cell Biol. 74:
     501-523.

14. Miller, E.K. and Dawson, R.M.C. (1972): Biochem. J. 126:805-821.

15. Pant, H.C., Pollard, H.B., Pappas, G.D., and Gainer, H. (1979):
     Proc. Natl. Acad. Sci. USA 76:6071-6075.

16. Pullarkat, R.K., Maddow, J., and Reha, H. (1976): Lipids 11:802-
     807.

17. Rubinson, K.A., and Baker, P.F. (1979): Proc. R. Soc. Lond. B. 205:
     323-345.

18. Schacht, J. (1978): J. Lipid Res. 19:1063-1067.

Phospholipids in the Nervous System, Vol. 1: Metabolism, edited by L. Horrocks, et al. Raven Press, New York © 1982.

Renewal of Phospholipids in Nerve Endings: Role of Axonal Transport and Local Incorporation

B. Droz, *M. Brunetti, H. L. Koenig, L. Di Giamberardino, and *G. Porcellati

*Département de Biologie, CEN Saclay, 91191 Gif-sur-Yvette Cedex, France; *Istituto di Chimica Biologica, Università di Perugia, 06100 Perugia, Italy*

The nerve endings are characterized by a complex architecture of membranous elements which circumscribe different synaptic compartments. For instance, mitochondria form independent and mobile organelles which supply the synapse with energy. In contrast, the axonal smooth endoplasmic reticulum appears as a continuous network of tubules which dispatches membrane constituents to the axon terminals (19). The population of synaptic vesicles and the specialized areas of the presynaptic plasma membrane are involved in the storage and release of neurotransmitters whereas endocytotic vacuoles and membranous bodies draw back synaptic material to the cell body (Fig. 1). These membranous organelles are made of components which are continuously renewed. These membranous elements must be considered as dynamic structures in which proteins, glycoproteins and phospholipids are continuously lost and replaced. It is the aim of this report to draw attention to particular aspects of the turnover of phospholipids in nerve endings. Presynaptic phospholipids may originate from two main sources : axonal transport from the nerve cell body in which phospholipids are synthesized and local incorporation of phospholipid precursors in nerve endings .

AXONAL TRANSPORT OF PHOSPHOLIPIDS TO NERVE ENDINGS

Axonal transport of phospholipids has been shown to occur in the central nervous system and in peripheral nerves (1, 3, 5, 7, 9, 11, 12, 13, 16, 21)). In the present study, the ciliary ganglion system of the chicken was chosen for the following reasons. 1. Labeled precursors of phospholipids were injected into the cerebral aqueduct with a stereotaxic apparatus; the tracer was therefore rapidly incorporated into the cell bodies of the preganglionic neurons which are located in the vicinity of the cerebral aqueduct. 2. Labeled phospholipids, which were conveyed with fast axonal flow along the preganglionic axons, were found to accumulate in the giant caliciform nerve endings of the ciliary ganglion. 3. The homogeneous length of the cholinergic preganglionic axons and the exceptional size of the nerve terminals facilitated the biochemical characterization and the radioautographic localization of the labeled material.

Technical procedure

In a first series of experiments, chickens were intracerebrally injected with (2-^{3}H) glycerol, (methyl-^{3}H) choline, (1-^{3}H) ethanolamine or myo (2 -^{3}H) inositol, then sacrificed at various time intervals. The left ciliary ganglion was removed to measure the radioactivity in the water-soluble fraction and in the chloroform-methanol extract. The right ciliary ganglion was processed for histology and the distribution of the labeled lipids was determined by quantitative light and electron microscope radioautography (8).

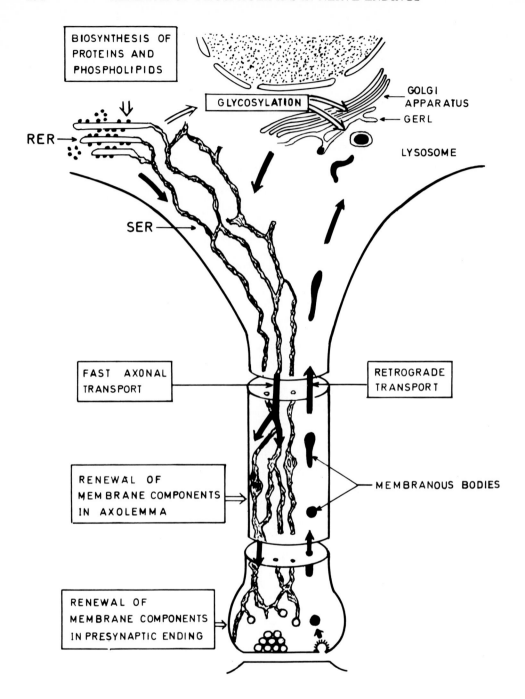

FIG.1. Pathways for fast and retrograde axonal transport of membrane components.

In the nerve cell body, proteins and phospholipids are synthesized in the rough endoplasmic reticulum (RER). Some of the proteins and phospholipids may enter directly the smooth endoplasmic reticulum (SER). Other proteins are directed towards the Golgi apparatus and/or GERL to complete their glycosylation. Later, they may be transferred to the smooth endoplasmic reticulum.

From the nerve cell body the rapidly transported membrane proteins, glycoproteins, and phospholipids are conveyed with the axonal smooth endoplasmic reticulum made up of longitudinal tubules and cisternae interconnected by oblique anastomoses. Just beneath the axolemma, the SER consists of a subaxolemmal meshwork in which membrane components destined to the axolemma may sojourn for some time. In the preterminal region of the axon, it expands into a preterminal network from which smaller tubules may originate to establish contact with the plasma membrane and give rise to vesicles, thereby providing anatomical pathways for the renewal of membrane components in presynaptic endings.

In contrast to the SER, the spherical or slightly elongated membranous bodies responsible for retrograde transport remain independent of each other and do not form a continuous structure. In the cell body, they may be found in the vicinity of the Golgi apparatus, intermingled with lysosomes (19).

TABLE 1. Time-dependent changes in labeling of the ciliary ganglia after an intracerebral injection of labeled precursors of phospholipid[a]

	Time interval after injection			
Injected precursor	45 min	18 h	40 h	7 d
	Water soluble fraction (dpm per ganglion x 10^{-3})			
$(2-{}^{3}H)$ glycerol	3.2	1.2	1.2	0.6
(methyl-${}^{3}H$) choline	14.3	11.4	7.8	3.7
$(1-{}^{3}H)$ ethanolamine	0.7	6.5	4.6	1.8
myo-$(2-{}^{3}H)$ inositol	6.1	15.0	10.4	7.4
	Lipid extract (dpm per ganglion x 10^{-3})			
$(2-{}^{3}H)$ glycerol	1.2	11.2	15.6	9.2
(methyl-${}^{3}H$) choline	2.6	34.8	41.0	36.7
$(1-{}^{3}H)$ ethanolamine	0.2	19.4	23.8	11.8
myo-$(2{}^{3}H)$ inositol	0.4	2.4	2.5	1.8
	Label concentration in nerve endings (number of silver grains per 100 μm^{2})			
$(2-{}^{3}H)$ glycerol	0.5	35.6	43.3	26.4
(methyl-${}^{3}H$) choline	0.5	42.9	55.8	27.7
$(1-{}^{3}H)$ ethanolamine	0.1	35.2	45.4	21.8
myo-$(2-{}^{3}H)$ inositol	0.5	2.3	3.7	2.0

[a]Each value is the mean of 3 animals.

In a second series, chickens were simultaneously given an intracerebral injection of both $(2-^3H)$ glycerol and $(methyl-^{14}C)$ choline. The ciliary ganglia were removed at three time intervals for analysis of the various classes of phospholipids and of water-soluble compounds by thin layer chromatography (4).

Analysis of the results

After the injection of each of the labeled precursors into the cerebral aqueduct, the lipid extract of the ciliary ganglia was practically devoid of label at 45 min. After a delay, the radioactivity of the lipid extract of the ciliary ganglia reached a maximum around 40 h and decreased by 7 days. With the labeled precursors, the light microscope radioautographs showed the progressive invasion of the preganglionic axons with radioactive lipids which dramatically piled up in the nerve endings (Figs. 2 and 3 and Table 1). Analysis of the label concentration in the axonal and presynaptic substructures pointed to the smooth endoplasmic reticulum as the first organelle associated with labeled phospholipids arriving in the axon terminals (7, 8). It thus may be assumed that fast axonally transported phospholipids are mainly conveyed to synapses along the tubular network of the smooth endoplasmic reticulum as it was shown for glycoproteins (15). After the rapid decline of the radioactivity associated with this organelle, the rise of label observed in the presynaptic plasma membrane and the synaptic vesicles suggests that labeled phospholipids are transferred from the smooth endoplasmic reticulum to presynaptic plasma membranes and synaptic vesicles (7). The late increase of radioactivity observed in synaptic mitochondria (Fig. 4) could result in part from the arrival of slowly moving mitochondria in which the tracer was incorporated when they were in the nerve cell body (3).

The composition of the labeled lipids recovered in the ciliary ganglion pointed to the choline phosphoglycerides as the most represented class of axonally transported phospholipids after injection of radioactive glycerol or choline (Table 2). In spite of the fact that the ethanolamine phosphoglycerides are especially abundant in the chicken ciliary ganglion, the small amount of ethanolamine phosphoglycerides labeled with $(2-^3H)$ glycerol is probably due to the loss of (^3H) label during the synthesis of ethanolamine plasmalogen through the dihydroxy-acetone pathway (17). The decrease of the (^3H) labeled glycerophospholipids between 40 h and 7 days and the delayed increase of labeled catabolic products such as (^{14}C) labeled glycerophosphorylcholine suggest a local breakdown of axonally transported phospholipids in the ciliary ganglion. Double labeling experiments with $(2-^3H)$ glycerol and $(methyl-^{14}C)$ choline showed a rapid loss of ^3H as compared to ^{14}C in labeled choline phosphoglycerides. The late rise of the isotopic ratio $^{14}C/^3H$ in choline phosphoglycerides results from the lack of recycling of the $(2-^3H)$ glycerol after lipid breakdown (2, 17) and from the extensive reincorporation of $(methyl-^{14}C)$ choline into new molecules of choline phosphoglycerides and sphingomyelin. The late increase of (^{14}C) radioactivity observed at 7 days in sphingomyelin (Table 2) corresponds mainly to a local reutilization of radioactive choline released from the preganglionic axons and reincorporated into phospholipids of the myelin sheath (4) and of postsynaptic ganglion cell bodies (14). Thus it is important to emphasize that the local breakdown of choline phosphoglycerides in these cholinergic nerve endings gives rise to free choline released from the axon terminals and reutilized by the postsynaptic ganglion cell for its own synthesis. Another possibility of choline reutilization is offered by the rapid base-exchange reaction (6, 18) which is discussed in the next section. It thus appears that the recycling of choline (20) plays a saving role in the economy of phospholipid and acetylcholine. Such a reutilization of the polar group was found to occur with $(1-^3H)$ ethanolamine-labeled phospholipids to a lesser degree. Fig. 2 which shows accumulations of label in nerve endings exhibits also scattered silver grains over the postsynaptic ganglion cell bodies. This fact results from a reincorporation of free ethanolamine released from presynaptically broken down phospholipids. As seen in Table 1, the release of labeled metabolites is supported by the moderate radioactivity found in the water-soluble fraction after injection of (methyl-^3H) choline or $(1-^3H)$ ethanolamine but very low radioactivity after injection of $(2-^3H)$ glycerol.

In the case of myo-$(2-^3H)$ inositol, axonal transport of labeled inositol-phosphoglycerides is more difficult to study because the relatively high radioactivity of the water-soluble fraction observed in the ciliary ganglia makes possible a local incorporation of the tracer (Table 1). It is probable that a part of the myo-$(2-^3H)$ inositol of the ciliary ganglion has diffused from the midbrain, a fact which was not observed with the other precursors (8). Thus Fig. 3 probably reflects both axonal transport of inositol phosphoglycerides and local incorporation of the tracer.

LOCAL INCORPORATION OF PHOSPHOLIPID PRECURSORS IN NERVE ENDING

As shown in the previous section, molecules forming the polar group of phospholipids may be locally recycled and reincorporated. To determine to what extent such a process takes place in nerve endings, ciliary ganglia of chickens were incubated <u>in vitro</u> with various labeled precursors of phospholipids.

Technical procedure

Ciliary ganglia were rapidly dissected and placed in an oxygenated medium at 38°C. One of the following precursors, $(2-^3H)$ glycerol, (methyl-^3H)choline, $(1-^3H)$ethanolamine or myo-$(2-^3H)$inositol was then added to reach a radioactivity concentration of 200 μ Ci/ml. After 15 or 60 min, the incubated ganglia were washed with a concentrated solution of cold precursor and processed for histology to detect radioactive lipids by light and electron microscope radioautography.

Analysis of the results

Each labeled precursor was found to be incorporated into the ganglion cell bodies and the Schwann cells. Yet the incorporation of the tracer into the presynaptic nerve endings showed clear differences according to the precursor used (9). With $(2-^3H)$ glycerol, only stray silver grains were observed over the axon terminal. The lack of a significant uptake of $(2-^3H)$glycerol by nerve endings indicates that no net biosynthesis of glycerophospholipids takes place in presynaptic elements. In contrast, myo-$(2-^3H)$inositol was found to be incorporated with a peculiar intensity into several nerve endings (Fig. 4a and b) whereas neighbouring axon terminals were not or poorly labeled. In the absence of a net synthesis of glycerophospholipids, the local incorporation of myo-$(2-^3H)$ inositol into certain nerve endings would correspond to the renewal of the inositol moiety of inositol phosphoglycerides, a process which seems to be enhanced in stimulated axon terminals (22). In the case of incubations with (methyl-^3H)choline or $(1-^3H)$ ethanolamine, the slight but definite incorporation of the tracer into the nerve endings could result from a substitution of labeled for unlabeled nitrogenous base of preexisting phospholipids. Looking for the subcellular location of the base-exchange reaction (18), analysis of electron microscope radioautographs suggests that this rapid process could take place preferentially in the area occupied by the presynaptic plasma membrane (7). However long incubation experiments do not preclude that a minimal part of the presynaptic labeling could derive from a

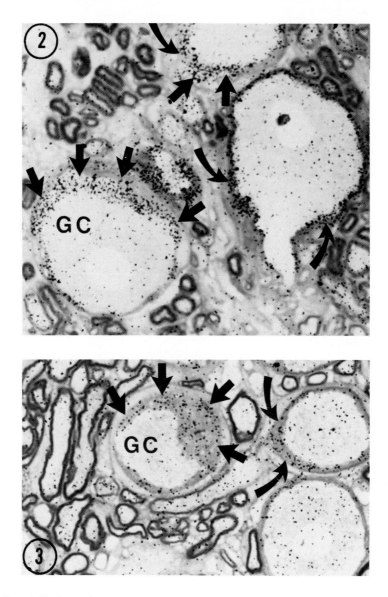

FIGS. 2 and 3. Axonal transport of labeled lipids to nerve endings of the ciliary ganglion after an intracerebral injection of (1-^{3}H) ethanolamine (Fig.2) or myo-(2-^{3}H) inositol (Fig.3).

By 40 h, light microscope radioautography points to the caliciform nerve endings (arrows) as the main site of label accumulation. Labeled preganglionic axons are intermingled with unlabeled postganglionic axons. Note that silver grains are scattered over the postsynaptic ganglion cell bodies (GC) which have reincorporated free tracers.

TABLE 2. Percentage distribution of lipid P and radioactivity in the ciliary ganglia at various times after an intracerebral injection of (2-^{3}H) glycerol and (methyl-^{14}C)choline

	Lipid P	12 h	40 h (^{3}H)	7 d
Ethanolamine phosphoglycerides	35.9	22	25	35
Choline phosphoglycerides	30.5	67	58	46
Serine phosphoglycerides	14.3	6	10	12
Inositol phosphoglycerides	11.4	5	7	8
Sphingomyelin	7.8			
			(^{14}C)	
Ethanolamine phosphoglycerides				
Choline phosphoglycerides		95	90	76
Serine phosphoglycerides				
Inositol phosphoglycerides				
Sphingomyelin		5	10	24

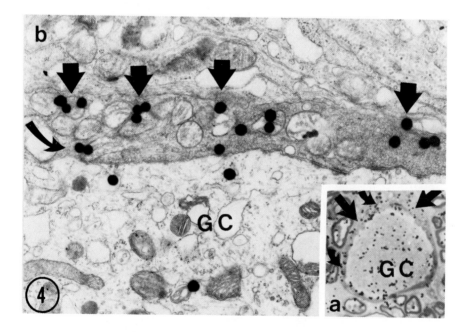

FIG. 4. Local incorporation of myo-(2-^{3}H)inositol into nerve endings.
After a 1-hour incubations with myo-(2-^{3}H)inositol, light (a) and electron (b) microscope radioautographs reveal a local incorporation of the tracer in axon terminals (arrows).

transcellular transfer of phospholipids synthesized in adjacent Schwann or ganglion cells. In any case, this process would be rather limited as compared with local incorporation of precursors or axonal transport of phospholipids.

DYNAMICS OF PRESYNAPTIC PHOSPHOLIPIDS

Like other membrane constituents, phospholipids are transported by fast axonal flow to nerve endings at rates of about 3$\overset{3}{}$0 mm per day. When axonally transported phospholipids were labeled with (2-^{3}H)glycerol, they were rapidly distributed from the smooth endoplasmic reticulum to synaptic vesicles and presynaptic plasma membranes in which they stayed for a mean time of sojourn of 7 and 9 days, respectively (9). In these presynaptic organelles, proteins or glycoproteins were found to stay for a mean time varying between 0.7 and 14 days. Thus it may be assumed that membranous presynaptic organelles are not renewed as a whole and that their components turn over independently.

Furthermore in presynaptic phospholipids, the rapid change of the polar group of glycerophospholipid, a process which bypasses de novo synthesis, could modify within a few minutes the local population and distribution of the classes of phospholipids. The substitution of one nitrogenous base for another base (18, 20) as well as the stimulated replacement of the inositol moiety in certain nerve endings and axons (10, 22) could indeed be used for a fast and local change of phospholipid class. However in spite of this flexible possibility, the renewal of the presynaptic phospholipids is mainly, if not exclusively, ensured by axonal transport. Fast axonal flow of membrane constituents along the tubular network of the axonal smooth endoplasmic reticulum as well as motion of mitochondria along the axon provide indeed the supply of phospholipids in nerve endings.

REFERENCES

1. Abe, T., Haga, T. and Kurokawa, M., (1973) : Rapid transport of phosphatidyl-choline occuring simultaneously with protein transport in the frog sciatic nerve, Biochem. J. 136 : 731-740.
2. Benjamins, J.A. and McKhann, G.M., (1973) : (2-^{3}H)Glycerol as a precursorof phospholipids in rat brain : evidence for lack of recycling. J.Neurochem., 20 : 1111-1120.
3. Blaker, W.D., Goodrum, J.F. and Morell, P. (1981) : Axonal transport of the mitochondria-specific lipid, diphosphatidylglycerol, in the rat visual system, J. Cell Biol. 89 : 579-584.
4. Brunetti, M., Di Giamberardino, L., Porcellati, G. and Droz, B. (1981) : Contribution of axonal transport to the renewal of myelin phospholipids in peripheral nerves. II. Biochemical study, Brain Res. 219 : 73-84.
5. Brunetti, M., Droz, B., Di Giamberardino, L. and Porcellati, G. (1978) : A study on the axonal flow of phospholipids in the ciliary ganglion of the chicken, Proc. Europ. Soc. Neurochem., 1 : 484.
6. Brunetti, M., Giuditta, A. and Porcellati, G. (1979) : The synthesis of choline phosphoglycerides in the giant fibre system of the squid, J. Neurochem., 32 : 319-324.
7. Droz, B., Brunetti, M., Di Giamberardino, L., Koenig, H.L., and Porcellati, G., (1981) : Axonal transport of phosphoglycerides to cholinergic synapses. In : Cholinergic mechanisms : Phylogenetic Aspects, Central and Peripheral Synapses, and Clinical Significance, edited by G. Pepeu, pp. 377-386, Plenum Press, New York.
8. Droz, B., Di Giamberardino, L. and Koenig, H.L. (1981) : Contribution of axonal transport to the renewal of myelin phospholipids in peripheral nerves. I. Quantitative radioautographic study, Brain Res. 219 : 57-72.

9. Droz, B., Koenig, H.L., Di Giamberardino, L., Couraud, J.Y., Chretien, M. and Souyri, F. (1979) : The importance of axonal transport and endoplasmic reticulum in the function of cholinergic synapse in normal and pathological conditions. In : The Cholinergic Synapse, edited by S. Tucek, Progr. Brain Res., vol 49, pp.23-44, Elsevier, Amsterdam.

10. Gould, R.M., Lasek, R.J. and Spencer, P.S. (1978): Phosphoinositide metabolism in peripheral axons. In Cyclitol and Phosphoinositides, pp. 535-547. Academic Press, New-York.

11. Gould, R.M., Sinatra, R.S., Spivack, W., Berti, M., Wisniewski, H.M.,Lindquist, R. and Ingoglia, N. (1979) : Axonal transport of phospholipids in rat sciatic nerve, Neurosci. Abstr., 5 : 60.

12. Grafstein, B., Miller, J.A., Ledeen, R.W., Haley, J. and Specht, S. (1975): Axonal transport of phospholipid in goldfish optic system. Exp. Neurol.46 : 261-281.

13. Haley, J.E., Tirri, L.J. and Ledeen, R.W. (1979) : Axonal transport of lipids in the rabbit optic system. J. Neurochem., 32 : 727-734.

14. Koenig, H.L. and Droz, B. (1980) : Pre and postsynaptic interactions in chick ciliary ganglion. In : Ontogenesis and Functional Mechanisms of Peripheral Synapses, edited by J. Taxi, pp. 41-52, Elsevier/North-Holland Biomedical Press, Amsterdam.

15. Markov, D., Rambourg, A. and Droz, B., (1976) : Smooth endoplasmic reticulum and fast axonal transport of glycoproteins : an electron microscope radioautographic study of thick sections after heavy metals impregnation, J. Microsc. Biol. Cell., 25 : 57-60.

16. Miani, N. (1963) : Analysis of the somato-axonal movement of phospholipids in the vagus and hypoglossal nerves, J. Neurochem., 10 : 859-874.

17. Miller, S. L., Benjamins, J.A. and Morell, P. (1977) : Metabolism of glycerophospholipids of myelin and microsomes in rat brain. Re-utilization of precursors, J. Biol. Chem., 252 : 4025-4037.

18. Porcellati, G., Arienti, G., Pirotta, M. and Giorgini, D., (1971) : Base-exchange reactions for the synthesis of phospholipids in nervous tissue. J. Neurochem., 18 (1971) 1395-1417.

19. Rambourg, A. and Droz, B. (1980) : Smooth endoplasmic reticulum and axonal transport, J. Neurochem., 35: 16-26.

20. Spanner, S. and Ansell, G.B. (1979) : Enzymes involved in the metabolism of lipid bases, Biochem. Soc. Trans. 7 : 338-341.

21. Toews, A.D., Goodrum, J.F. and Morell, P., (1979) : Axonal transport of phospholipids in rat visual system, J. Neurochem., 32 : 1165-1173.

22. Yandrasitz, J.R. and Segal, S. (1979) : The effect of $MnCl_2$ on the basal and acetylcholine-stimulated turnover of phosphatidyl-inositol in synaptosomes. FEBS Letters, 108 : 279-282.

Phospholipids in the Nervous System, Vol. 1: Metabolism, edited by L. Horrocks, et al. Raven Press, New York © 1982.

The Hydrolysis of Phosphatidylinositol in Nervous Tissue

R. M. C. Dawson, R. F. Irvine, and K. Hirasawa

Biochemistry Department, ARC Institute of Animal Physiology, Babraham, Cambridge CB2 4AT, United Kingdom

There is no doubt that in brain and peripheral nerve in vivo the simplest and most abundant of the phosphoinositides, phosphatidylinositol, is much more metabolically active in terms of its phosphorus turnover than are the bulk of the other phospholipids (4,40). Such activity may be above that to be expected from the normal dynamic turnover of all membranes because it has other physiological functions in addition to a need to maintain membrane vitality, e.g., synaptic transmission connected perhaps with receptor function and calcium gating (22,35), prostaglandin release (17,34,42) and its involvement in polyphosphoinositide metabolism with other possible physiological implications (13,1,21). In all these instances the catabolism of phosphatidylinositol plays an important and perhaps primary central role in the biochemical events associated with the physiological activity.

If calcium is available to support its enzymic activity, the phosphodiesterase liberating diglyceride and inositol monophosphate or its cyclic analogue is probably the predominant route of phosphatidylinositol degradation. Brain is one of the richest sources of this enzyme, its specific activity on a protein basis in the rat being much higher than liver or kidney. While there are suggestions that a fairly specific deacylation of phosphatidylinositol may occur in certain physiological conditions (27), the specificity of phosphatidylinositol phosphodiesterase, its ubiquitous distribution in animal cells, and its formidable activity, advance it as the most likely candidate for initiating stimulated phosphatidylinositol turnover. In one case, namely the enhanced turnover of phosphatidylinositol in the blowfly gland triggered by 5-hydroxytryptamine, the typical products of the phosphodiesterase, namely inositol monophosphate and its cyclic analogue, have been observed to accumulate (19).

It can be calculated that in cerebral cells the potential of the phosphodiesterase for degrading phosphatidylinositol is theoretically sufficient for hydrolysing the membrane complement of this phospholipid within seconds. The enzyme, which our measurements show is almost exclusively cytoplasmic (28), is presumably in contact with the membrane complement, yet until the reaction is initiated in some way the substrate remains substantially or totally immune. The question which becomes of paramount importance, therefore, is how the activity of the enzyme is controlled. Without a detailed knowledge of the molecular biology of the enzyme-substrate interaction and the factors involved in its initiation and suppression, it is difficult to see how the connection between the physiological events and the chain of biochemical reactions started can be fully understood.

The soluble phosphatidylinositol phosphodiesterase in brain tissue was first studied by Thompson (43), Friedel et al. (20) and Keough and Thompson (31). It was shown that, using an enzyme preparation purified by ammonium sulphate fractionation, it had an absolute requirement for Ca^{2+} and that the pH optimum was in the region of 5.4 - 5.9 with little activity above pH 7 (Fig.1). However, if a simple 0.32 M sucrose supernatant fraction from brain tissue is used we have shown that the phosphodiesterase can show considerable activity in the alkaline range up to pH 8.5. At low pH values inositol 1:2-cyclic phosphate is the main

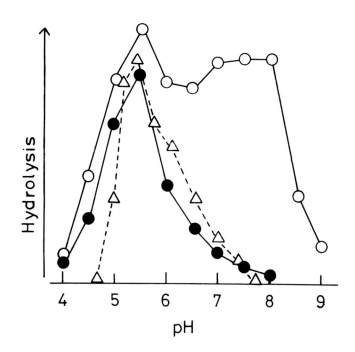

FIG.1   pH/activity profiles of the phosphatidylinositol phosphodiesterase in a rat brain supernatant fraction

  0   original supernatant.
  ●   enzyme purified by ammonium sulphate fractionation according to Thompson (43).
  △   published results of Thompson (43) using ammonium sulphate purified enzyme.
Hydrolysis of substrate denoted in arbitrary units.

product while at pH 7 inositol-1-phosphate becomes predominant. Similar changes in the balance of these metabolites have been observed for phosphatidylinositol phosphodiesterase in pancreas and thyroid gland (15,18) and could suggest that a cyclysing intramolecular phospho-transferase is the main activity until the free hydroxyl ions accumulating in the buffer at higher pH values favour true hydrolysis of the substrate. The alkaline pH optimum of inositol-1:2-cyclic phosphate-2-phosphodiesterase could also be a contributing factor (14).

At low Ca^{2+} concentrations (0.8 μM) there is very small liberation of lysophosphatidylinositol around pH 8, with the phosphodiesterase forming a single peak at pH 6. The deacylating enzyme involved is a phospho-lipase A_1 which unlike the phosphodiesterase does not require Ca^{2+} as an obligatory cofactor for hydrolysing phosphatidylinositol. Consequently, if a pH/activity profile is carried out in the presence of EDTA, then this becomes the sole phosphatidylinositol-degrading enzyme with a small secondary deacylation of the released lysophosphatidylinositol into glycerophosphoinositol. A similar result is obtained using a microsomal membrane fraction isolated from rat brain where, in the presence of Ca^{2+}, the typical phosphodiesterase pattern is seen with inositol cyclic phosphate predominating below pH 7 and inositol monophosphate above. We presume, of course, such activity is due mainly to entrapped cytoplasm (28). Diglyceride is the main neutral lipid formed throughout the pH range. Although some fatty acid is lost from the 2-acyl position, the preparation contains diglyceride lipase (8, 9) which we have shown is active under the present incubation conditions. We have not obtained any evidence for the brain phospholipase A_2 active against phosphatidyl-inositol described by Shum et al. (39).

The reasons for our obtaining considerable activity of the enzyme at higher pH values are not immediately obvious. However, it is clear from our very recent studies that the enzyme in crude supernatant fractions exists in a number of forms which can fairly readily be separated by isoelectric focussing and all of which have somewhat differing pH profiles. When ammonium sulphate fractionation is used to enrich the enzyme (43,20,31), it has been found that the activity at higher pH values virtually disappears and there is a single distinct optimum at about pH 5.5 - 6.0 (Fig.1). Thus, it would appear that either the activity apparent at higher pH values is lost or it is converted to a form with a lower pH optimum. It is relevant to mention at this point the detrimental effect of Tris buffers on the enzyme. Tris-HCl and Tris-maleate have often been used to assess activity at higher pH values. Yet they can be very inhibitory to the enzyme, especially at low Ca^{2+} concentrations. Thus, for example, at pH 8.3 the true activity can only be measured by using low Tris buffer concentrations and high Ca^{2+} (Fig.2). Presumably, the excess of Tris ion which is, to a limited degree, surface active, may compete with Ca^{2+} for essential sites on the substrate or enzyme molecules. The detrimental effect that Tris can have on other enzyme systems has been reported on many occasions (e.g., 41, 3).

We have been interested for some time in the observation that high activity preparations of cerebral Ca-activated phosphodiesterase, although active against pure phosphatidylinositol dispersed as a liposome, are almost totally inactive against the lipid incorporated in a membrane preparation, e.g., endoplasmic reticulum or plasma membrane (28,30). If steps are taken to disrupt the structure and organisation of the membrane, e.g., addition of deoxycholate or sonication, some break-down can be detected (32) and this could be the explanation for the ability of high concentrations of fatty acid to induce membrane

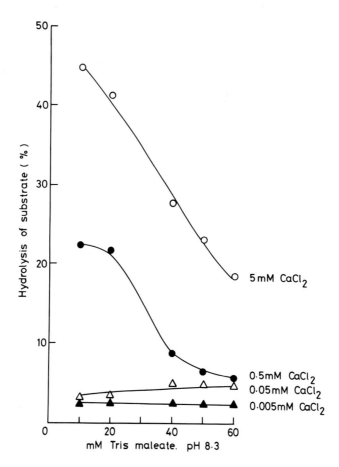

FIG.2 Hydrolysis of phosphatidylinositol by a rat brain cytoplasmic phosphodiesterase showing dependence on calcium and tris-maleate pH 8.3 buffer concentration

phosphatidylinositol hydrolysis (30). Some of the lipid in a membrane would appear to be reasonably accessible at the surface since it can be degraded by the lysosomal Ca-independent phosphatidylinositol phospho-diesterase (38) and at least part of it can readily exchange with phosphatidylinositol liposomes in the presence of an exchange protein (23, 7).

There are a number of factors which could contribute to the normal resistance of the membrane-bound phosphatidylinositol to the cytoplasmic enzyme. The intracellular conditions under which the enzyme would be operating have high K^+ and Mg^{2+} concentrations, and the cerebral enzyme is substantially inhibited at a physiological pH (6.8) by such ions. Positively-charged proteins which undoubtedly exist in membranes can also be extremely inhibitory to the 'test-tube' activity of the enzyme (29). In this connection it has been shown that the basic experimental allergic encephalitogenic protein isolated from brain membranes forms definite proteolipid complexes with phosphatidylinositol (37). The studies of

Brophy et al. (7) have clearly shown that a substantial portion of the phosphatidylinositol in microsomal membranes is not accessible to exchange protein, and the authors suggest it is firmly bound to membrane proteins.

In the course of our research we were also surprised to find that the phosphatidylinositol within liposomes prepared from the mixed lipids extracted from tissue membranes was not hydrolysed by preparations of the phosphodiesterase. Investigations soon proved this was caused by the phosphatidylcholine present in such preparations. In fact, phospholipids containing a phosphorylcholine hydrophilic head group (e.g., phosphatidylcholine, lysophosphatidylcholine, sphingomyelin) proved to be powerful inhibitors of phosphatidylinositol hydrolysis. In a liposome in which they were mixed in equimolecular proportions, 90% or greater inhibition occurred (29). We do not yet understand why a phosphorylcholine head group in juxtaposition to a phosphorylinositol head group should prove such an anathema to the enzyme. Certainly, an organised water-lipid interface is essential for the inhibition, since, whereas saturated lecithins with chain lengths down to C_8 were inhibitors of the reaction; dihexanoyl lecithin was, in marked contrast, an excellent activator. The latter short-acyl chain lecithin caused a substantial break-up of the bilayer structure of the mixed liposomes as far as could be judged from electron microscopic and centrifugal studies (16). When the phenomenon was studied using a surface monolayer film technique, we observed that quite small percentages of lecithin drastically reduced the limiting pressure at which the enzyme can catalyse the hydrolysis and presumably therefore penetrate into a ^{32}P-phosphatidylinositol monolayer (25). Whereas the enzyme could hydrolyse the pure phosphatidylinositol film as it was compressed up to a limiting surface pressure of 33 dynes/cm, if 20% molar lecithin was added this limiting pressure decreased to 26 dynes/cm, and at 40% molar to 20 dynes/cm. This means that as the lecithin content is increased the kinetic energy of individual molecules of enzyme is less able to overcome the potential energy barriers preventing access to the susceptible ester bond of the substrate. Even if the enzyme could penetrate at a given pressure, there was always a substantial reduction in the rate of the hydrolysis compared with that occurring in the absence of lecithin. We have shown that in vitro, the hydrolysis of phosphatidylinositol liposomes by the phosphodiesterase can be effectively inhibited by adding a sonicated suspension of lecithin rather than by forming mixed liposomes, and a similar effect is seen by adding serum, plasma or the lecithin-rich blood lipoproteins (16). Presumably, the lecithin in all these can rapidly exchange and enter into the phosphatidylinositol liposomes, possibly assisted by any exchange protein present in the enzyme preparation. The phenomenon of phosphatidylcholine inhibition of the phosphodiesterase appears not to be specific to brain, since we have also observed it with the soluble phosphatidylinositol phosphodiesterase enzyme from human blood platelets.

In contrast to the inhibitory action of choline-containing phospholipids, virtually all other membrane phospholipids were, to a greater or lesser degree, activators of the phosphodiesterase (29). Although in our test system phosphatidylserine and phosphatidylethanolamine produced a 2.5 - 3.5 fold activation at 50% molar concentration, both phosphatidic acid and phosphatidylglycerol produced a similar stimulation in much lower proportions (10 - 15%). It was evident from monolayer experiments that phosphatidic acid and phosphatidylglycerol were acting in a reverse way to phosphatidylcholine - they were dramatically increasing the maximum film pressure of $[^{32}P]$phosphatidylinositol films at which penetration of the enzyme could take place (25).

In contrast, phosphatidylethanolamine did not increase this threshold pressure for enzyme penetration, but, nevertheless, at any given pressure below the threshold it dramatically increased the rate of hydrolysis of the monolayer. The same sort of phenomenon was observed with oleic acid, which we had shown earlier was also an activator of phosphodiesterase action (30). Again, the rate of hydrolysis was dramatically increased at any pressure below the threshold pressure, but the value of this cut-off pressure was not changed. In contrast to oleic acid, however, octadec-9-en-1-ol showed a marked ability to increase the threshold pressure. Clearly, therefore, increasing the threshold pressure of hydrolysis is not always a question of introducing a negatively charged head group into the surface; the octadec-9-en-1-ol is presumably intro-ducing discontinuities in the film's molecular packing, or changing its fluidity to allow penetration of the enzyme's active centre even at high film pressures. The complexities of the steric factors involved must be rather precise since neither octadecan-1-ol nor stearic acid are significant activators. Thus, it seems that the perturbation in the orderly packing of the film induced by the unsaturated kink in the hydrocarbon chain is more important than the nature of the hydrophilic head group. In general, the activators seem to represent wedge-shaped molecules, with larger effective hydrophobic regions, i.e., the sort of molecules, which if in sufficient concentration could cause a bilayer structure to convert to micelles or transform to a hexagonal phase (11). However, the physiochemical explanation of these phenomena must be very complex since two activators operating at their maximum effect can show synergy, particularly in overcoming the inhibitory action of phosphatidyl-choline (29).

If one considers a membrane, ignoring for the time-being the possible effects of protein-phosphatidylinositol interactions, it is obvious from the preceding paragraphs that the phosphatidylinositol in the membrane will be in a balanced sensitive state as regards susceptibility to phosphodiesterase action. In most membranes of the cell there will be a preponderance of choline-containing phospholipids, and assuming relatively symmetric distribution of phosphatidylinositol in the lipid bilayer it will remain immune to the enzyme. However, if one considers the inner lamella of the plasma membrane bilayer, the only analysis which we have available (for liver sinusoidal plasma membrane (24)) suggests a far higher concentration of activating phospholipids (phosphatidyl-ethanolamine 24.0%; phosphatidylserine 23.1%) than inhibitory phospho-lipids (phosphatidylcholine 13.0%; sphingomyelin 16.0%). Indeed, we found that if we made liposomes of such a composition containing $[^{32}P]$phosphatidylinositol at the concentration at which it occurs in the plasma membrane, then the introduction of one or two molar per cent phosphatidic acid caused a substantial enhancement of phosphodiesterase activity (16). Extrapolating this to the membrane in vivo it is quite possible that a local metabolic production of phosphatidic acid could cause a stimulation of phosphatidylinositol phosphodiesterase. Since the diglyceride formed from the hydrolysis of phosphatidylinositol is often rapidly rephosphorylated to phosphatidic acid by the enzyme diglyceride kinase (33,26) then the system would have the potentiality for self-amplification. Furthermore, liberation of fatty acid by diglyceride lipase (29) could cause a synergistic combination with phosphatidate (29) thus amplifying the hydrolysis still further.

It is possible that these studies on the suppression and activation of phosphatidylinositol phosphodiesterase could therefore provide a basis for understanding the sudden turn-on of phosphatidylinositol breakdown when a responsive cell is stimulated by an agonist and the equally rapid turn-off when the latter is removed. There is now good evidence that the receptors in a plasma membrane are intimately connected with the phospholipids in the membrane; indeed, some evidence would suggest that phosphatidylinositol is directly associated with agonist receptor interaction (10,2). The receptor proteins presumably span the lipid bilayer, and when the agonist interacts with the exposed extracellular side of the protein it is likely there would be a complimentary change on the intracellular side. This could be a conformation change altering the hydrophobicity of the exposed surface, or the distribution and balance of its charged groups. Such changes could in turn cause a phase separation in the inner lamella of the bilayer lipids adjacent to the receptor protein, so that the phosphatidylinositol molecules cluster around the receptor protein and become separated from the inhibitory molecules in the bulk-domain. In model systems these clustering responses of acidic phospholipids are well known and can be induced by hydrophobic or highly-charged proteins (5,6). Once the cluster is attacked by the cytoplasmic phosphodiesterase, the self-amplification mechanisms discussed above would come into operation, leading to a rapid breakdown of phosphatidylinositol. This would continue until either all available substrate was exhausted or until the agonist was removed, the transmembrane receptor protein reverted to its resting conformation, and the inhibitory phospholipids flooded back to damp down phosphatidylinositol hydrolysis.

The process envisaged may seem speculative, but before much further progress can be made we need to understand the molecular biology of how agonist-receptor interaction can often by followed within seconds by a turn on of phosphatidylinositol hydrolysis and how, and if, this causes changes in the properties of the plasma membrane adjacent to the receptor. There is no evidence that calcium entering into the cell causes the increased phosphatidylinositol breakdown, and already phase changes in the lipids adjacent to receptors have been noted after stimulation by agonists (36,12) although at this stage it is not possible to deduce whether it is the cause or effect of the lipid hydrolysis which undoubtedly occurs.

REFERENCES

1. Abdel-Latif, A.A., Akhtar, R.A. and Hawthorne, J.N. (1977): Biochem. J., 162:61-73.

2. Aloj, S.M., Lee, G., Grollman, E.F., Beguinot, F., Consiglio, E. and Kohn, L.D. (1979): J. biol. Chem., 254:9040-9049.

3. Alonso, G.L., Arrigó, D.M. and de Fermani, S.T. (1979): Arch. Biochem. Biophys., 198:131-136.

4. Ansell, G.B. and Dohmen, H. (1957): J. Neurochem., 2:1-10.

5. Boggs, J.M., Moscarello, M. and Papahadjopoulos, D. (1977): Biochemistry, 16:5420-5426.

6. Boggs, J.M., Wood, D.D., Moscarello, M.A. and Papahadjopoulos, D. (1977): Biochemistry, 16:2325-2329.

7. Brophy, P.J., Burbach, P., Nelemans, S.A., Westerman, J., Wirtz, K.W.A. and van Deenen, L.L.M. (1978): Biochem. J., 174:413-420.

8. Cabot, M.C. and Gatt, S. (1976): Biochim. biophys. Acta., 431: 105-115.

9. Cabot, M.C. and Gatt, S. (1977): Biochemistry, 16:2330-2334.

10. Chang, H.W. and Bock, E. (1979): Biochemistry, 18:172-179.

11. Cullis, P.R. and DeKruijff, B. (1979): Biochim. biophys. Acta., 559: 399-420.

12. Curtain, C.C., Looney, F.D. and Smelstorius, J.A. (1980): Biochim. biophys. Acta., 596:43-56.

13. Dawson, R.M.C. (1969): Ann. N.Y. Acad. Sci., 165:774-783.

14. Dawson, R.M.C. and Clarke, N. (1972): Biochem. J., 127:113-118.

15. Dawson, R.M.C., Freinkel, N., Jungalwala, F.B. and Clarke, N. (1971): Biochem. J., 122:605-607.

16. Dawson, R.M.C., Hemington, N. and Irvine, R.F. (1980): Eur. J. Biochem., 112:33-38.

17. Dawson, R.M.C. and Irvine, R.F. (1978): Adv. Prostaglandin Thromboxane Res., 3:47-54.

18. Dawson, R.M.C., Irvine, R.F., Hirasawa, K. and Hemington, N. (1982): Biochim. biophys. Acta. (submitted for publication)

19. Fain, J.N. and Berridge, M.J. (1979): Biochem. J., 178:45-58.

20. Friedel, R.O., Brown, J.D. and Durrell, J. (1967): Biochim. biophys. Acta., 144:684-686.

21. Griffin, H.D. and Hawthorne, J.N. (1978): Biochem. J., 176:541-552.

22. Hawthorne, J.N. (1973): In: Form and Function of Phospholipids, edited by G.B. Ansell, J.N. Hawthorne and R.M.C. Dawson, pp 423-440. Elsevier, Amsterdam.

23. Helmkamp, G.M., Harvey, M.S., Wirtz, K.W.A. and van Deenen, L.L.M. (1974): J. biol. Chem., 249:6382-6389.

24. Higgins, J.A. and Evans, W.H. (1978): Biochem. J., 174:563-567.

25. Hirasawa, K., Irvine, R.F. and Dawson, R.M.C. (1981): Biochem. J., 193:607-614.

26. Hokin-Neaverson, M. (1977): Adv. Exp. Med. Biol., 83:429-446.

27. Hong, S.L. and Deykin, D. (1981): J. biol. Chem., 256:5215-5219.

28. Irvine, R.F. and Dawson, R.M.C. (1978): J. Neurochem., 31:1427-1434.

29. Irvine, R.F., Hemington, N. and Dawson, R.M.C. (1979): Eur. J. Biochem., 99:525-530.

30. Irvine, R.F., Letcher, A.J. and Dawson, R.M.C. (1979): Biochem. J., 178:497-500.

31. Keough, K.M.W. and Thompson, W. (1972): Biochim. biophys. Acta., 270:324-336.

32. Lapetina, E.G. and Michell, R.H. (1973): Biochem. J., 131:433-442.

33. Lloyd, J.V., Nishizawa, E.E., Joist, J.H. and Mustard, J.F. (1973): Brit. J. Haemat., 24:589-604.

34. Marion, J., Pappius, H.M. and Wolfe, L.S. (1979): Biochim. biophys. Acta., 573:229-237.

35. Michell, R.H. (1975): Biochim. biophys. Acta., 415:81-147.

36. Nathan, I., Fleischer, G., Livne, A., Dvilansky, A. and Parola, A.H. (1979): J. biol. Chem., 254:9822-9828.

37. Palmer, F.B. and Dawson, R.M.C. (1969): Biochem. J., 111:637-646.

38. Richards, D.E., Irvine, R.F. and Dawson, R.M.C. (1979): Biochem. J., 182:599-606.

39. Shum, T.Y.P., Gray, N.C.C. and Strickland, K.P. (1979): Can. J. Biochem., 57:1359-1367.

40. Sheltawy, A. and Dawson, R.M.C. (1969): Biochem. J., 111:157-165.

41. Slein, M.W. (1955): J. Am. chem. Soc., 77:1663-1667.

42. Sun, G.Y., Su, K.L., Der, O.M. and Tang, W. (1979): Lipids, 14: 229-235.

43. Thompson, W. (1967): Can. J. Biochem., 45:853-861.

*Phospholipids in the Nervous System, Vol. 1:
Metabolism*, edited by L. Horrocks, et al. Raven
Press, New York © 1982.

Cations and the Acetycholine-Stimulated ^{32}P-Labelling of Phosphoinositides in the Rabbit Iris

Ata A. Abdel-Latif and Rashid A. Akhtar

Department of Cell and Molecular Biology, Medical College of Georgia, Augusta, Georgia 30912

Until recently most of the reports which have appeared on the phosphoinositide effect (refers to both PI and poly PI effects) have dealt with studies of its characteristics in a variety of tissues and some speculations on its molecular mechanism(s) and physiological significance. The latter studies were hampered by two major problems: (a) lack of experimental evidence showing the biochemical site of this phenomenon in the stimulated cell. (b) lack of information on how phosphoinositide turnover is actually coupled to receptor activation.

It is well established now that the phosphoinositide effect is mediated through muscarinic-cholinergic and α-adrenergic receptors, and that activation of these receptors leads to an increase in cell-surface cationic permeability. In this communication we summarize our recent studies on the possible interrelationship between the ionic permeability changes, in particular Ca^{2+} and Na^+, subsequent to neurotransmitter-receptor interaction, and the enhanced phosphoinositide turnover in the rabbit iris smooth muscle.

CALCIUM ION AND THE PHOSPHOINOSITIDE EFFECT

Calcium ion is known to play a key role as a regulatory ion controlling a wide variety of membrane and intracellular functions, and thus it has been a particular interest of many investigators. In the early 1970's it was shown that in most systems which have been tested enhanced PI turnover was found to be somewhat insensitive to omission of Ca^{2+} from the incubation medium (for review see ref. 30). Thus it was reported that Ca^{2+} is not required for PI and/or PA turnover in response to various stimuli in adrenal medulla (36), parotid gland (32,25,36), guinea-pig ileum (23), and synaptosomes (33,37). In contrast Ca^{2+} was reported to be required for "maximal" PI and/or PA turnover in response to ACh in the pancreas (21), thyroid-stimulating hormone in the thyroid (39), ACh and norepinephrine in the iris muscle (1). There is also evidence which has been interpreted as indicating that in muscle severe and prolonged depletion of Ca^{2+} can depress the 'resting' rate of PI turnover (29).

[1]Abbreviations used: PI, phosphatidylinositol; Poly PI, phosphatidyl-inositol-4-P (diphosphoinositide, DPI) plus phosphatidyl-inositol-4,5-bisphosphate (triphosphoinositide, TPI); PA, phosphatidic acid; PC, phosphatidylcholine; ACh, acetylcholine; S.A., specific radioactivity.

In 1978, we reported that in rabbit iris smooth muscle which was prelabelled with ^{32}Pi and its Ca^{2+} content depleted with EGTA, the ACh-stimulated breakdown of polyphosphoinositides and [^{32}P] labelling of PA and to a much lesser extent PI is dependent on the presence of extracellular Ca^{2+} (8). Thus as can be seen from Table 1, addition of EGTA to the incubation medium abolished the ACh-stimulated breakdown of TPI and PA labelling in [^{32}P]labelled iris muscle. The effect on PI was less pronounced. Abolition of the phosphoinositide effect by EGTA was reversed when excess Ca^{2+} was added to the incubation medium. This suggests to us that in order to show dependence of the phosphoinositide effect on Ca^{2+}, extracellular Ca^{2+} must be effectively chelated. Later it was found that in iris muscle which was prelabelled with ^{3}H-<u>myo</u>-inositol, ACh stimulated the release of water-soluble inositol mono-phosphate and inositol triphosphate from tissue phosphoinositides, and again this was found to be dependent on the presence of extracellular Ca^{2+} (10). Thus as shown in Table 2, ACh alone increased the labelling of PI but had little effect on the labelling of TPI and the water-soluble inositol phosphates. In contrast, Ca^{2+} alone had no effect on the labelling of PI but increased the breakdown of TPI by 8% and increased the labelling of inositol triphosphate and inositol monophos-phate by 40 and 57% respectively. When both ACh and Ca^{2+} were added there was a 32% increase in PI labelling and 30% increase in the break-down of TPI and a concomitant increase of 96 and 153% in those of inositol triphosphate and inositol monophosphate respectively. The radioactivities of DPI and inositol diphosphate were unchanged under all experimental conditions. The marked increase observed in the production of inositol monophosphate could result from Ca^{2+} activation of PI-phosphodiesterase and/or enzymic degradation of inositol triphos-phate to inositol monophosphate.

In light of these findings it was suggested that the interaction of the neurotransmitter with its receptor results in an activated complex, which in turn could lead to the enhanced phosphoinositide breakdown via a Ca^{2+}-mediated step and consequently to muscle response (8,10,18). In this tissue ACh and norepinephrine act to increase intracellular concentration of calcium ion (9), and both PI and poly PI phosphodiesterases are stimulated by this cation (3,7). Furthermore, kinetic studies on dose-phosphoinositide and dose-contraction responses revealed a close relationship between the biochemical and pharmaco-logical responses (18). The dependency of the phosphoinositide effect on the presence of extracellular Ca^{2+} has also been demonstrated in synaptosomes in response to ACh (16,17,31), in dispersed pancreatic fragments when stimulated by ionophore A23187 and carbachol (15), in rat pancreatic islets when stimulated by glucose (13) and in rabbit neutrophils when stimulated by the synthetic peptide f-MetLeuPhe (14).

From the above studies it can be concluded that while in some tissues the phosphoinositide effect appears to be Ca^{2+} independent, there is accumulating evidence in more recent years to suggest that in certain tissues this cation could play a key role in this phenomenon.

TABLE 1

Requirement for Ca^{2+} in ACh-Stimulated Breakdown of TPI and
Labelling of PA in Rabbit Iris Muscle Labelled with ^{32}Pi in vitro*

| Additions | | | ^{32}P-Radioactivity in individual phospholipids (% of control) | | | |
Ca^{2+} (1.25 mM)	ACh (0.05 mM)	EGTA (0.25 mM)	PA	PI	DPI	TPI
-	-	+	89 ± 10 (NS)	101 ± 7 (NS)	98 ± 6 (NS)	102 ± 6 (NS)
-	+	-	156 ± 6 (p 0.01)	117 ± 4 (p 0.05)	106 ± 10 (NS)	84 ± 7 (p 0.05)
-	+	+	107 ± 8 (NS)	111 ± 4 (p 0.05)	104 ± 5 (NS)	98 ± 4 (p 0.02)
+	+	-	198 ± 9 (p 0.01)	117 ± 8 (p 0.05)	102 ± 7 (NS)	71 ± 8 (p 0.02)
+	+	+	211 ± 8 (p 0.01)	112 ± 3 (p 0.05)	108 ± 9 (NS)	70 ± 9 (p 0.02)

Irises, in pairs, were incubated for 30 min in a Ca^{2+}-free medium which contained 30 µCi ^{32}Pi/ ml. At the end of incubation the irises were washed in non-radioactive Ca^{2+}-free medium that contained 10 mM 2-deoxyglucose and 0.25 mM EGTA. The irises were then incubated singly for 10 min in the presence or absence of Ca^{2+}, ACh and/or EGTA as shown in the table. Phospholipids were extracted and separated by means of two-dimensional TLC.

*Taken from Ref. 8 with permission

TABLE 2

Effects of Ca^{2+} and ACh on the Radioactivity of Phosphoinositides
and Inositol Phosphates in Rabbit Iris Muscle Labelled with [³H] Myo-Inositol in vitro*

Additions		^{3}H-Radioactivity in Phospholipids and inositol phosphates (dpm)					
Ca^{2+} (0.75 mM)	ACh (0.05 mM)	PI	DPI	TPI	Inositol monophosphate	Inositol diphosphate	Inositol triphosphate
–	–	26382 ± 1760	4114 ± 232	11560 ± 263	987 ± 113	136 ± 15	198 ± 7
–	+	33722 ± 1790 (p<0.05)	4454 ± 216 (NS)	11055 ± 619 (NS)	1079 ± 190 (NS)	123 ± 12 (NS)	213 ± 21 (NS)
+	–	27411 ± 1976 (NS)	3970 ± 321 (NS)	10586 ± 256 (p<0.05)	1546 ± 66 (p<0.01)	131 ± 18 (NS)	277 ± 18 (p<0.01)
+	+	34951 ± 922 (p<0.02)	4130 ± 230 (NS)	8144 ± 263 (p<0.01)	2498 ± 115 (p<0.01)	124 ± 23 (NS)	389 ± 21 (p<0.01)

In general incubation conditions were the same as described in Table 1, except that the labelling medium contained 10 μCi of [³H]myo-inositol and the prelabelling period was 60 min. At the end of incubation the irises were homogenized in 10% (w/v) TCA and the homogenate centrifuged. The resulting pellet and supernatant were then analyzed for phospholipids and water-soluble inositol phosphates respectively. The inositol phosphate were separated by means of low-voltage paper electrophoresis in pyridine-acetic acid buffer (pH 3.2) at 40 V/cm for 8 h.

*Taken from Ref. 10 with permission.

SODIUM ION AND THE PHOSPHOINOSITIDE EFFECT

Activation of muscarinic cholinergic and α-adrenergic receptors also leads to increases in cell-surface permeability to Na^+ and K^+ in addition to Ca^{2+}. Brossard and Quastel (11), working with rat brain slices, reported that ACh stimulation of ^{32}Pi incorporation into total phospholipids is dependent on the presence of Na^+. More recently Keryer et al. (27) reported that in rat parotid glands cholinergic stimulation of ^3H-myo-inositol into PI is dependent on extracellular Na^+. In the iris muscle (2,4, Tables 3 and 4), studies on the effects of monovalent cations on the phosphoinositide effect revealed the following: 1. The neurotransmitter-stimulated $[^{32}]P$ labelling of PA, PI and PC is dependent on the presence of extracellular Na^+ (Table 3). This is also true in rat brain synaptosomes (10a). 2. The monovalent cation requirement for Na^+ is specific. Of the monovalent cations Li^+, NH_4^+, K^+, choline$^+$ and Tris, only Li^+ partially substituted for Na^+ (Table 4). 3. A significant decrease in $[^{32}P]$ labelling of phospholipids in response to ACh was observed when Ca^{2+} and/or K^+ were added to an isoosmotic medium deficient of Na^+. 4. Ouabain, which blocks the Na^+-pump, inhibited the basal ^{32}Pi incorporation into PC and the ACh-stimulated $[^{32}P]$ labelling of PA, PI and PC. Incubation of synaptosomes (19) or fragments of guinea pig ileum smooth muscle (24) in medium containing of an elevated extracellular K^+ concentration, which causes an increase in cell-surface permeability to Ca^{2+}, caused a marked increase in ^{32}Pi incorporation into PI. The administration of LiCl (3.6 mg/Kg/day) to adult male rats for 9 days resulted in an increase in the cerebral cortex level of myo-inositol-1-P to 4.43 ± 0.52 µmol/ kg (dry wt) compared to a control level of 0.24 ± 0.02 µmol/ Kg (34). About 90% of the increase is due to the D-enantiomer, evidence that Li is largely producing this effect via phospholipase C mediated phosphoinositide metabolism.

In view of the profound effects of Na^+ in the iris, it was of interest to show whether the effects of this cation and ACh on phospholipid $[^{32}P]$ labelling are secondary to changes in the S.A. of $[^{32}P]ATP$. In general the ATP contents of the iris muscle was about 7.18 nmoles/ iris (the wet wt. of one iris muscle is about 35 mg). In the complete incubation medium, ACh lowered the ATP content of the iris muscle by 15%, and had no effect on the S.A. of $[^{32}P]ATP$ (Table 3). In contrast, ACh increased the $[^{32}P]$ labelling of PA and PI by 121% and 109%, respectively, and decreased that of poly-PI by 22%. Omission of Na^+ from the incubation medium reduced considerably the S.A. of ATP and the $[^{32}P]$ labelling of phospholipids in the iris (Table 3). Furthermore, the ACh-stimulated $[^{32}P]$ labelling of phospholipids was almost abolished. Thus in the absence of Na^+ the content and S.A. of ATP in the unstimulated iris were reduced by 43% and 80%, respectively, and the $[^{32}P]$ labelling of PA, PI, poly-PI and PC were reduced by 74%, 68%, 75% and 85%, respectively. Dose-response studies revealed that as low as 2 mM Na^+ can significantly increase the S.A. of ATP and the ^{32}P labelling of phospholipids, and that these effects increased with Na^+ concentration (data not shown).

TABLE 3

Effect of Omission of Na^+ on the Acetycholine-Stimulated ^{32}P-labelling of Phospholipids and on the Specific Radioactivity of [^{32}P]ATP of Rabbit Iris Muscle

Medium	Additions	$[^{32}P]$Radioactivity incorporated into phospholipids (dpm x 10^3/iris)				Content and specific radioactivity of ATP	
		PA	PI	Poly PI	PC	Content (nmol/iris)	S.A. (dpm/pmol ATP)
Complete	None	24.6 ± 4.6	52.7 ± 6.2	128.1 ± 10.0	55.8 ± 4.8	7.76 ± 0.23	124 ± 4.8
Complete	ACh (50 µM)	54.5 ± 4.0*	110.0 ± 8.0*	100.0 ± 6.3	63.5 ± 2.8*	6.58 ± 0.28*	121 ± 4.6
Na^+-Free	None	6.3 ± 0.5	16.6 ± 3.1	18.6 ± 1.1	8.6 ± 0.9	4.40 ± 0.61	25 ± 1.5
Na^+-Free†	ACh (50 µM)	7.8 ± 0.3*	22.5 ± 2.0	17.8 ± 0.5	6.7 ± 0.4	5.07 ± 0.64	28 ± 0.8

Irises (one of a pair) were preincubated in a medium containing 50 µCi ^{32}P Pi/ml for 30 min, then acetyl-choline (50 µM) + eserine (50 µM) were added and incubation continued for an additional 30 min. At the end of incubation the tissues were processed and analyzed for phospholipids and ATP. The results are mean ± SEM of three separate experiments conducted in triplicate. P values were calculated by Student's t test for paired data.

*Significantly different (P<0.02) from corresponding control in the absence of acetylcholine.
†Isoosmolar substitution of NaCl by sucrose.

TABLE 4

Effects of Monovalent Cations on ^{32}P-Labelling of Iris
Phospholipids in Presence and Absence of ACh*

Cation (125 mM)	^{32}P labelling of phospholipids (cpm x 10^{-2})/iris					
	PA	%	PI	%	PC	%
None	11 (12.9)†	117	15.6 (16.2)	104	7 (8)	114
NaCl	126 (390)	310	397 (698)	176	486 (594)	122
LiCl	64.7 (100)	155	55.9 (50)	89	63.9 (69)	108
NH$_4$Cl	13.9 (13.6)	98	6 (7)	117	1.6 (1.8)	113
KCl	12.9 (14)	109	9.5 (11.6)	122	3.9 (2.9)	74
Choline Cl	1.5 (1.2)	80	1.8 (2)	111	1.3 (1.1)	85
Tris-HCl	8.2 (8.1)	99	3.7 (4.5)	122	1.3 (1.5)	115

Irises were incubated for 30 min in isoosmotic medium that contained 10 µCi ^{32}Pi and
the cations as shown in the table. ACh plus eserine (0.05 mM each) was then added and
incubation continued for an additional 30 min.

*Taken from Ref. 4 with permission.

†In the presence of ACh + eserine

Neurotransmitters increase the permeability of the plasma membrane to Na^+. To maintain the steady state, the monovalent cation is extruded from the cell by an energy requiring process mediated by Na^+, K^+-ATPase. This is followed by compensatory resynthesis of $[\gamma-^{32}P]ATP$ from ^{32}Pi and ADP, thus resulting in an overall transitory increase in the S.A. of $[^{32}P]ATP$. This $[\gamma-^{32}P]ATP$ is utilized in phosphorylation of diacylglycerol, which results from the ACh-stimulated breakdown of phosphoinositides, to PA and subsequently to the phosphoinositides.

The precise mechanism underlying the observed changes in the S.A. of $[^{32}P]ATP$ remains to be investigated. Our studies point to an important role for Na^+ in these changes, which is undoubtedly related to the Na^+-pump. The possibility that as a consequence of Na^+ omission the transport of D-glucose and/or phosphate across the plasma membrane is impaired is now under investigation in our laboratory.

THE PHOSPHOINOSITIDE EFFECT AND THE MICROSOMAL FRACTION

Although activation of muscarinic-cholinergic and α-adrenergic receptors leads to phosphoinositide breakdown there is no convincing evidence at this time to show that this phenomenon does indeed occur at the plasma membrane of the cell. Radioautographic studies of pancreas (22), sympathetic ganglia (20) and subcellular fractionation of cerebral cortex (6,28) and sympathetic ganglia (12) revealed that the stimulated labelling of phosphoinositides is distributed throughout the cell.

Phospholipid synthesis occurs mainly at the endoplasmic reticulum, and furthermore in the iris muscle, as in other excitable tissues, muscarinic-cholinergic and α-adrenergic receptors are concentrated in the microsomal fraction (35). It must also be emphasized that this fraction contains plasma membrane fragments (5). Efforts to demonstrate an effect of ACh on ^{32}Pi incorporation into phospholipids of iris muscle homogenates were unsuccessful. This observation is supported by the fact that with the exception of synaptosomes (33,38) there is no experimental evidence to suggest that this phenomenon does occur in a cell-free homogenate. This could be interpreted as follows: (a) that the phosphoinositide effect is coupled to muscarinic-cholinergic and α-adrenergic receptors through Ca^{2+} as we have suggested previously (*), and that tissue homogenization leads to disruption of this coupling mechanism; or (b) that muscarinic and α-adrenergic receptor properties are altered by the homogenization process. Comparative studies on the binding characteristics of $[^3H]QNB$ to muscarinic sites and of $[^3H]WB-4101$ to α-adrenergic sites in microsomal fractions and in iris muscle revealed them to be comparable (35). Thus the findings of comparable binding patterns for $[^3H]QNB$ and $[^3H]$-WB-4101 binding to microsomal fractions and muscle argue against the possibility of alterations in receptor properties following tissue disruption. It was concluded from these studies that the differences in receptor-mediated biochemical responses that are seen between intact tissue and cell-free homogenates, such as the phosphoinositide effect

TABLE 5

Effects of ACh and Atropine on ^{32}Pi Incorporation into
Phospholipids of Microsomes Isolated from Incubated Iris Muscle*

Additions	^{32}P-Radioactivity in microsomal phospholipids (cpm x 10^{-3}/mg microsomal protein)				
	PA	PI	Poly PI	PC	
None	9.96	86.45	91.07	86.69	
ACh (50 μM)	30.66 (308%)*	230.42 (267%)	115.92 (127%)	118.81 (137%)	
Atropine (20 μM)	9.53	103.24	95.19	97.11	
ACh + Atropine (50 μM each)	7.62 (80%)	96.42 (93%)	83.13 (87%)	90.66 (93%)	

*Ten irises (one of a pair) were preincubated in an isoosmotic medium containing ^{32}Pi for 15 min at 37°C; atropine was then added and incubation continued for 15 min, ACh + eserine were added as indicated and incubation conducted for an additional 30 min. Reaction was stopped by briefly washing the tissue in cold 0.25 M sucrose, 10 mM Tris-HCl, 2 mM EDTA (pH 7.4). The tissue was then homogenized and microsomes isolated by means of differential centrifugation. Phospholipids were extracted from microsomes, separated and analyzed by two-dimensional TLC.

*% of control

are more likely to be due to alterations in receptor function, e.g. changes in ionic permeabilities, rather than to actual changes in receptor properties (35).

This conclusion is supported by the following findings: (1) Prior incubation of the iris muscle with ACh caused an increase in ^{32}P incorporation into PA and PI of the tissue microsomes by 208% and 167% respectively and this increase was blocked by atropine (Table 5). Under the same experimental conditions ACh induced a slight increase in the ^{32}P labelling of poly PI and PC. These data could suggest that at least in situ, the phosphoinositide effect is associated with membranes of the microsomal fraction. (2) Acetylcholine had no effect on the breakdown of ^{32}P-labelled phosphoinositides of microsomes isolated from labelled iris muscle (Table 6). Thus after 10 min of incubation, the loss of ^{32}P radioactivity from PI and poly PI was 28% and 17% respectively, and this hydrolysis was not affected by ACh. (3) Acetylcholine had little effect on the incorporation of ^{32}Pi from [^{32}P]ATP into PA and poly PI of iris muscle microsomes (Table 7). These data clearly suggest that the stimulatory effect of ACh on [^{32}P] labelling of phosphoinositides is not a result of a direct action of the neurotransmitter on the enzymes involved in their metabolism.

TABLE 6

Effect of ACh on ^{32}P-labelled Phospholipids of
Microsomes Isolated from Incubated Iris Muscle*

Time of incubation (min)	Additions	^{32}P-Radioactivity in microsomes (cpm/100 ug microsomal protein)			
		PA	PI	Poly PI	PC
Zero	None	1710	15021	8980	13958
10	None	1614	10748	7451	14434
10	ACh + eserine (50 M each)	1578 (98%)*	11129 (104%)	6863 (92%)	14008 (97%)

*Irises were incubated in an isoosmotic medium containing 50 µCi ^{32}Pi/ml for 60 min at 37°C. After incubation the irises were washed with buffer, homogenized and ^{32}P-labelled microsomes isolated by differential centrifugation. The effect of ACh on hydrolysis of phospholipids of ^{32}P-labelled microsomes was carried out as follows: ^{32}P-labelled microsomes (equivalent to 100 µg protein) were incubated at 37°C in a medium containing $CaCl_2$ (2 mM), $MgCl_2$ (5 mM), and Na-acetate buffer (50 mM), pH 6.8, in a final volume of 50 µl. The reaction was terminated by addition of 10% TCA. Phospholipids were extracted and analyzed by two dimensional TLC.

*% of Control

TABLE 7

Effect of ACh on the In Vitro Incorporation of ^{32}Pi
from [^{32}P]ATP into Phosphoinositides of Rabbit
Iris Muscle Microsomes

Additions	^{32}P-Radioactivity Incorporated (cpm)		
	PA	DPI	TPI
None	848	5778	1354
ACh (50 µM)	762	5823	1222

Iris muscle microsomes (equivalent to 50 µg protein) were
incubated in 50 mM sodium acetate buffer (pH 6.8) containing
10 mM Mg acetate, 20 µCi [^{32}P]ATP, 200 µM ATP in a final
volume of 50 µl for 1 min at 37°C. The reaction was terminated by the addition of 10% TCA (final conc.). Phospholipids
were extracted, separated by one-dimensional TLC and analyzed
for radioactivity. Values are means of two determinations

It can be concluded from the above that in certain tissues,
including the iris muscle, ACh-induced phosphoinositide breakdown into
diacylglycerol and inositol phosphates and its subsequent resynthesis
is probably a consequence of the neurotransmitter-induced ionic
changes. A plausible model as to how Ca^{2+} and Na^+ could be involved in
the phosphoinositide effect in the iris smooth muscle is given in
Fig. 1.

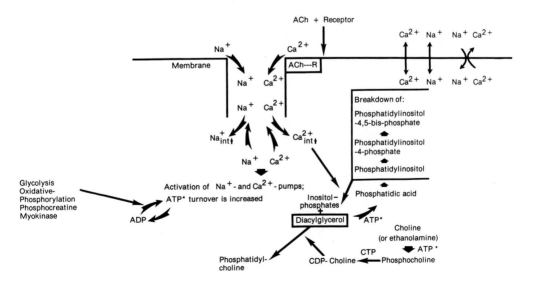

FIG. 1. Probable roles of Ca^{2+} and Na^+ in the phosphoinositide effect
in the iris muscle (Taken from Ref. 2a with permission).

According to this hypothesis the Ca^{2+} entering the cell in response to receptor activation could activate the enzymes involved in phosphoinositide breakdown, which are stimulated by Ca^{2+}, to diacylglyerol and inositol phosphates. Removal of the polar head groups from these phospholipids could facilitate the cationic fluxes through the Na^+-Ca^{2+} channels. The Na^+ entering the cell, through passive flux and in response to ACh, leads to an increase in intracellular Na^+ concentration which, in turn, stimulates the Na^+-pump activity and ATP turnover. Restoration of the polar head groups to the diacylglyerol backbone at the Na^+-Ca^{2+} channels, which is reflected in the enhanced $[^{32}P]$-labelling from $[^{32}P]ATP$, could be associated with the extrusion of Na^+ and Ca^{2+}, presumably via the Na^+- and Ca^{2+}-pumps. In more recent studies we have shown that ACh stimulated the $[^{32}P]$labelling of PA and PI and the breakdown of poly PI_2 in ^{32}P-labelled iris muscle only in the presence of both Na^+ and Ca^{2+} (R.A. Akhtar and A.A. Abdel-Latif, unpublished work).

CONCLUSIONS

The effects of Ca^{2+}, Na^+, other cations and the neurotransmitter, acetylcholine on phosphoinositide and ATP metabolism in the rabbit iris smooth muscle were investigated. Calcium ion was found to be required for the acetylcholine-stimulated phosphodiesteratic cleavage of triphosphoinositide and the water-soluble inositol triphosphate and inositol monophosphate. The production of the latter could result from Ca^{2+} activation of phosphatidylinositol phosphodiesterase. The acetylcholine-stimulated $[^{32}P]$labelling of phosphoinositides is dependent on the presence of extracellular Na^+, and the monovalent cation requirement is specific for this cation. Addition of acetylcholine did not alter the specific radioactivity of $[^{32}P]ATP$, however in the absence of Na^+ the neurotransmitter-stimulated $[^{32}P]$labelling of phosphoinositides was either abolished or drastically reduced. Acetylcholine increased $[^{32}P]$ incorporation into phosphatidic acid and phosphatidyl inositol of microsomes isolated from incubated iris muscle by 208% and 167%, and this was blocked by atropine. Acetylcholine had no effect on the breakdown of $[^{32}P]$labelled phosphoinositides of microsomes isolated from labelled iris muscle. Acetylcholine had no effect on the incorporation of $[^{32}P]$ from $[^{32}P]ATP$ into phosphoinositides of iris muscle microsomes. It was concluded that the stimulatory effect of acetylcholine on $[^{32}P]$labelling of phosphoinositides in the rabbit iris is not a result of a direct action of the neurotransmitter on the lipolytic enzymes involved in their metabolism, but probably is a consequence of the neurotransmitter-induced ionic changes.

ACKNOWLEDGEMENTS

This work was supported from U.S. Public Health Service Grants EY-04171 and EY-04387. This paper is contribution No. 0677 from the Department of Cell and Molecular Biology, Medical College of Georgia.

REFERENCES

1. Abdel-Latif, A.A. (1976): In: Function and Metabolism of Phospholipids in CNS and PNS, edited by G. Porcellati, L. Amaducci, and C. Galli, pp. 227-256, Plenum Press, New York.

2. Abdel-Latif, A.A. (1981): Biochem. Pharmacol., 30:1371-1374.
2a. Abdel-Latif, A.A. (1982): In: Handbook of Neurochemistry, edited by A. Lajtha, Vol. 3, In Press, Plenum Press, New York.
3. Abdel-Latif, A.A., Luke, B. and Smith, J.P. (1980): Biochim. Biophys. Acta, 614:424-434.
4. Abdel-Latif, A.A. and Luke, B. (1981): Biochim. Biophys. Acta, 673:64-74.
5. Abdel-Latif, A.A. and Smith, J.P. (1976): Biochem. Pharmacol. 25: 1697-1704.
6. Abdel-Latif, A.A., Yau, S-J., and Smith, J.P. (1974): J.Neurochem. 22:383-393.
7. Akhtar, R.A., and Abdel-Latif, A.A. (1978): Biochim. Biophys. Acta, 527:159-170.
8. Akhtar, R.A., and Abdel-Latif, A.A. (1978): J. Pharmacol. Exp. Ther., 204:655-668.
9. Akhtar, R.A., and Abdel-Latif, A.A. (1979): Gen. Pharmacol., 10: 445-450.
10. Akhtar, R.A., and Abdel-Latif, A.A. (1980): Biochem. J., 192:785-791.
10a. Aly, M.I. and Abdel-Latif, A.A. (1982): Neurochem. Res., 7: 159-169.
11. Brossard, M. and Quastel, J.H. (1963): Can. J. Biochem. Physiol., 41:1243-1256.
12. Burt, D.R. And Larrabee, M.A. (1973): J. Neurochem., 21: 255-272.
13. Clements, R.S., Evans, M.H., and Pace, C.S. (1981): Biochim. Biophys. Acta, 674:1-9.
14. Crockroft, S., Bennett, J.P., and Gomperts, B.D. (1980): FEBS Letters, 110:115-118.
15. Farese, R.V., Larson, R.E., and Sabir, M.A. (1980): Biochim. Biophys. Acta, 633:479-484.
16. Fisher, S.K. and Agranoff, B.W. (1980): J. Neurochem. 34:1231-1240.
17. Griffin, H.D., Hawthorne, J.N. and Sykes, M. (1979): Biochem. Pharmacol., 28:1143-1147.
18. Grimes, M.J., Abdel-Latif, A.A. and Carrier, G.O. (1979): Biochem. Pharmacol., 28:3213-3219.
19. Hawthorne, J.N. and Bleasdale, J.E. (1975): Mol. Cell Biochem. 8: 83-87.
20. Hokin, L.E. (1965): Proc. Natl. Acad. Sci. USA, 53:1369-1370.
21. Hokin, L.E. (1966): Biochim. Biophys. Acta, 115:219-221.
22. Hokin, L.E. and Huebner, D. (1969): J. Cell Biol., 33:521-530.
23. Jafferji, S.S. and Michell, R.H. (1976): Biochem. J., 160:163-169.
24. Jafferji, S.S. and Michell, R.H. (1976): Biochem. J., 160-397-399.
25. Jones, L.M. and Michell, R.H. (1976): Biochem. J., 158:505-507.
26. Jones, L.M. and Michell, R.H. (1975): Biochem. J., 148:479-485.
27. Keryer, G., Herman, G. and Rossignol, G. (1979): FEBS Letters, 102:4-8.
28. Lapetina, E.G. and Michell, R.H. (1972): Biochem. J., 126:1141-1146.
29. Lennon, A.M. and Steinberg, H.R. (1973): J. Neurochem., 20:337-345.
30. Michell, R.H. (1975): Biochim. Biophys. Acta, 415:81-147.
31. Miller, J.C. and Leung, I. (1979): Biochem. J., 178:9-13.
32. Oron, Y., Lowe, M. and Sellinger, Z. (1975): Mol. Pharmacol., 11: 79-86.

33. Schacht, J. and Agranoff, B.W. (1972): J. Biol. Chem., 247: 771-777.

34. Sherman, W.R., Leavitt, A.L., Honchar, M.P., Hallcher, L.M. and Phillips, B.E. (1981): J. Neurochem., 36:1947-1951.

35. Taft, W.C., Abdel-Latif, A.A. and Akhtar, R.A. (1980): Biochem. Pharmacol., 29:2713-2720.

36. Trifaro, J.M. (1969): Mol. Pharmacol., 5: 424-427.

37. Yagihara, Y., Bleasdale, J.E. and Hawthorne, J.N. (1973): J. Neurochem., 21:173-190.

38. Yagihara, Y. and Hawthorne, J.N. (1972): J. Neurochem., 19:355-367.

39. Zor, Y., Low, I.P., Bloom, G. and Field, J.B. (1968): Biochem. Biophys. Res. Commun., 33: 649-658.

Phospholipids in the Nervous System, Vol. 1:
Metabolism, edited by L. Horrocks, et al. Raven
Press, New York © 1982.

Phosphatidylinositol and Calcium Gating:
Some Difficulties

J. N. Hawthorne and N. Azila

Department of Biochemistry, University Hospital and Medical School, Nottingham NG7 2UH,
United Kingdom

Michell et al. (6,7) have proposed that phosphatidylinositol
hydrolysis is an essential part of the mechanism by which activation of
certain cell surface receptors increases influx of calcium ions. If the
proposal is correct, the phosphatidylinositol sensitive to receptor
activation should be located in the plasma membrane. However, Kirk et
al. (4) observed loss of labelled phosphatidylinositol from all
membrane fractions of rat hepatocytes in response to vasopressin. We
have obtained similar results with perfused bovine adrenal medulla,
where catecholamine secretion induced by carbachol is accompanied by
phosphatidylinositol breakdown.

PHOSPHATIDYLINOSITOL CHANGES IN PERFUSED ADRENAL MEDULLA

Perfusion and Subcellular Fractionation

Bovine adrenal glands were obtained within 15 min of the death of the
animal and kept on ice for 30 min until perfusion began. Connective
tissue and fat were removed and two incisions made in the cortical
tissue so that perfusion fluid could flow out. A tapered polythene
canula was inserted into the central vein opening and tied in place.
Through it, the gland was perfused with Locke's solution at a flow rate
of 4 ml per min. The solution was maintained at 30°C and continuously
gassed with 95:5 oxygen-carbon dioxide. A control gland was perfused
simultaneously.

Adrenal phospholipids were labelled by perfusion for 1 h in this way
with Locke's solution containing carrier-free [^{32}P]orthophosphate
(total of 1 mCi per gland). A further 15 min perfusion with Locke's
solution without ^{32}P removed excess radioactivity and after this 2 min-
samples of perfusion fluid were collected for catecholamine estimation.
After 8 min, four 1 ml injections of 15 mM carbachol in Locke's fluid
into the tubing carrying Locke's solution into the gland were made at
30 sec intervals. The process was repeated 10 min later. Similar
injections of Locke's fluid without carbachol were made into the control
adrenal. After a further 12 min the glands were removed for
subcellular fractionation.

Figs. 1a and 1b outline the preparation of subcellular fractions and
Table 1 gives some marker enzyme results.

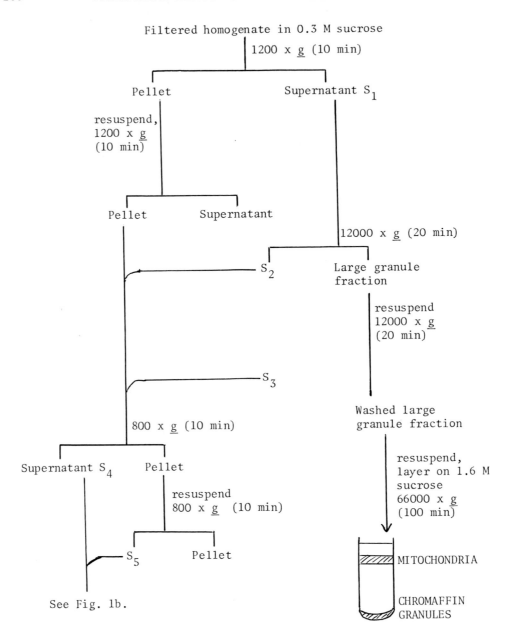

FIG. 1a. Subcellular fractionation of adrenal medulla

The chromaffin granule fraction contained the greatest proportion of catecholamine and dopamine β-hydroxylase, as expected. Though only about 2% of the homogenate protein appeared in the plasma membrane fraction, it was enriched in both calcium-activated ATPase and acetylcholinesterase.

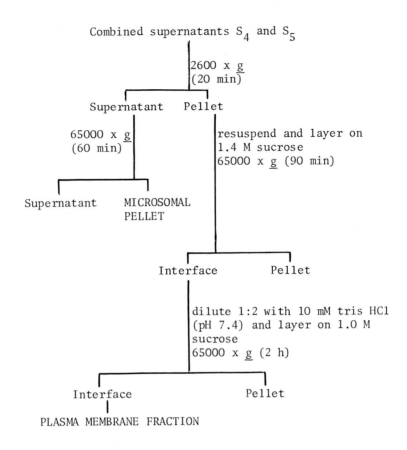

FIG. 1b. Subcellular fractionation of adrenal medulla (contd.)

TABLE 1. Markers for selected subcellular fractions of adrenal medulla

Fraction	Protein	Cytochrome oxidase	Catecholamine	Calcium ATPase	Arylesterase
Mitochondrial	7.7	77.8	4.6	11.6	8.5
Chromaffin granule	9.2	0.9	45.1	2.8	1.8
Plasma membrane	1.8	-	-	20.3	0.7
Microsomal	5.5	4.4	3.3	12.1	26.4

Each result is the mean from 4 fractionations and represents % of homogenate activity.

Effect of secretagogues on phospholipid labelling

As described earlier, carbachol was administered to the perfused gland. It provoked catecholamine secretion, the quantity secreted being much less during the second stimulation. Secretion was accompanied by a reduction in the specific radioactivity of phosphatidate and phosphatidylinositol (Table 2). Other phospholipids were unaffected. The loss of label was seen in all the subcellular fractions studied and was significantly greater in the chromaffin granule and microsomal fractions when glands were stimulated twice. After only one period of stimulation the loss was much the same in each fraction.

TABLE 2. Effect of carbachol on specific radioactivity (^{32}P) of adrenal phospholipids

	PHOSPHATIDYLINOSITOL (% decrease)		PHOSPHATIDATE (% decrease)	
	Stimulated twice	Stimulated once	Stimulated twice	Stimulated once
Homogenate	47.4±23.7	55.7±21.8	47.6±11.8	51.2±17.1
Chromaffin granule	64.9±12.9*	45.2±13.7	61.7±21.0^{+}	41.4±16.7
Plasma membrane	40.8±11.5	45.3±16.5	35.0±16.1	43.5±12.4
Microsomal	59.1±15.3^{+}	53.3±14.4	64.1±12.6*	57.1±17.2
Mitochondrial	50.0± 8.9	48.7±13.4	46.3±12.2	44.9±12.0

Figures are means ± S.D. of 8 results from two perfusions in each case. Significantly different from plasma membrane result: *P <0.001; $^{+}$P <0.01.

Stimulation of the adrenal once in calcium-free Locke's solution containing 0.1 mM EGTA produced the same phospholipid effects but there was no secretion of catecholamine. Instead of 15 mM carbachol, 56 mM KCl was also used to stimulate catecholamine secretion. In this case, the Locke's solution contained 10^{-4}M atropine and 2 mM hexamethonium to exclude stimulation of cholinergic receptors. Secretion induced by KCl was not accompanied by a phosphatidylinositol effect.

DISCUSSION

We have shown elsewhere (8) that the phosphatidylinositol response in bovine adrenal medulla is associated with muscarinic and not nicotinic receptors. The present study indicates that KCl depolarization, which presumably allows Ca^{2+} entry through voltage-dependent channels, causes catecholamine secretion but no loss of prelabelled phosphatidylinositol. Carbachol stimulation in a Ca^{2+}-free medium produced the opposite, loss of phosphatidylinositol without catecholamine secretion. Both results are consistent with Michell's theory that phosphatidylinositol hydrolysis is associated with Ca^{2+}

entry in response to activation of muscarinic receptors.

The loss of labelled phosphatidylinositol from all the subcellular fractions studied is not easy to reconcile with the calcium gating theory, which requires loss of the lipid from plasma membrane only. Kirk et al. (4) obtained a similar generalised loss of phosphatidylinositol in isolated hepatocytes stimulated by vasopressin. This was explained by the action of exchange proteins in replacing phosphatidylinositol initially lost from the plasma membrane by transfer from other cell membranes. The hepatocytes (4) were obtained from rats injected with [^{3}H]inositol 20 h before death and most of the radioactive phosphatidylinositol was located in microsomal membranes. Since the lipid is synthesised in the endoplasmic reticulum, this microsomal fraction might well have been more highly labelled than other subcellular fractions. Exchange proteins would be likely to transfer this phosphatidylinositol to make good the proposed loss from plasma membrane. If the exchange protein explanation is correct, a plasma membrane fraction should show a smaller loss of radioactivity than the other fractions, or even a net gain. However, preparation of plasma membrane from isolated hepatocytes presents considerable problems. Our results (Table 2) do not show a significant difference between plasma membrane and the other fractions after one stimulation. After two stimulations loss from plasma membrane is less than that from microsomal or chromaffin granule membranes.

An alternative explanation for the general loss of membrane phosphatidylinositol is that the cytoplasmic phospholipase C responsible for its hydrolysis is activated throughout the cell. Increased free Ca^{2+} in the cytosol might provide a mechanism, but it is not at all clear (7) whether calcium ionophores can induce phosphatidylinositol hydrolysis. Nevertheless, it seems peculiarly inappropriate that the key enzyme of Michell's calcium gating theory should be soluble, rather than being located along with the relevant receptors in the plasma membrane.

Another major difficulty is that the biochemical events associated with phosphatidylinositol hydrolysis and resynthesis are unusually complex for a simple gating phenomenon. The reactions and possible locations are as follows:

1. phosphatidylinositol + H_2O → diacylglycerol + inositol 1,2-cyclic phosphate (cytosol)

2. diacylglycerol + ATP → phosphatidate + ADP (plasma membrane?)

3. phosphatidate + CTP → CDP-diacylglycerol + pyrophosphate (endoplasmic reticulum)

4. CDP-diacylglycerol + inositol → phosphatidylinositol + CMP (endoplasmic reticulum)

Initial loss of phosphatidylinositol from the plasma membrane would require an exchange protein to return the lipid there from the endoplasmic reticulum and another to transfer phosphatidate from plasma membrane to endoplasmic reticulum. The whole process involves loss of three high-energy phosphate bonds.

One of Michell's arguments for his theory is that the phosphatidylinositol response is independent of external calcium (5). Several systems are now known in which this is not the case. Farese et al. (2) have shown, contrary to earlier work, that the carbachol-induced phosphatidylinositol loss in rat pancreas is abolished in a calcium-free medium. Calcium entry induced by ionophore A23187 caused phosphatidylinositol breakdown. Both results suggest that loss of the lipid is a consequence rather than the cause of calcium entry. The increased labelling of phosphatidylinositol by ^{32}P in synaptosomes is a muscarinic effect also dependent on external calcium (3). Finally, Cockroft et al. (1) found that the breakdown of phosphatidylinositol accompanying secretion of lysosomal enzymes by activated rabbit neutrophils is dependent on calcium. These authors concluded that the phosphatidylinositol and phosphatidate changes were consequences, not causes of a rise in intracellular Ca^{2+}.

If there is a universal role of phosphatidylinositol in response to surface receptor activation, these results and the more general considerations above exclude the control of calcium entry.

REFERENCES

1. Cockroft, S., Bennett, J.P., and Gomperts, B.D. (1980): Nature, 288: 275-277.
2. Farese, R.V., Larson, R.E., and Sabir, M.A. (1980): Biochim. Biophys. Acta, 633:479-484.
3. Griffin, H.D., Hawthorne, J.N., Sykes, M., and Orlacchio, A. (1979): Biochem. Pharmacol., 28:1143-1147.
4. Kirk, C.J., Michell, R.H., and Hems, D.A. (1981): Biochem. J., 194: 155-165.
5. Michell, R.H. (1975): Biochim. Biophys. Acta, 415:81-147.
6. Michell, R.H., Jafferji, S.S., and Jones, L.M. (1977): Adv. exp. Med. Biol., 83:447-464.
7. Michell, R.H., and Kirk, C.J. (1981): Trends Pharmacol. Sci., 2:86-89.
8. Mohd. Adnan, N.A., and Hawthorne, J.N. (1981): J. Neurochem., 36: 1858-1860.

Phospholipids in the Nervous System, Vol. 1:
Metabolism, edited by L. Horrocks, et al. Raven
Press, New York © 1982.

Metabolism of Polyphosphoinositides and Other Phospholipids in Peripheral Nerve of Normal and Streptozotocin Diabetic Rats

Joseph Eichberg, Margaret E. Bell, and *Richard G. Peterson

Department of Biochemical and Biophysical Sciences, University of Houston, Houston, Texas 77004;
Department of Anatomy, Indiana University School of Medicine, Indianapolis, Indiana 46223

Alterations in the metabolism of phosphoinositides accompany and appear to constitute a part of the mechanism which underlies a variety of receptor-mediated cellular events. Thus, considerable evidence has accumulated that accelerated catabolism of phosphatidylinositol which is triggered by a number of hormones and other environmental stimuli acting at receptors is often associated with calcium mobilization within the cell(23,24). In the case of polyphosphoinositides, the rapid metabolism of the monoesterified phosphate moieties of these compounds has led to speculation that their turnover is also an integral part of dynamic cellular phenomena which involve cation movements(1,17,20). One long-standing suggestion is that polyphosphoinositide metabolism in the axonal membrane might be integral to some facet of nerve impulse propagation along the axon(16). To date, the evidence for this hypothesis is tenuous and is based on the metabolic lability of these substances, their localization in part in neuronal and glial membranes(10) and their ability to bind divalent cations(5,9). In addition, under proper incubation conditions, electrical stimulation of poorly myelinated nerves has produced either increased incorporation of ^{32}P into di-and triphosphoinositide or accelerated loss of radioactivity from prelabeled triphosphoinositide(3,34,35). These results are consistent with the concept that enhanced triphosphoinositide turnover is associated with the conduction process but fails to link these two phenomena directly.

Recently, we have initiated studies on phospholipid metabolism in experimental diabetic neuropathy, a disease state in which the velocity of nerve impulse conduction is impaired. The aims of this investigation were twofold: to determine whether abnormalities in the metabolism of peripheral nerve phospholipids are manifested in the disorder and if so to utilize the disease state as a system in which a possible biochemical role of polyphosphoinositides in axonal function may be further examined.

DIABETIC NEUROPATHY AND INOSITOL-CONTAINING PHOSPHOLIPIDS

Overt distal symmetrical polyneuropathy is an important medical problem which afflicts about 25% of all patients with diabetes mellitus. Abnormal electrophysiological behavior, particularly reduced peripheral nerve conduction velocites, is even more widely apparent among diabetic individuals. In rats made diabetic by injection of streptozotocin, similar electrophysiological changes are detectable as early as 1 to 2 weeks following drug administration(4,13). Biochemical alterations which appear in experimental diabetic neuropathy include an accumulation of sorbitol within the nerve(11,33) and a decrease in the incorporation of lipid and protein precursors into the major molecular components of myelin(31).

A reduction in inositol content of sciatic nerve in rats with streptozotocin-induced diabetes was first observed by Greene et al.(13) and has since been amply confirmed(6,28). The distributon space of the cyclitol within the nerve has been reported to be decreased(7), a finding which suggests that an abnormality of myo-inositol transport or of its accessibility to nerve structures may be involved. The level of lipid-bound inositol in peripheral nerve was found to be depressed in acute but not chronic streptozotocin diabetes(28) and the incorporation of [^{3}H]-inositol into sciatic nerve lipids was also reported to be reduced both in vivo and in vitro(7,18). Assay of several enzymes of inositol lipid metabolism has revealed that the disease is accompanied by a substantial decline in the activity of CDP-diacylglycerol:inositol phosphatidyltransferase in liver and sciatic nerve (21,36,37).

These findings prompted us to examine the incorporation of [^{32}P]-orthophosphate into the phosphoinositides and other phospholipids in normal and diabetic sciatic nerve and to correlate these observationss with measurements of peripheral nerve conduction velocities and examination of nerve ultrastructure.

INCORPORATION OF ^{32}P INTO PHOSPHOLIPIDS OF NORMAL RAT SCIATIC NERVE

When nerve segments were incubated in Krebs-Ringer bicarbonate medium which contained 5.5 mM glucose and isotope, the principal labeled phospholipids were triphosphoinositide and phosphatidylcholine (FIGURE 1 and TABLE 1). Several other lipids, including the ethanolamine phosphoglycerides, sphingomyelin and phosphatidylserine (which cochromatographed with phosphatidic acid in the solvent system used) contained negligible radioactivity. The time course of labeling was essentially linear for up to 2 hours except for a lag in isotope incorporation into phosphatidylcholine(2). The pattern of labeling was not altered when the concentration of glucose in the medium was raised six to ten times above the physiological level (TABLE 1). The inclusion of cytidine and inositol in the incubation medium was also without effect.

ALTERATIONS IN PHOSPHOLIPID METABOLISM IN SCIATIC NERVE FROM STREPTOZOTOCIN-DIABETIC RATS

Most rats injected intraperitoneally with streptozotocin developed diabetes as judged by serum glucose levels which ranged from 400 to 500 mg per 100 ml serum at the time of sacrifice. A small propor-

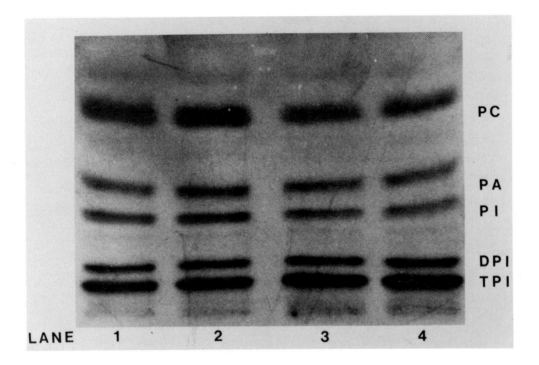

FIGURE 1. Autoradiogram of a developed high performance thin layer chromatogram of sciatic nerve phospholipids labeled with ^{32}P by incubation as described in the legend to TABLE 1. Lipids were extracted with acidified chloroform-methanol and duplicate portions of the contents of the washed extract were chromatographed in chloroform-methanol-20% methylamine (60:36:10) as described elsewhere(2). Lanes 1 and 2: control nerve; Lanes 3 and 4: diabetic nerve.

tion of rats which received the drug failed to become diabetic. These animals comprised an additional "streptozotocin control" group and were included in the experimental protocol to evaluate possible effects of streptozotocin which were unrelated to the induction of diabetes.

At successive time intervals from 2 to 20 weeks following the onset of the disease, the pattern of incorporation of ^{32}P into lipids of sciatic nerve incubated in vitro was determined and compared to that of weight-matched controls. The overall quantity of isotope which entered phospholipids was quite variable. However, at all times examined, there was a specific and significant increase of from 48 to 67% in the amount of label present in triphosphoinositide (TABLE 2). A small decrease in the labeling of phosphatidylcholine was seen only after 20 weeks duration of chronic diabetes. The quantity of isotope incorporated into each lipid in nerves of "streptozotocin control" animals was indistinguishable from values obtained for normal rats.

TABLE 1. Effect of glucose and other additions on incorporation of ^{32}P into phospholipids of rat sciatic nerve

Phospholipid	5.5 mM glucose (N=5)	30-50 mM glucose (N=4)	5.5 mM glucose 1 mM cytidine 1 mM inositol (N=2)
	% of ^{32}P incorporated into total phospholipids		
Triphosphoinositide	27 ± 2	25 ± 2	25,26
Diphosphoinositide	14 ± 1	13 ± 1	15,16
Phosphatidylinositol	12 ± 1	13 ± 1	15,15
Phosphatidic Acid	10 ± 3	12 ± 1	10,11
Phosphatidylcholine	29 ± 2	29 ± 3	27,27
Other phospholipids	8 ± 1	8 ± 1	6,7

[a]Excised sciatic nerves from female Sprague-Dawley rats were divided into four pieces, pairs of segments were combined and incubated for 2 hours in Krebs-Ringer bicarbonate medium which contained 15-30 µCi ^{32}P-orthophosphate and additions as indicated. Lipids were extracted and chromatographed as described in the legend to FIGURE 1. N=number of incubations. Values are means ± S.E.M.

TABLE 2. Incorporation of ^{32}P into phospholipids in sciatic nerve from normal and streptozotocin diabetic rats

	Control			Diabetic		
Weeks after injection	2	10	20	2	10	20
Number of incubations	8	16	4	12	11	4
Number of rats	4	6	2	6	6	2
Phospholipid	nmol ^{32}P incorporated/g wet weight nerve					
Triphosphoinositide	35±6	18±2	94±7	56±7[b]	30±5[a]	139±10[d]
Diphosphoinositide	23±2	12±1	44±3	27±2	15±2	51±4
Phosphatidylinositol	36±2	9±1	55±4	38±2	9±1	45±3
Phosphatidic Acid	42±3	8±1	47±3	45±2	10±2	45±3
Phosphatidylcholine	64±3	20±4	97±2	67±4	19±2	74±5[c]

Weight-matched rats were injected intraperitonally either with streptozotocin (60 mg/kg) or with the citrate buffer vehicle. Incubations of control and diabetic nerves were performed as described in the legend to Table 1. Values are expressed as means ± S.E.M. Differences from respective controls: [a]p<0.02, [b]p<0.01, [c]p<0.005, [d]p<0.001.

Since these experiments were performed using intact nerve, the metabolic differences observed might reflect changes in the connective tissue sheath which could affect the accessibility of precursor in the medium to the nerve. This possibility was partially excluded as a result of incubations performed using control and 10 week diabetic nerves from which the epineurium had been removed. In the desheathed diabetic nerve, increases in triphosphoinositide labeling were evident which were similar to those obtained with the intact preparation.

A reduction in peripheral nerve myelin content has been reported to occur in chronic streptozotocin diabetes(32). In order to determine whether the level of triphosphoinositide was decreased in this tissue in chronic diabetes, measurements of the concentration of this lipid were made in sciatic nerves which had been frozen in liquid nitrogen within 10 seconds after removal from anesthetized rats. Triphosphoinositide was quantified by a densitometric method for P content involving separation of lipids by high performance thin layer chromatography followed by derivatization by means of a molybdate-containing spray(14,22). The level of triphosphoinositide in normal animals (0.44±0.05 nmol P/mg wet weight) was indistinguishable from that for animals which had been diabetic for over 20 weeks (0.41±0.05 nmol P/mg wet weight) (average of five determinations ± S.E.M.).

CONDUCTION VELOCITIES IN NERVES FROM NORMAL AND DIABETIC RATS

To verify that electrophysiological alterations indeed accompanied the metabolic changes in peripheral nerve from chronic streptozotocin diabetic rats, measurements of conduction velocities were performed 10 and 20 weeks after onset of the disease. As seen in TABLE 3, a greater than 20% decrease was observed in conduction velocities for both the motor and sensory components of rat sciatic and caudal nerve in 10 week diabetic as compared to control animals. Similar results were obtained using 20 week diabetic animals.

TABLE 3. Conduction velocities in peripheral nerves of control and 10-week diabetic rats

	Control	Diabetic
Number of rats	5	4
	Meters per second	
Nerve:		
Motor sciatic [37°C]	53.8 ± 5.1	40.9 ± 1.7 (p<0.01)
Sensory sciatic [37°C]	56.5 ± 4.3	45.2 ± 1.8 (p<0.01)
Motor caudal [30°C]	27.0 ± 1.6	19.8 ± 2.8 (p<0.01)
Sensory caudal [29°C]	38.2 ± 2.2	30.9 ± 2.1 (p<0.01)

Measurements were performed essentially as described in (25). Values are presented as means ± S.E.M.; p values different from controls are given in parentheses. Temperatures at which measurements were taken are given in brackets.

ULTRASTRUCTURAL CHANGES IN NERVES FROM DIABETIC RATS

To characterize morphological alterations which might accompany the electrophysiological and biochemical changes, tibial nerves from animals which had been diabetic for 10 and 20 weeks were embedded and examined by electron microscopy according to the procedure of Moore et al. (26). Ultrastructural evaluation of the tissues revealed no gross neuropathological changes in the myelin sheath. Some accumulation of glycogen-like granules was noted in the Schwann cells which otherwise appeared normal. Much larger deposits of electron-dense glycogen-like material were observed consistently in perineurial cells from all diabetic nerves, but were absent from control nerves (Figure 2).

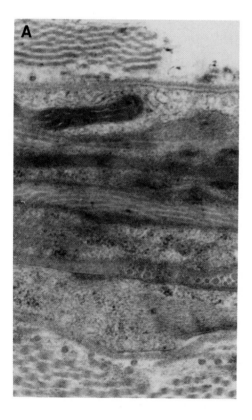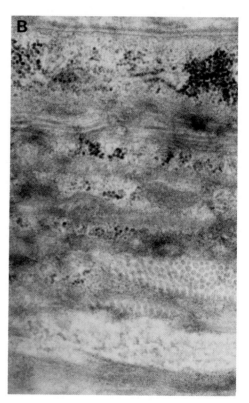

FIGURE 2. Electron micrographs of small segments of perineurium from control rats (A) and rats that had been diabetic for 10 weeks (B). Note the accumulation of glycogen (dark spots) in the perineurium from the diabetic animals. 37,000X.

EFFECT OF CALCIUM DEPLETION ON INCORPORATION OF ^{32}P INTO
SCIATIC NERVE PHOSPHOLIPIDS OF NORMAL AND DIABETIC ANIMALS

In view of the importance of Ca^{2+} in the maintenance of many membrane functions including nerve impulse transmission and the capacity of polyphosphoinositides to bind this ion and possibly to regulate Ca^{2+} flux, we examined the effects of lowering the level of Ca^{2+} in the sciatic nerve incubation medium on the incorporation pattern. Simply omitting Ca^{2+} from the medium had a negligible effect on the extent of labeling of individual phospholipids. However, when EGTA was also present, a marked alteration in the pattern of incorporated radioactivity resulted (TABLE 4). In incubations of normal nerves, the removal of Ca^{2+} caused a 67% increase in isotope incorporation into triphosphoinositide, a rise which was identical to that seen when diabetic nerve was incubated in Ca^{2+}-containing medium. Diphosphoinositide labeling was also stimulated. In contrast, the amount of isotope which entered phosphatidic acid fell by 60% and the labeling of phosphatidylinositol and phosphatidylcholine registered smaller decreases.

TABLE 4. Comparison of effects of calcium depletion and streptozotocin diabetes on incorporation of ^{32}P into phospholipids of rat sciatic nerve.

Lipid	Control		Diabetic	
	$+Ca^{2+}$	$-Ca^{2+}$	$+Ca^{2+}$	$-Ca^{2+}$
	nmol ^{32}P incorporated/g wet weight nerve			
Triphosphoinositide	35 ± 6	56 ± 4[a]	56 ± 7[b]	84 ± 14[a,b]
Diphosphoinositide	23 ± 2	39 ± 3[a]	27 ± 2	49 ± 4[a,b]
Phosphatidylinositol	36 ± 2	28 ± 2[a]	38 ± 2	27 ± 1[a]
Phosphatidic acid	42 ± 3	17 ± 1[a]	45 ± 2	21 ± 1[a]
Phosphatidylcholine	64 ± 3	48 ± 3[a]	67 ± 4	48 ± 3[a]
Other phospholipids	21 ± 1	18 ± 4	21 ± 1	17 ± 1

Incubations were performed as described in the legend to TABLE 1. To bring about Ca^{2+} depletion, the ion was omitted from the incubation medium and 2 mM EGTA was present. Nerves from diabetic animals were used two weeks after injection of streptozotocin. Values given as means of incubations ± S.E.M. Number of incubations: 8-12; number of rats: 4-6. [a]different from Ca^{2+} containing control [b]different from Ca^{2+} depleted control: p<0.005 based on number of incubations.

As previously noted, none of these phospholipids in diabetic nerve incubated in Ca^{2+}-containing medium except triphosphoinositide exhibited a change in isotope incorporation. Under conditions of Ca^{2+} depletion, diabetic nerves displayed a substantial further increase in the labeling of triphosphoinositide and a small increase in the quantity of isotope present in diphosphoinositide above that seen for normal nerve. The extent of labeling of other phospholipids was unchanged from that in Ca^{2+}-depleted controls.

INFLUENCE OF SORBINIL ON THE LABELING OF PHOSPHOLIPIDS IN NORMAL AND DIABETIC SCIATIC NERVE

Sorbinil (CP-45,634; d-6-fluoro-spiro(chroman-4,4'-imidazoline-2', 5'-dione) is a recently described uncompetitive inhibitor of aldose reductase(29). This drug when given to streptozotocin diabetic rats was reported to markedly lower the concentration in sciatic nerve of sorbitol which accumulates in peripheral nerve and other tissues due to excessive reduction of glucose via the polyol pathway. Moreover, 10 μM sorbinil almost completely prevented the accumulation of sorbitol which otherwise occurred when rat sciatic nerve was incubated with 50 mM glucose in vitro. Consequently, it was of interest to establish whether this compound was able to affect the metabolism of phospholipids in diabetic sciatic nerve.

As shown in TABLE 5, sorbinil had no effect on the labeling pattern of phospholipids in normal nerve incubated in medium which contained 5.5 mM glucose. In the case of nerve from diabetic animals, the

TABLE 5. Effect of sorbinil on the distribution of radioactive label in phospholipids of control and 10-week diabetic nerve

Lipid	Control		Diabetic	
	No Additions	Sorbinil (10 μM)	No Additions	Sorbinil (10 μM)
	% of ^{32}P incorporated into total phospholipids			
Triphosphoinositide	23 ± 3	22 ± 1	33 ± 3[a]	28 ± 1[b]
Diphosphoinositide	14 ± 3	12 ± 1	13 ± 1	11 ± 2
Phosphatidylinositol	11 ± 3	15 ± 0.5	13 ± 1	14 ± 0.5
Phosphatidic acid	14 ± 2	16 ± 0.5	15 ± 0.5	15 ± 1
Phosphatidylcholine	25 ± 1	24 ± 1	18 ± 2[a]	21 ± 1
Other phospholipids	13 ± 1	12 ± 2	10 ± 1	11 ± 1

Values are expressed as means ± S.E.M. determined from three to six incubations.

[a]Different from no addition control: p<0.005;

[b]Different from no addition diabetic: p<0.05.

proportion of label in triphosphoinositide rose nearly 50%, whereas that in phosphatidylcholine decreased by 25%. Both these effects appeared to be at least partially reversed when 10 µM sorbinil was present in the medium.

DISCUSSION

Current knowledge concerning polyphosphoinositides makes it attractive to postulate that metabolic transformations of these lipids are part of the molecular mechanism which underlies axonal conduction. In the brain, the portion of polyphosphoinositides associated with extra-myelin membranes appears metabolically more active than the bulk of these substances in myelin. Thus the fraction of these compounds in myelin-deficient regions undergoes the most rapid breakdown within minutes after death (15). In addition, polyphosphoinositide P equilibrates more rapidly with acid-soluble P in myelin-poor as compared to myelin-rich areas(12). It may be hypothesized that a discrete compartment of these compounds, presumably located in the axonal membrane, can undergo rapid metabolic turnover associated with cation movements during nerve impulse propagation. The results reported in this communication suggest that changes in the metabolism of triphosphoinositide phosphate groups in peripheral nerve occur in conjunction with reduced nerve conduction velocity in streptozotocin-induced diabetic neuropathy and that further studies employing this model may be useful in ascertaining whether polyphosphoinositides in fact play a role in axonal conduction.

The increased incorporation of ^{32}P into triphosphoinositide in diabetic nerve was invariably seen at all time intervals examined after the induction of diabetes. Natarajan et al.(27) have also reported changes in the metabolism of inositol-containing phospholipids in sciatic nerve from streptozotocin diabetic rats, but their results are substantially different from ours(2).

The biochemical mechanism responsible for the effect could involve either increased synthesis or decreased breakdown of triphospho-inositide and can only be elucidated by further experimentation. Examination of the activities of enzymes in the polyphosphoinositide metabolic pathways has thus far revealed a marginal decrease in diphosphoinositide kinase activity and no change in phospha-tidylinositol kinase and triphosphoinositide phosphomonoesterase activities in diabetic nerve (37). These results provide little basis for a plausible mechanism concerning the metabolic changes.

Since the labeling of sciatic nerve phospholipids is not affected by incubation in the presence of high glucose concentrations, it is likely that an elevated glucose level is not the immediate cause of alterations in phospholipid metabolism in diabetic nerve. Instead, gradual structural changes which irreversibly and adversely affect aspects of peripheral nerve function may accompany the appearance of abnormal polyphosphoinositide metabolism. In this connection, it is noteworthy that Dyck et al.(8) observed that production of acute hyperosmolar hyperglycemia in cats gave rise to axonal shrinkage and reduced nerve conduction velocity. The authors suggest that less elevated glucose concentrations may bring about these changes over a sufficiently long time span.

The accumulation of granules, tentatively identified as glycogen, in the perineureum and to a lesser extent in Schwann cells in tibial nerves from streptozotocin-diabetic animals constitutes a further abnormality associated with the disease. Whether or not the deposits are involved in either the reduction of conduction velocity or the changes in polyphosphoinositide metabolism remains to be investigated. However, it is possible that glycogen accumulation results from a metabolic derangement which could in turn affect the barrier function of perineurial and Schwann cells to ions and small molecules. The consequent alterations in endoneurial and axonal environments could have adverse effects on peripheral nerve function.

The well-documented accumulation of sorbitol in streptozotocin diabetic nerve may well be involved in one structural change, namely, the increase in endoneurial space which occurs as a consequence of a rise in nerve water content(19). Moreover, administration of aldose reductase inhibitors to galactose-fed rats delayed the onset of decreased peripheral nerve conduction velocity. The hypothesis that increased polyol pathway activity plays a role in the development of deficient nerve metabolism is consistent with our observation that addition of sorbinil to the incubation medium appeared to prevent in part the increase in triphosphoinositide labeling seen in diabetic nerve. However, a complete interpretation of this finding must await a demonstration that the aldose reductase inhibitor effectively reduces the level of previously accumulated sorbitol during incubation of diabetic nerve.

It may be noteworthy that Ca^{2+} depletion of normal nerve increased the incorporation of isotope into triphosphoinositide to the same extent seen in diabetic nerve incubated in complete medium. Since several enzymatic reactions in phosphoinositide metabolism either require or are affected by Ca^{2+}, this finding suggests that the availability of the ion might somehow be altered in nerves from diabetic animals. It is clear however that the removal of Ca^{2+} causes other changes which amount to a considerable disruption of the metabolism of other major phospholipids as well, alterations which are not observed in the disease state. Moreover, depletion of Ca^{2+} from diabetic nerve further increases the labeling of triphosphoinositide in an additive manner and this might mean that the effects of diabetic neuropathy and cation removal are independent. Nonetheless, it remains possible that the long-term changes in peripheral nerve as a consequence of diabetes could influence a specific Ca^{2+} compartment, perhaps that associated with the axonal membrane, which is not readily depleted by EGTA. In this regard, it would be desirable to determine whether the activity of triphosphoinositide phosphodiesterase, a Ca^{2+}-requiring enzyme, is reduced in diabetic nerve, since this would tend to cause an increase in labeled substrate.

Our results show that a normal concentration of triphosphoinositide was maintained in sciatic nerve from rats which had been diabetic for nearly 6 months. Hence the observed metabolic alterations are not likely to be associated with a gross disturbance of the bulk of this predominantly myelin-associated lipid and could be restricted to a small fraction which continues to be rapidly renewed in vitro.

Finally, although an abnormality in peripheral triphosphoinositide metabolism appears to be a characteristic early feature of chronic streptozotocin diabetes, it may not be unique to this disorder. Thus an increase in the specific radioactivity of $[^{32}P]$-triphosphoinositide in chicken sciatic nerve in vivo was seen starting 24 hours after the administration of tri-orthocresyl phosphate to the animals(30). The organophosphorus compound failed to affect the metabolism of other phospholipids. This observation taken together with our findings suggests that alterations in triphosphoinositide metabolism may be a sensitive indicator of abnormal nerve function in more than one neuropathy.

Acknowledgements

We wish to thank Mr. Ioannis Galetas for expert technical assistance and Mr. C. A. Harrington for performing triphosphoinositide determinations. This work was supported by NIH grants NS-12493, RR-07147 and RR-0531, Grant E-675 from Robert A. Welch Foundation and a grant from the American Diabetes Association.

REFERENCES

1. Akhtar, R. A. and Abdel-Latif, A. A. (1978): J. Pharmacol. Exp. Ther., 204:655-668.
2. Bell, M. E., Peterson, R. G., and Eichberg, J. J. Neurochem (in press).
3. Birnberger, A. C., Birnberger, K. L., Eliasson, S. G., and Simpson, P. C. (1971): J. Neurochem., 18:1291-1298.
4. Bisby, M. A. (1980): Exp. Neurol. 69:74-84.
5. Buckley, J. T. and Hawthorne, J. N. (1972): J. Biol. Chem. 247:7218-7223.
6. Clements, R. S., Jr. (1979): Diabetes 28:604-611.
7. Clements, R. S., Jr. and Stockard, C. R. (1980): Diabetes 29: 227-235.
8. Dyck, P. J., Lambert, E. H., Windebank, A. J., Lais, A. A., Sparks, M. F., Karnes, J., Sherman, W. R., Hallcher, L. M., Low, P. A., and Service, F. J. (1981): Exp. Neurol. 71:507-514.
9. Eichberg, J. and Dawson, R. M. C. (1965): Biochem. J. 96: 644-650.
10. Eichberg, J. and Hauser, G. (1973): Biochim. Biophys. Acta. 326:210-223.
11. Gabbay, K. H. (1973): In: Vascular and Neurological Changes in Early Diabetes, edited by R. A. Camenni-Davalos and H. S. Cole, pp. 417-432. Academic Press, New York.
12. Gonzalez-Sastre, F., Eichberg, J., and Hauser, G. (1971): Biochim. Biophys. Acta. 248:96-104.

13. Greene, D. A., De Jesus, P. V., Jr., and Winegrad, A. (1975): J. Clin. Invest. 55:1325-1336.
14. Harrington, C. A., Fenimore, D. C., and Eichberg, J. (1980): Anal. Biochem. 106:307-313.
15. Hauser, G., Gonzalez-Sastre, F., and Eichberg, J. (1971): Biochim. Biophys. Acta. 248:87-95.
16. Hawthorne, J. N. and Kai, M. (1970): In: Handbook of Neurochemistry, edited by A. Lajtha, volume 3, pp. 491-508. Plenum Press, New York.
17. Hendrickson, H. S. and Reinertson, J. L. (1971): Biochem. Biophys. Res. Commun. 44:1258-1264.
18. Hothersall, J. S. and McLean, P. (1979): Biochem. Biophys. Res. Commun. 88:477-484.
19. Jakobsen, J. (1978): Diabetologia 14:113-119.
20. Kai, M. and Hawthorne, J. N. (1969): Ann. N.Y. Acad. Sci. 165 Art. 2: 761-773.
21. Kumara-Siri, M. H. and Gould, R. M. (1980): Brain Res. 180: 315-330.
22. Kundu, S. S., Chakravarty, S., Bhaduri, N., and Saha, H. K. (1977): J. Lipid Res. 18:128-130.
23. Michell, R. H. (1975): Biochim. Biophys. Acta. 415:81-147.
24. Michell, R. H. and Kirk, C. J. (1981): Trends Pharmacol. Sci. 2:86-90.
25. Moore, S. A., Peterson, R. G., Felten, D. L., and O'Connor, B. L. (1980): J. Neurol. Sci. 48:133-152.
26. Moore, S. A., Peterson, R. G., Felten, D. L., and O'Connor, B. L. (1981): J. Neurol Sci. 32:289-303.
27. Natarajan, V., Dyck, P. J., and Schmid, H. H. O. (1981): J. Neurochem. 36:413-419.
28. Palmano, K. P., Whiting, P. H., and Hawthorne, J. N. (1977): Biochem. J. 167:229-235.
29. Peterson, M. J., Sarges, R., Aldinger, C. E., and MacDonald, D. P. (1979): Metabolism 28:456-461.
30. Sheltawy, A. and Dawson, R. M. C. (1969): Biochem. J. 111:157-165.
31. Spritz, N., Singh, H., and Marinan, B. (1975): J. Clin. Invest. 55:1049-1056.
32. Spritz, N., Singh, H., and Marinan, B. (1975): Diabetes 24:680-683.
33. Stewart, M. A., Sherman, W. R., Kunen, M. M., Moonsammy, G. I., and Wisgerhof, M. (1967): J. Neurochem. 14:1057-1066.
34. Tret'jak, A. G., Limatenko, I. M., Kossova, G. V., Gulak, P. V., and Kozlov, Yu. P. (1977): J. Neurochem. 28:199-205.
35. White, G. L., Schellhase, H. U., and Hawthorne, J. N. (1974): J. Neurochem. 22:149-158.
36. Whiting, P. H., Bowley, M., Sturton, R. G., Pritchard, P. H., Brindley, D. N., and Hawthorne, J. N. (1977): Biochem. J. 168:147-153.
37. Whiting, P. H., Palmano, K. P., and Hawthorne, J. N. (1979): Biochem. J. 179:549-553.

Phospholipids in the Nervous System, Vol. 1:
Metabolism, edited by L. Horrocks, et al. Raven
Press, New York © 1982.

Effects of Propranolol and Other Cationic Amphiphilic Drugs on Phospholipid Metabolism

George Hauser and *Anuradha S. Pappu

Ralph Lowell Laboratories, Mailman Research Center, McLean Hospital, Belmont, Massachusetts 02178, and Department of Biological Chemistry, Harvard Medical School, Boston, Massachusetts 02115

In the course of studying the nature of the receptors involved in the stimulation of phospholipid metabolism in rat pineal gland by norepinephrine, we discovered that propranolol, which we were using as a β-receptor blocking agent, had a characteristic effect on the incorporation of $^{32}P_i$ (18,19). In contrast to the norepinephrine-induced alterations of the phospholipid labeling pattern, this effect turned out not to be stereospecific (19) or mediated through α-receptors, as shown through the inability of α-receptor blocking agents to prevent its occurrence (26). In pursuing these observations in pineal glands, we noted particularly an accumulation of phosphatidyl-CMP, the liponucleotide intermediate for phosphatidylinositol (PhI) and phosphatidylglycerol (PhG) biosynthesis (15,24,25), increased incorporation of $^{32}P_i$ into acidic phospholipids as well as a pronounced decrease in labeling of phosphatidylcholine (PhC) and -ethanolamine (PhE). These studies have been published during the past several years (15-19,24-26,42,43).

Similar investigations with propranolol and a number of other compounds in peripheral tissues have been reported and reveal an analogous redirection of phospholipid metabolism from neutral into acidic compounds (1-3,10). However, information on the response to the action of these drugs by the phospholipid metabolism of nervous tissue in vitro is scarce (5,6,30,42,43).

CHARACTERISTICS OF PHOSPHOLIPIDOSIS INDUCED BY CATIONIC AMPHIPHILIC DRUGS

Propranolol can be considered to belong to a group of substances which share the characteristics of being cationic amphiphilic drugs (CADs). They possess a hydrophobic region consisting of an aromatic ring or ring system and a hydrophilic region which usually is a short side chain with a positively charged amino nitrogen. They have pK_as considerably above 7.4 so that they are mostly in the protonated form at physiological pH. Although a number of experimental compounds have been used in studies with CADs, most of them have clinical applications covering a wide variety of conditions. Thus they include drugs used as anorectics, antianginals, antihistaminics, antimalarials, antirheumatics and cholesterol synthesis inhibitors as well as antidepressants and neuroleptics.

Present address of A.S.P.: Veterans Administration Hospital, La Jolla, California 92161.

The reason that CADs have aroused the interest of the clinician, apart from their therapeutic efficacy, is the observation that chronic treatment with some of these drugs can lead to a phospholipidosis and to characteristic cellular lesions (for detailed reviews and references, see 9, 14,35,37). These lesions, which can also be induced in experimental animals by treatment with the same drugs and also with a considerable number of other CADs, can occur in peripheral as well as nervous tissues (14). They consist of membrane-bound cytoplasmic inclusion bodies of either lamellated or crystalline-like structure having the biochemical and morphological characteristics of secondary lysosomes. Cytochemical studies have shown the presence of acid phosphatase in these inclusions and have contributed to the identification of the accumulated material as largely phospholipids. Cellular phospholipid content can rise up to fourfold, but the excess material is exclusively concentrated in the inclusion bodies which increase in size with continued treatment and can reach diameters greater than 10 μm. The pattern of the stored phospholipids varies with the drug, the tissue and the animal species, but PhC is usually the most prominent class, just as it is in normal cells. Bis(monoacylglycero)phosphate, suggested to occur typically in lysosomes (12,52), is usually present in markedly elevated amounts. The lamellar or crystalloid nature of the inclusion bodies may be determined by the phase preference of the accumulated lipid which, in vitro, may assume either a lamellated or hexagonal (H_{II} phase) pattern. Together with the phospholipids the administered drug is concentrated in the lysosomes. When the drug is discontinued, the lipid and drug accumulation gradually disappears, although the reversal and cessation of symptoms in humans may take several months.

CATIONIC DRUG EFFECTS ON PHOSPHOLIPID METABOLISM IN RAT TISSUE MINCES

Propranolol does not fall into the group of CADs capable of causing lysosomal phospholipidosis as a result of chronic treatment. This may be the result of relatively rapid metabolic transformation and elimination of the drug. In the rat propranolol is cleared from blood with a half time of about an hour, although it can persist in certain brain regions up to seven times as long (7) (Table 1). However, the accumulation, and the levels at any time point after injection, are about an order of magnitude higher in brain than in blood or liver (21).

TABLE 1. Clearance of (±)propranolol from rat brain

Tissue	$t_{1/2}$ (min)
Blood, whole brain, anterior cortex, hippocampus, amygdala	52- 71
Hypothalamus	149-174
Medulla	385-440

5 mg propranolol/kg were injected i.v. Tissue levels were measured by gas-liquid chromatography. From Elghozi et al. (21).

Alteration by Propranolol of Precursor Incorporation Patterns

Despite the prompt removal of propranolol from tissues in vivo, its ability to alter phospholipid metabolism, observed previously in pineal gland (18,19), iris smooth muscle (1,2) and retina (5,6), is also manifest in cerebral cortex (27). In labeling studies with $^{32}P_i$ the most prominent changes in phospholipids, extractable with neutral solvents, in a mince prepared from cerebral cortex slices are an increase in phosphatidic acid (PhA) and a decrease in PhC (Fig. 1A). Total incorporation is more than doubled, a high percentage of the incorporation occurring in polyphosphoinositides (PPI), as discussed in greater detail below. A deficiency of water-soluble precursors does not appear to be involved in these effects (42).

That the stimulation of lipid metabolism involves increased <u>de novo</u> synthesis, rather than merely enhanced turnover as do the receptor-mediated changes, is seen in experiments with [2-^{3}H]glycerol as precursor (Fig. 1B). Here too total incorporation is doubled and analogous changes in the incorporation of radioactivity into acidic, most prominently PhA, and neutral phospholipids are obtained.

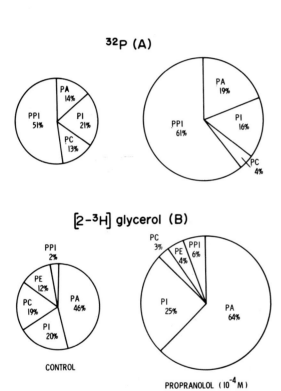

FIG. 1. Isotope distribution patterns in cerebral cortex phospholipids. The sources of materials and the methods for preparing rat tissue minces, incubations with isotope, extraction of lipids with neutral and acidified solvents, washing of lipid extracts, separation of lipids by thin-layer chromatography, identification of phospholipid-containing areas by radioautography and counting of phospholipid classes have been described in previous publications (23,42,49) and are identical for this figure and subsequent figures and tables. Data were normalized to 10^7 cpm of isotope added to the medium.

The area of the circles represents the total incorporation which was, in cpm x 10^{-3}/10 mg mince/hr, for ^{32}P (A): 31 ± 2 without and 67 ± 5 with propranolol; for [2-^{3}H]glycerol (B): 29 ± 1 without and 62 ± 1 with propranolol. (±)propranolol·HCl was 0.1 mM. The percentages of incorporation are means from 12 incubations; standard deviations were in general less than 10%.

In contrast with cerebral cortex, the bulk of the incorporation of $^{32}P_i$ in rat kidney cortex mince is into PhC (Fig. 2A). Propranolol addition results in only a small increase in total incorporation but alters the incorporation pattern. In this case the increased labeling appears in PhI, whereas the percentage of radioactivity in PhC is reduced by one-third. In liver mince, on the other hand, the two neutral phospholipids, PhC and PhE, are labeled equally, and the decrease in both brought about by propranolol is substantial (Fig. 2B). A fourfold increase in PhA labeling also results. From the data on these tissues as well as on others (pineal, iris, retina), it appears that the most consistent finding is a shift in the incorporation pattern away from neutral and into acidic phospholipids. However, the phospholipid class in which radioactivity accumulates probably depends on the metabolic capabilities of the individual tissues.

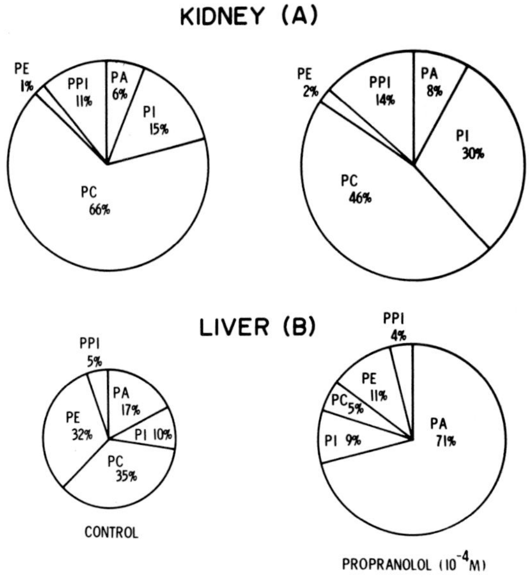

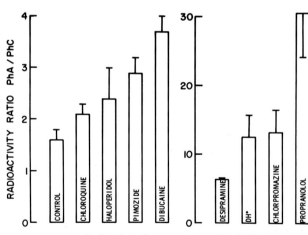

KIDNEY (A)

FIG. 2. Isotope distribution patterns in kidney and liver phospholipids. Kidney (A) or liver (B) mince (10 mg) was incubated with $^{32}P_i$. Basal incorporation in cpm x 10^{-3} was 181 ± 27 in kidney and 7 ± 3 in liver. The area of the circles represents the relative total incorporation in basal and 0.1 mM propranolol-containing incubations. The percentages of incorporation are means from six incubations; standard deviations were 10% or less except up to 20% for PPI.

FIG. 3. Relative potencies of CADs. Results are the mean ratios of $^{32}P_i$ incorporated into PhA and PhC in incubations of cerebral cortex minces from three determinations ± S.D. All drugs were 0.2 mM. *4,4'-bis(diethylaminoethoxy)α,β-diethyldiphenylethane.

Relative Potencies of Different Cationic Drugs

In view of the characteristic changes in phospholipid metabolism induced by propranolol, the radioactivity ratio PhA/PhC seems a useful indication of the potential of a given compound to induce phospholipidosis. When a number of CADs with varied clinical uses were screened to determine their ability to alter labeling patterns, chloroquine, haloperidol and pimozide changed the ratio relatively little. Dibucaine and desmethylimipramine were of intermediate effectiveness, and 4,4'-bis(diethylaminoethoxy)α,β-diethyldiphenylethane and chlorpromazine were markedly more potent, but propranolol was the compound with the highest potency among those tested (Fig. 3). Among several other CADs, none shifted phospholipid metabolism as much as did propranolol (42).

Effects on Phosphoinositide Metabolism

In our original studies we examined only phospholipids which could be extracted with neutral chloroform-methanol. Radioautograms of two-dimensional thin-layer chromatograms of the washed lipid extract showed a substantial unidentified radioactive area near the origin which was eventually identified through chromatographic and chemical techniques as being due to PPI with phosphatidylinositol-4-phosphate (PhIP) predominating (43). This was traced to the fact that, owing to the nature of the tissue preparation, the extracted residue was not removed before equilibration of the lipid extract with dilute aqueous HCl. Using acidified solvents for extractions (23), we found that with $^{32}P_i$ as precursor half of the incorporation occurred in PPI and was increased further in the presence of propranolol (Fig. 1A), another characteristic of the action of the drug in cerebral cortex. Similar stimulation was seen in minces from other brain areas (brain stem, hypothalamus), but not from peripheral tissues (kidney, liver, lung) (Figs. 2, 4), where a much smaller percentage of the incorporated radioactivity appeared in PPI.

Although very little label of [2-^{3}H]glycerol went into PPI, the stimulation by propranolol could nonetheless be obtained (Fig. 1B). A measure of drug effectiveness, similar to the PhA/PhC radioactivity ratio, is that for PPI/PhI. When [2-^{3}H]inositol was used as precursor, the ratio changed by a factor of 3 upon addition of propranolol to the cortex mince incubation mixture. When several CADs were screened by this criterion, their order of potency was not appreciably different from that given by the earlier measure discussed above (Fig. 5).

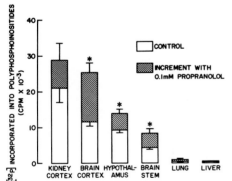

FIG. 4. Propranolol effect on polyphosphoinositide labeling in vitro. After incubation of tissue minces with $^{32}P_i$ neutral and acidified solvent extracts were obtained and washed. PPI were separated on silica gel HL (Analtech) or 60 (Merck) thin-layer plates using the solvent system chloroform-methanol-conc. NH₄OH-water (45:45:11:5.5, by volume). Means ± S.D. from three incubations are shown. * = significant increase, P < 0.02.

Pulse-Chase Experiments

In order to determine whether the effect of the drug is primarily on biosynthetic or degradative reactions, cerebral cortex minces were pulse labeled with $^{32}P_i$ or [2-^{3}H]glycerol, thoroughly washed and reincubated with or without propranolol. Although unlabeled precursor was present during the washing and chase, some additional incorporation took place during the second incubation. Propranolol caused either an increase in label in PhA (Fig. 6) and PPI (41) or a diminished decrease. In contrast, it reduced radioactivity in PhC compared with control, in line with expectations based on earlier results. These experiments led to the conclusion that the action of propranolol is largely an inhibition of acidic phospholipid breakdown which is consonant with the observation in other tissues and that described further on, that phosphatidate phosphohydrolase action is impaired by the drug (3,11,15,16,32,50).

PROPRANOLOL EFFECT ON ^{32}P INCORPORATION AFTER TREATMENT WITH PHOSPHOLIPASES

The integrity of the cell membrane may be an essential factor in permitting the entry both of drug and of radioactive precursor and may also serve to control some of the metabolic reactions insofar as they are localized in this membrane. Further, CADs are known to stabilize membranes (discussed in 9). In an attempt to obtain information on the effect of altering lipid constituents located in the external leaflet, cerebral cortex minces were treated with phospholipases before being incubated with ^{32}P$_i$ and propranolol (Table 2).

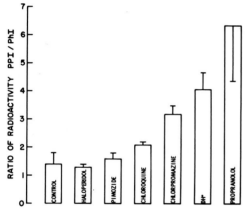

FIG. 5. Effects of CADs on phosphoinositide biosynthesis. Results are the mean ratios of ^{32}P$_i$ incorporated into total PPI and PhI in incubations of cerebral cortex minces ± S.D. from three determinations. All drugs were 0.2 mM. *4,4'-(bis)-diethylaminoethoxy)α,β-diethyldiphenylethane.

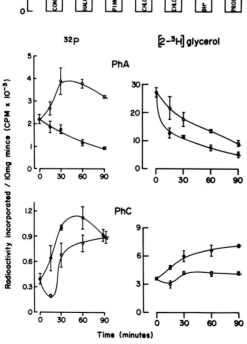

FIG. 6. Pulse-chase experiments. Cerebral cortex mince was labeled for 15 min with 10 µCi of ^{32}P$_i$ or 20 µCi of [2-^{3}H]glycerol per mg tissue, washed three times with ice-cold medium containing 2 mM precursor and reincubated in the same medium, including precursor, with or without 0.1 mM propranolol. The zero time point indicates the amount of radioactivity in the washed mince before the second incubation. Results are means ± S.D. from three determinations. ● = control; o = propranolol. Adapted from (42) and reproduced by permission of the copyright owner, the International Society for Neurochemistry.

TABLE 2. Effect of propranolol on ^{32}Pi incorporation into phospholipids of brain cortex mince treated with phospholipases

Conditions		PhA	PhC	PhI	PPI	Total
		(^{32}Pi incorporated [cpm x 10^{-3}/10 mg mince])				
No enzyme, pH 8.0	Control	3.5 ± 1.0	2.8 ± 0.8	4.2 ± 0.8	11.2 ± 3.0	22.1 ± 4.8
	Propranolol	11.5 ± 1.0[a]	1.8 ± 0.2[a]	7.5 ± 0.6[a]	25.3 ± 0.8[a]	46.3 ± 0.9[a]
Phospholipase A$_2$	Control	1.5 ± 0.0	0.3 ± 0.1	0.8 ± 0.1	5.4 ± 0.3	8.1 ± 0.4
	Propranolol	5.6 ± 0.8[a]	0.1 ± 0.1[a]	1.9 ± 0.2[a]	11.7 ± 1.2[a]	19.2 ± 2.2[a]
No enzyme, pH 7.4	Control	4.6 ± 0.3	4.4 ± 0.7	5.7 ± 0.7	14.1 ± 3.1	29.4 ± 3.8
	Propranolol	8.0 ± 1.0[a]	2.0 ± 1.0[a]	5.0 ± 0.4	21.8 ± 2.0[a]	37.2 ± 1.1[a]
Phospholipase C	Control	4.4 ± 0.7	4.1 ± 0.4	5.5 ± 1.1	19.8 ± 3.9	34.4 ± 5.3
	Propranolol	13.0 ± 2.7[a]	2.2 ± 0.6[a]	8.4 ± 1.2[a]	38.7 ± 5.3[a]	62.6 ± 9.3[a]
No enzyme, pH 7.4	Control	6.2 ± 0.5	7.4 ± 0.8	5.2 ± 1.7	9.8 ± 0.6	28.6 ± 2.2
	Propranolol	8.0 ± 0.7[a]	2.1 ± 0.6[a]	6.5 ± 1.8	12.9 ± 2.5[a]	29.5 ± 1.2
PhI-specific phospholipase C	Control	7.2 ± 0.7	7.4 ± 1.5	5.4 ± 0.6	11.0 ± 1.1	31.0 ± 2.4
	Propranolol	15.6 ± 1.6[a]	4.3 ± 0.6[a]	11.8 ± 2.3[a]	17.9 ± 2.7[a]	49.6 ± 6.8[a]
No enzyme, pH 6.5	Control	6.8 ± 1.6	8.8 ± 2.1	8.5 ± 0.3	15.1 ± 4.8	39.7 ± 8.2
	Propranolol	14.2 ± 3.0[a]	2.6 ± 0.2[a]	8.8 ± 0.3	28.5 ± 4.7[a]	54.6 ± 6.2[a]
Phospholipase D	Control	8.5 ± 0.5	11.2 ± 0.5	11.7 ± 0.6	17.9 ± 0.6	50.1 ± 0.8
	Propranolol	14.8 ± 3.4[a]	2.3 ± 0.3[a]	7.8 ± 1.8[a]	29.4 ± 2.1[a]	54.3 ± 4.6

Rat brain mince (120 mg) was incubated with enzymes for 30 min at 37° as follows: phospholipase A$_2$ from Naja naja venom (0.05 units) at pH 8; phospholipase C from C. perfringens (0.05 units) at pH 7.4; PhI-specific phospholipase C from S. aureus (30 μg) at pH 7.4; phospholipase D from cabbage (3 units) at pH 6.5. Control tissue was incubated in parallel without enzyme at the same pH. After the first incubation the mince was washed twice with cold HEPES-buffered medium (pH 7.4), resuspended and 10 mg per tube were incubated in the same medium containing 5-10 μCi of ^{32}P$_i$ for 60 min at 37°. Propranolol was 0.1 mM. The results are means ± S.D. from three to six determinations.

[a] P < 0.05 compared with corresponding control.

Mild treatment of brain cortex with a low concentration of phospholipase A_2 from snake venom which yields lysophospholipid with detergent
properties decreased the ability of the mince to incorporate $^{32}P_i$ into
total phospholipids markedly and caused some shift in the labeling pattern. It had no effect on the direction of the propranolol-induced
changes. There were no similarities between lipid alterations brought
about by the enzyme and propranolol, suggesting that the effect of the
drug is not mediated by activation of membrane-bound phospholipase A_2.
The enzyme does, however, cause considerable disruption of the membrane,
and the free fatty acids liberated may inhibit oxidative phosphorylation
and thus account for the lower isotope incorporation.

Phospholipase C from C. perfringens splits only PhC and PhE into phos-
phorylester and diacylglycerol (DAG); the latter remains in the membrane
and the former dissolves in the aqueous medium. Incubation of the cerebral cortex mince with low concentrations of the enzyme had virtually no
effect on the $^{32}P_i$ incorporation total or pattern. A combination of enzyme treatment and propranolol increased the labeling in acidic lipids
much more than propranolol alone, possibly owing to the greater availability of DAG within the membrane and the presence of an active DAG
kinase.

A similar amplification of the propranolol effect was caused by treatment with PhI-specific phospholipase C from S. aureus, even though PhI
constitutes only about 5% of the membrane phospholipids. It is unlikely
that in this instance the observed magnification is due to the liberated
DAG. In both cases of phospholipase C action the isotope may be gaining
access to the cell interior more readily and be available for phosphorylation reactions resulting from the presence of propranolol. Despite possibly higher levels of DAG, PhC labeling was reduced as it was in untreated tissues.

Phospholipase D from cabbage converts phospholipids into PhA and
water-soluble base, thereby conferring a more negative charge on the
phospholipids. Mild phospholipase-D treatment increased the ability of
the mince to incorporate $^{32}P_i$ into phospholipids somewhat, without altering the labeling pattern. Incubation with enzyme probably enhances the
availability of PhA for lipid biosynthesis, but propranolol did not ele-
vate the total radioactivity incorporated nor change the characteristic
labeling pattern despite the added PhA available.

In light of these findings, further modifications of the cell surface
with phospholipases and other enzymes may prove fruitful in contributing
to the clarification of the typical CAD effects.

$^{32}P_i$ INCORPORATION IN VITRO AFTER PROPRANOLOL INJECTIONS

With the intent of examining the possible clinical implications of the
redirection of phospholipid metabolism, a number of experiments were carried out in which minces were prepared and incubated with $^{32}P_i$ at various
times after injections of propranolol into rats (Table 3). The maximal
decrease in total incorporation was seen when 15 mg/kg were given and the
animals were used 0.5-1.5 hr later, but no effect on the total incorporation or the pattern was obtained in young animals. By 3 hours in rats
weighing 300 g or more, incorporation was the same as in sham-injected
controls. Raising the dose to 45 mg/kg did not result in a further decrease of incorporation, but the distribution of ^{32}P was shifted progressively towards acidic lipids (40).

When multiple injections at a lower dose were used over a period of
several days, total incorporation was lower, but changes in pattern were

small and a decrease in percent labeling of PhC was notably absent (Table 3). At 15 mg/kg, given repeatedly, the effects seen a half hour after a single injection were not extended to 5 hr as might have been expected if a build-up of drug in cerebral cortex occurs with chronic treatment.

In peripheral tissues, propranolol injections lowered the ability of kidney mince to incorporate $^{32}P_i$ into phospholipids, altering the pattern only at high doses (45 mg/kg). Liver mince, at this dose, showed reduction in total labeling without variations in individual phospholipids.* Liver and kidney have a low capacity to concentrate and retain propranolol, as compared with brain (7,45).

The time course of total incorporation into cerebral cortex mince is parallel with the levels of propranolol in brain after injection, although different regions apparently clear the drug at different rates (Table 1). In young animals this may happen at even greater speed and thus account for the failure to see any remaining propranolol effect even as early as one-half hour after injection.

The reduction in total label incorporated seems to precede changes in labeling pattern as evidenced by the dose-response curves both in brain and in peripheral tissues.* It may be due to an effect of propranolol in lowering the cerebral metabolic rate, resulting in decreased availability of ATP and intermediates for phospholipid biosynthesis (29).

The relatively less pronounced changes in phospholipid metabolism after propranolol injection as compared with those after addition of the drug in vitro can thus be ascribed to the pharmacodynamics of the compound. The relative susceptibility of the tissues is in agreement with the distribution of the drug, and the findings after multiple injections are consonant with only a gradual increase in tissue concentration (45) and hence capacity to affect metabolic processes. Since the effects are readily reversible as drug disappears from the tissues, no permanent adverse effects would be expected even on prolonged treatment with propranolol. However, the high doses used over long periods in the treatment of schizophrenia (44,48) can lead to abnormalities in phospholipid metabolism, especially in older patients and those with impaired liver function and thus lowered drug metabolizing ability. This may in part be responsible for some of the toxic side effects that have been observed (4,54). It would be prudent to bear this possibility in mind.

EXPERIMENTS BEARING ON THE MECHANISM OF THE EFFECT

The descriptive discussion of the data has emphasized that cationic amphiphilic drugs in general and propranolol in particular can cause specific and characteristic dislocations of phospholipid metabolism. It is not clear to date from experiments in our laboratory or by others by what mechanism the compounds in question achieve these particular consequences. Some approaches are detailed below.

Incorporation of $^{32}P_i$ in Brain Cortex Homogenates

In view of the changes in total incorporation induced by propranolol it was of interest to examine whether they are due to an influence on the cell membrane or on enzymatic reactions. When homogenates rather than minces were incubated under identical conditions, considerably less radioactivity was incorporated into phospholipids, and, in addition, propranolol did not cause increased labeling (Table 4). The basal

*Pappu, A.S. and Hauser, G., submitted for publication.

TABLE 3. ^{32}Pi incorporation into phospholipids of brain cortex mince after propranolol injections

Age of rats	Propranolol injected i.p.	Total radio-activity incorporated	PhA	PhC	PhI	PPI
		(cpm x 10^{-3}/10 mg mince^a/h)		(percent)		
5-6 weeks	none	29.8 ± 0.3	17.1 ± 1.3	18.2 ± 0.8	24.7 ± 0.2	37.8 ± 1.5
	15 mg/kg	32.2 ± 5.3	18.4 ± 0.7	17.3 ± 0.4	25.6 ± 1.1	37.9 ± 2.0
>6 months	none	15.5 ± 1.5	21.2 ± 1.6	11.6 ± 1.5	22.0 ± 1.1	43.5 ± 2.5
	15 mg/kg$_b$	7.5 ± 0.3^c	23.8 ± 1.2	5.8 ± 1.0^c	17.0 ± 3.1^c	56.4 ± 1.1^c
	15 mg/kg^b	16.5 ± 0.3	21.6 ± 0.8	10.6 ± 0.8	21.1 ± 1.2	44.8 ± 1.5
	15 mg/kg, once daily, 4 days$_b$	14.4 ± 1.9	20.5 ± 0.6	13.1 ± 1.1	19.2 ± 1.1	45.5 ± 2.3
	7.5 mg/kg, twice daily, 8 days	6.7 ± 2.2^c	27.7 ± 0.5^c	10.2 ± 1.9	18.9 ± 1.2^c	42.9 ± 4.1

^{a}Cerebral cortex mince was prepared 0.5 h after injection, except where (^{b}) indicates that 5 hr were allowed to elapse. The results are means ± S.D. from six determinations.

^{c}P < 0.05 compared with corresponding control.

TABLE 4. Effect of homogenization of mince on propranolol-induced alterations of brain cortex phospholipid labeling

Conditions	Total radio-activity incorporated	PhA	PhC	PhE	PhI	PPI
	(cpm x 10^{-3}/10 mg tissue/h)			(percent)		
Control	6.9 ± 0.5	39.8 ± 1.7	2.5 ± 0.4	0.7 ± 0.2	9.9 ± 0.3	47.0 ± 1.6
Propranolol	7.8 ± 0.5	34.6 ± 1.1^a	0.8 ± 0.2^a	0.3 ± 0.1^a	5.2 ± 0.3^a	59.0 ± 1.7^a
No Ca^{2+} + EGTA	10.9 ± 0.5	17.8 ± 0.6	1.6 ± 0.1	0.3 ± 0.1	5.1 ± 0.1	75.1 ± 0.6
No Ca^{2+} + EGTA and propranolol	10.9 ± 1.5	20.2 ± 1.5^a	0.3 ± 0.1^a	0.1 ± 0.0^a	3.4 ± 0.3^a	75.8 ± 1.7

^{a}P < 0.01 compared with corresponding control.

Rat brain homogenate was prepared in the incubation medium with a Potter-Elvehjem homogenizer at a concentration of 40 mg tissue/ml. Ca^{2+}, EGTA, and propranolol, when added, were respectively 2.5 mM, 0.2 mM and 0.1 mM. Incubations were identical with those of minces. The results are means ± S.D. from three determinations.

distribution of isotope was different with increased amounts appearing in PhA at the expense of PhC and PhI. Reduction in neutral phospholipids and elevation in PPI did occur in response to drug addition and is therefore not contingent upon an intact plasma membrane. The extent of labeling does, however, seem to be regulated by the entry of precursor which in turn seems to be affected by cationic drug action. How permeability is modified in membranes said to be stabilized (47) is unclear.

Modification of Calcium Levels

Since the cationic group of propranolol can compete for cation binding sites, displace membrane-bound Ca^{2+} (22,39) and interfere with cellular Ca^{2+} pools which in turn regulate a number of cellular events, incubations were modified so as to change calcium fluxes and availability. This was done in an effort to detect to what extent disturbances of normal calcium levels are involved in the action of propranolol and included elevated extracellular calcium, addition of ionophore A23187, verapamil which blocks calcium influx, or veratridine which causes membrane depolarization followed by calcium influx, as well as omission of calcium with or without added EGTA. Some of these conditions caused specific changes either in total incorporation or in the labeling pattern (Table 5). However, in each instance propranolol inclusion produced the characteristic decrease in the labeling of neutral phospholipids and an increase in PhA (except in PPI with veratridine). A shift from phosphatidylinositol-4,5-bisphosphate towards phosphatidylinositol-4-phosphate occurred with propranolol when calcium displacement was facilitated by EGTA or ionophore. Thus whatever dislocations of calcium metabolism were induced by the manipulations employed, none was by itself able to produce a shift as did propranolol or to prevent the interference of the drug with phospholipid metabolism.

When the conceivably confounding influence of the plasma membrane and hence of calcium fluxes was removed by homogenization, and calcium levels were reduced with EGTA, propranolol still significantly reduced incorporation into neutral lipids and increased that into PhA (Table 4). It is noteworthy that under these conditions three-quarters of the $^{32}P_i$ appeared in PPI.

Propranolol Effects on Phosphatidate Phosphohydrolase

As mentioned earlier, in pineal gland and in liver cationic drugs, including propranolol, have been found to be able to inhibit phosphatidate phosphohydrolase (3,11,15,32,50), which provides at least a partial explanation for the observations made in isotope incorporation experiments. In the present studies with brain tissue, propranolol was similarly tested to see whether this inhibition is a general phenomenon. Indeed progressive reduction of activity of the soluble brain enzyme occurred with increasing drug concentration and was virtually complete at 0.1 mM (Fig. 7).

From these data it was not certain whether propranolol formed an ionic complex with PhA which was resistant to enzyme attack or whether it inactivated the enzyme directly. To address this question, membrane-bound, ^{32}P-labeled PhA was exposed to the enzyme in the cytosolic fraction of cerebral cortex mince which had been incubated with or without propranolol. No difference was seen in the extent of hydrolysis by the two enzyme preparations (Table 6). In contrast, if the substrate was derived

TABLE 5. Effects of altered calcium availability on ^{32}Pi incorporation into phospholipids of brain cortex mince

Conditions	Total radio- activity incorporated (cpm × 10^{-4}/10 mg mince/h)	PhA	PhC (percent)	PhE	PhI	PPI	Ratio of radioactivity PhIP[b]/PhIPP
Control	3.1 ± 0.2	14.0 ± 0.3	12.5 ± 0.4	1.4 ± 0.1	21.2 ± 3.9	50.9 ± 1.7	2.2 ± 0.2
Propranolol	6.7 ± 0.5[a]	18.9 ± 0.9[a]	3.7 ± 0.4[a]	0.3 ± 0.1[a]	16.1 ± 2.0	61.0 ± 2.3[a]	2.5 ± 0.5
Ionophore A23187	2.4 ± 0.2	25.4 ± 2.3	13.0 ± 0.9	0.9 ± 0.2	18.1 ± 1.3	42.6 ± 2.2	1.9 ± 0.5
Ionophore A23187 + Pr[c]	2.6 ± 0.3	34.6 ± 1.0[a]	6.2 ± 0.7[a]	0.3 ± 0.1[a]	21.1 ± 2.0	37.8 ± 4.5	4.7 ± 0.3[a]
Ca^{2+} (10 mM)	3.1 ± 0.2	12.9 ± 0.7	15.4 ± 3.6	1.4 ± 0.0	19.1 ± 1.7	51.2 ± 5.0	1.7 ± 0.2
Ca^{2+} (10 mM) + Pr	5.7 ± 0.3[a]	21.6 ± 0.9[a]	5.8 ± 0.6[a]	0.1 ± 0.0[a]	16.9 ± 0.6	55.6 ± 3.0	2.2 ± 0.3
Veratridine	0.4 ± 0.1	40.9 ± 1.8	14.2 ± 7.0	0.2 ± 0.0	24.1 ± 2.2	20.6 ± 3.4	1.0 ± 0.3
Veratridine + Pr	5.5 ± 0.2[a]	25.6 ± 1.0[a]	4.9 ± 0.2[a]	0.4 ± 0.0[a]	21.5 ± 1.7	47.6 ± 1.9	2.7 ± 0.3[a]
No Ca^{2+}	3.1 ± 0.4	12.9 ± 1.2	9.6 ± 1.1	1.2 ± 0.3	15.5 ± 5.1	60.5 ± 4.6	2.6 ± 0.1
No Ca^{2+} + Pr	6.8 ± 0.1	18.4 ± 0.4	4.1 ± 0.1	0.3 ± 0.0	16.8 ± 0.4	60.2 ± 1.5	4.8 ± 0.9[a]
No Ca^{2+} + EGTA	2.2 ± 0.4	11.6 ± 1.2	7.9 ± 0.8	1.1 ± 0.2	19.3 ± 1.9	60.1 ± 4.0	5.4 ± 1.1
No Ca^{2+} + EGTA + Pr	4.4 ± 0.3	18.5 ± 1.3	2.9 ± 0.1	0.1 ± 0.1	13.1 ± 0.5	63.4 ± 2.0	7.8 ± 0.5[a]
Verapamil	3.6 ± 0.2	16.6 ± 2.0	13.1 ± 1.3	1.3 ± 0.1	19.5 ± 1.2	49.5 ± 2.1	1.6 ± 0.3
Verapamil + Pr	8.5 ± 0.3[a]	22.1 ± 0.7[a]	5.7 ± 0.6[a]	0.1 ± 0.0[a]	20.0 ± 1.7	52.1 ± 2.2	2.1 ± 0.6

Incubations contained 2.5 mM CaCl$_2$ except where indicated otherwise. Concentrations of additions were: propranolol, 0.1 mM; ionophore A23187, 0.01 mM; EGTA, 0.2 mM; verapamil, 0.05 mM; and veratridine, 0.1 mM. The results are means ± S.D. from three to six observations.

[a] $p < 0.001$ compared with corresponding control.

[b] PhIP = phosphatidylinositol-4-phosphate, PhIPP = phosphatidylinositol-4,5-bisphosphate

[c] Pr = propranolol

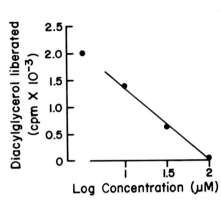

FIG. 7. Effect of increasing concentrations of propranolol on the activity of rat brain soluble phosphatidate phosphohydrolase. The enzyme activity in the 105,000 x g cytosolic fraction was assayed according to the method of Bleasdale et al. (8) using membrane-bound phosphatidic acid, prepared by incubating liver microsomes with glycero-3-phosphate and [1-^{14}C]oleate as substrates. The liberated DAG was isolated by thin-layer chromatography and counted. In the absence of propranolol about 5% of the substrate was hydrolyzed in 30 min. The results are means from three determinations. S.D.s were less than 10%.

TABLE 6. Brain phosphatidate phosphohydrolase activity: enzyme-drug or substrate-drug complex?

Source of ^{32}P-labeled particulate fraction[a]	Source of 1.05 x 10^6 x g supernatant fraction	
	Untreated mince	Propranolol-treated mince
Untreated mince	8.39 ± 0.16[b]	8.66 ± 0.66
Propranolol-treated mince	1.21 ± 0.22	1.06 ± 0.03
% Inhibition	86	88

Brain cortex mince was incubated 1 h with or without ^{32}P$_i$ (10 µCi) and with or without propranolol (0.1 mM). After three washes with P$_i$-containing buffer, subcellular fractions were prepared and the assay performed according to Bleasdale et al. (8). For counting, phosphatidic acid was isolated from the lipid extract by tlc. The numbers represent the difference between the radioactivity in phosphatidic acid in the particulate fraction before and after incubation. About 28% of the added substrate was hydrolyzed when both particulate and supernatant fractions were obtained from untreated mince. The results are means ± S.D. from triplicate incubations.
[a]Heated for 2 min at 100° C.
[b]Phosphatidic acid hydrolyzed/mg particulate protein/mg supernatant protein/30 min expressed as cpm x 10^{-4}.

from an incubation with propranolol very little hydrolysis took place and was not further prevented when the enzyme source was also obtained from a propranolol-containing incubation. These results clearly show that the enzyme is not affected by exposure to propranolol, but that the substrate is made unavailable for the action of the phosphohydrolase, presumably owing to complex formation. Such complexes are, in fact, readily formed (28,36,46). The immediate consequence of this inhibition would be greater availability of PhA and decreased levels of DAG, which can to some extent account for the observed shift in labeling towards acidic and away from neutral phospholipids.

Propranolol Effects on Phosphatidylcholine Biosynthesis

A possibility that needed to be considered is interference with reactions concerned with the biosynthesis of PhC and PhE resulting in the characteristic lower labeling of these lipids, which has already been discussed (Fig. 1). Although this occurs when either $^{32}P_i$ or [2-^{3}H]glycerol is used, incorporation of the more specific precursor [^{14}C]choline is reduced by only 20% in the presence of propranolol (Table 7). If a lack of DAG were responsible for these reductions, one would expect them to be of approximately equal magnitude. However, a DAG deficiency may still be the main defect, and the fact that the incorporation of choline is decreased less by the drug than the incorporation of the other precursors could be due to an active exchange reaction, mediated by a PhC-specific enzyme (34). Attempts to provide additional DAG through treatment of the tissue preparation with phospholipase C were unsuccessful in preventing the decreased PhC labeling (Table 2), possibly owing to an inability of the liberated DAG to reach the site of phosphocholine transferase activity.

As far as the biosynthetic enzymes are concerned, choline kinase is not only not inhibited, but even increasingly activated by propranolol (Table 8). It is unlikely that the other two enzymes required for PhC biosynthesis, the pacemaker enzyme cytidylyl transferase and phosphocholine transferase, are specifically affected, by analogy with the functioning of comparable enzymes in the biosynthesis of PhI and PPI from PhA as evidenced by the data cited (Fig. 1). This hypothesis will, however, have to be experimentally confirmed.

Propranolol Effects on Phospholipid Degradation

In addition to the inhibition of phosphatidate phosphohydrolase, inhibition of other phospholipases has been considered as possibly participating in the mechanism of CAD action, particularly in lysosomes (31,38, 46). To test the effectiveness of propranolol against several phospholipases, three brain enzymes, localized in different cell fractions, were assayed (Table 9). Phospholipase A_1, almost exclusively located in microsomes (53), phospholipase A_2, predominantly in mitochondria (53), and phospholipase C, a soluble enzyme specific for PhI (33) were all inhibited progressively by increasing concentrations of the drug. The differences in extent of hydrolysis can at least in part be ascribed to the pH of the assay mixture which was 8.4, 6.8 and 5.6 for phospholipase A_2, A_1, and C, respectively, and which would alter the degree of protonation of both drug and substrate and perhaps also the availability of Ca^{2+} where this ion is an important factor.

When lysosomal phospholipases from liver were tested against PhC at pH 4.4 for inhibition by propranolol, the concentration which resulted in 50% inhibition was 0.25 mM for phospholipase A and 0.38 mM for phospholipase C (31). Other cationic drugs exert this effect at similar concentrations (31,38). Phospholipase C was not tested against PhC in our study, because this activity is thought not to exist in brain.

As in the case of phosphatidate phosphohydrolase, the mechanism of inhibition is likely to be to a large extent formation of a phospholipid-drug complex which cannot be readily hydrolyzed. Through feedback inhibition the accumulated PhC and PhE could contribute to the reduced incorporation of precursors into neutral phospholipids.

TABLE 7. Effect of propranolol on the incorporation in vitro of radioactive precursors into PhC of brain cortex mince

Labeled precursor	Control	Propranolol	Reduction
	(radioactivity incorporated [cpm x 10^{-3}/mg mince])		(percent)
$^{32}P_i$	3.5 ± 0.6	1.1 ± 0.1	71
[2-^{3}H]glycerol	5.5 ± 0.5	1.6 ± 0.2	71
[1,2-^{14}C]choline	24.0 ± 0.6	19.7 ± 1.0	20

Brain cortex mince (10 mg) was incubated with $^{32}P_i$ (5 µCi), [2-^{3}H]glycerol (10 µCi) or [1,2-^{14}C]choline (2 µCi) with or without 0.1 mM propranolol. The results are means ± S.D. from three determinations.

TABLE 8. Choline kinase activity

Propranolol concentration	Choline phosphorylated
µM	(nmol/mg protein/20 min)
0	119 ± 3
10	134 ± 6
33	147 ± 9
100	175 ± 1

Choline kinase activity in rat brain 105,000 x g supernatant fraction was assayed according to the method of Weinhold et al. (51) using [1,2-^{14}C] choline as substrate. The results are means ± S.D. from three determinations.

TABLE 9. Effects of propranolol on some phospholipid hydrolyzing enzymes

Enzyme source	activity	Propranolol (µM) 10	33	100
		(percent inhibition)		
Mitochondria	Phospholipase A	46	95	100
Microsomes	Phospholipase A	21	35	45
105,000 x g supernatant	Phospholipase C	8	22	58

Rat brain subcellular fractions were prepared from a 10% homogenate in 0.32 M sucrose according to the procedure of De Robertis et al. (13). Phospholipase A in mitochondria or microsomes was assayed according to the method of Woelk and Porcellati (53), using [^{32}P]PhC, prepared in kidney mince, as substrate. Phospholipase C was assayed according to the method of Eichberg et al. (20), using [^{32}P]PhI, prepared in brain mince, as substrate.

CONCLUSIONS

In sum, the observations reported here extend previous observations on the effects of CADs including propranolol. They confirm the general nature of the induced changes in shifting precursor incorporation towards acidic and away from neutral phospholipids. This redirection can occur in preparations from brain as well as from peripheral tissues, but in vivo brain is apparently more susceptible than either kidney or liver owing to the pharmacodynamics of propranolol and especially the relative clearing rates. Nonetheless, side effects related to disturbance of phospholipid metabolism are a possibility, especially during therapy with large doses in elderly patients with impaired liver function. However, a phospholipidosis with multilamellar, phospholipid- and drug-filled cytoplasmic inclusion bodies as seen with other CADs in chronic use is not likely to occur with propranolol.

As to the mechanisms by which propranolol brings about changes in phospholipid metabolism, several factors seem to be involved. One is the plasma membrane which is apparently made more permeable by the drug. The nature of its action in reducing the integrity of the membrane is unclear but may involve interactions either of the positively charged side chain with negatively charged groups or of the hydrophobic ring system with non-polar domains to lessen resistance to the entry of ionic polar substances such as phosphate. Phospholipase treatment can facilitate this action. The cationic moiety may furthermore compete at calcium binding sites, although this possibility is not likely to play a major role in the shift in isotope incorporation.

The main area of interference is presumably degradation of phospholipids by phospholipases. Among these phosphatidate phosphohydrolase is a prime candidate as determinant of the direction of $^{32}P_i$ incorporation by controlling the availability of DAG. If complex formation with PhA and other phospholipid species is indeed the reason for the inability of the enzyme(s) to act, it is puzzling that biosynthetic reactions for the generation of acidic lipids can proceed normally. The potential for the biosynthesis of neutral lipids is probably also not impaired. The further elucidation of the processes involved could not only be useful for dealing with drug side effects and especially phospholipidosis, but also provide information on cell membrane function and regulation of phospholipid metabolism. CADs could be useful tools in this effort.

Acknowledgment: These studies were supported by research grants from the U.S. Public Health Service (NS06399) and the National Science Foundation (PCM7824387). We are grateful to Dr. Martin Low for a sample of PhI-specific phospholipase C.

REFERENCES

1.   Abdel-Latif, A.A. (1976): Adv. Exp. Biol. Med., 72:227-256.
2.   Abdel-Latif, A.A., and Smith, J.P. (1976): Biochem. Pharmacol., 25: 1697-1704.
3.   Allan, D., and Michell, R.H. (1975): Biochem. J., 148:470-478.
4.   Atsmon, A., and Blum, I. (1978): In: Propranolol and Schizophrenia, edited by E. Roberts and P. Amacher, pp. 5-38. Alan R. Liss, Inc., New York.
5.   Bazán, N.G., Ilincheta de Boschero, M.G., and Giusto, N.M. (1977): Adv. Exp. Biol. Med., 83:377-388.

6. Bazán, N.G., Ilincheta de Boschero, M.G., Giusto, N.M., and Pascual de Bazán, H.E. (1976): Adv. Exp. Biol. Med., 72:139-148.
7. Bianchetti, G., Elghozi, J.L., Gomeni, R., Meyer, P., and Morselli, P.L. (1980): J. Pharmacol. Exp. Ther., 214:682-687.
8. Bleasdale, J.E., Davis, C.S., Hajra, A.K., and Agranoff, B.W. (1978): Anal. Biochem., 87:19-27.
9. Blohm, T.R. (1979): Pharmacol. Rev., 30:593-603.
10. Brindley, D.N., Allan, D., and Michell, R.H. (1975): J. Pharm. Pharmacol., 27:462-464.
11. Brindley, D.N., and Bowley, M. (1975): Biochem. J., 148:461-469.
12. Brotherus, J., and Renkonen, O. (1977): J. Lipid Res., 18:191-202.
13. De Robertis, E., Pellegrino de Iraldi, A., Rodriguez de Lores Arnaiz, G., and Salganicoff, L. (1962): J. Neurochem., 9:23-35.
14. Drenckhahn, T.R., and Lüllmann-Rauch, R. (1979): Neuroscience, 4: 697-712.
15. Eichberg, J., Gates, J., and Hauser, G. (1979): Biochim. Biophys. Acta, 573:90-106.
16. Eichberg, J., and Hauser, G. (1974): Biochem. Biophys. Res. Commun., 60:1460-1467.
17. Eichberg, J., Killion, J., Guerrant, G., and Hauser, G. (1978): In: Cyclitols and Phosphoinositides, edited by F. Eisenberg, Jr., and W. W. Wells, pp. 183-199. Academic Press, New York.
18. Eichberg, J., Shein, H., and Hauser, G. (1973): Biochem. Soc. Transact., 1:352-359.
19. Eichberg, J., Shein, H., Schwartz, M., and Hauser, G. (1973): J. Biol. Chem., 248:3615-3622.
20. Eichberg, J., Zetusky, W.J., Bell, M.E., and Cavanagh, E. (1981): J. Neurochem., 36:1868-1871.
21. Elghozi, J.-L., Bianchetti, G., Morselli, P.L., and Meyer, P. (1979): Eur. J. Pharmacol., 55:319-322.
22. Feldman, D.A., and Weinhold, P.A. (1977): Biochem. Pharmacol., 26: 2283-2289.
23. Hauser, G., and Eichberg, J. (1973): Biochim. Biophys. Acta, 326: 201-209.
24. Hauser, G., and Eichberg, J. (1975): J. Biol. Chem., 250:105-112.
25. Hauser, G., and Eichberg, J. (1976): Adv. Exp. Biol. Med., 72:149-158.
26. Hauser, G., Shein, H.M., and Eichberg, J. (1974): Nature, 252:482-483.
27. Hauser, G., Pappu, A.S., Smith, T.L., and Eichberg, J. (1980): Progr. Clin. Biol. Res., 39:469.
28. Hauser, H., Penkett, S.A., and Chapman, D. (1969): Biochim. Biophys. Acta, 183:466-475.
29. Hemingsen, R., Hertz, M.M., and Barry, D.I. (1979): Acta Physiol. Scand., 105:274-281.
30. Hokin-Neaverson, M. (1980): Biochem. Pharmacol., 29:2697-2700.
31. Hostetler, K.Y., and Matsuzawa, Y. (1981): Biochem. Pharmacol., 30: 1121-1126.
32. Ide, H., and Nakazawa, Y. (1980): Biochem. Pharmacol., 29:789-793.
33. Irvine, R.F., and Dawson, R.M.C. (1978): J. Neurochem., 31:1427-1434.
34. Kanfer, J.N. (1982): This volume.
35. Lüllmann, H., Lüllmann-Rauch, R., and Wassermann, O. (1978): Biochem. Pharmacol., 27:1103-1108.
36. Lüllmann, H., and Wehling, M. (1979): Biochem. Pharmacol., 28: 3409-3415.

37. Lüllmann-Rauch, R. (1979): In: Lysosomes in Applied Biology and Therapeutics, edited by J.T. Dingle, P.J. Jacques, and I.H. Shaw, pp. 49-130. North Holland Publishing Co., Amsterdam.

38. Matsuzawa, Y., and Hostetler, K.Y. (1980): J. Biol. Chem., 255: 5190-5194.

39. Noack, G., Kurzmack, M., Verjovski-Almeida, S., and Inesi, G. (1978): J. Pharmacol. Exp. Ther., 206:281-288.

40. Pappu, A.S., and Hauser, G. (1981): Trans. Am. Soc. Neurochem., 12:104.

41. Pappu, A.S., and Hauser, G. (1981): Abstr. 8th Internat. Meeting, Internat. Soc. Neurochem., 330.

42. Pappu, A.S., and Hauser, G. (1981): J. Neurochem., 37:1006-1014.

43. Pappu, A.S., and Hauser, G. (1981): Biochem.Pharmacol.,30:3243-3246.

44. Roberts, E., and Amacher, P., editors (1978): Propranolol and Schizophrenia, Alan R. Liss, Inc., New York.

45. Schneck, D.W., Pritchard, F., and Hayes, A.H. (1977): J. Pharmacol. Exp. Ther., 203:621-629.

46. Seydel, J.K., and Wassermann, O. (1976): Biochem. Pharmacol., 25: 2357-2364.

47. Sheetz, M.P., and Singer, S.J. (1974): Proc. Natl. Acad. Sci. USA, 71:4457-4461.

48. Sheppard, G.P. (1979): Brit. J. Psychiat., 134:470-476.

49. Smith, T.L., and Hauser, G. (1979): Biochem. Pharmacol., 28:1759-1763.

50. Sturton, R.G., and Brindley, D.N. (1977): Biochem. J., 162:25-32.

51. Weinhold, P.A., Skinner, R.S., and Roberts, R.D. (1973): Biochim. Biophys. Acta, 326:43-51.

52. Wherrett, J.R., and Huterer, S. (1972): J. Biol. Chem., 247:4114-4120.

53. Woelk, H., and Porcellati, G. (1973): Hoppe-Seyler's Z. Physiol. Chem., 354:90-100.

54. Yorkston, N.J., Zaki, S.A., and Havard, C.W.H. (1978): In: Propranolol and Schizophrenia, edited by E. Roberts and P. Amacher, pp. 83-97. Alan R. Liss, Inc., New York.

Phospholipids in the Nervous System, Vol. 1: Metabolism, edited by L. Horrocks, et al. Raven Press, New York © 1982.

Stimulated Phospholipid Labeling in Nerve Ending Preparations: Studies on Localization and Biochemical Mechanism

Bernard W. Agranoff and Stephen K. Fisher

Neuroscience Laboratory, Mental Health Research Institute, and Department of Biological Chemistry, The University of Michigan, Ann Arbor, Michigan 48109

It has now been some 28 years (32) since Hokin and Hokin observed that the addition of acetylcholine (ACh) to pancreas slices stimulates the incorporation of exogenously added $^{32}P_i$ into two quantitatively minor membrane phospholipids--phosphatidate (PhA) and phosphatidylinositol (PhI). At the time the metabolic interrelationship of the two lipids was not yet understood, and there was even some question as to whether PhA could be considered a naturally occurring lipid. The role of PhA as an intermediate in phospholipid formation has since been well-established. It occupies an important branch point in lipid biosynthesis, since it can be either dephosphorylated to diglyceride prior to synthesis of phosphatidylcholine and phosphatidylethanolamine, or alternatively can retain its phosphomonoester moiety for the synthesis of phosphatidylglycerols and the phosphoinositides via CDP-diglyceride. In contrast to the progress in elucidation of the metabolic interrelationship of the phospholipids, the nature of the stimulated labeling effect and its physiological significance has largely remained an unsolved mystery. The number of well-documented circumstances under which lipid labeling of tissue preparations can be stimulated by either receptor-specific ligands, secretagogues or drugs has grown considerably and the widespread occurrence of the phenomenon has prompted the suggestion that the response may be a reflection of a common cellular event (43). Recently, considerable effort has been directed at understanding receptor-mediated stimulation of phospholipid labeling in a number of simple cell systems, particularly in thrombin-stimulated platelets (9) and in neutrophils stimulated by the addition of a chemotactic peptide (17). In both of these preparations there is reason to believe that the labeling may be part of a mechanism whereby arachidonate is released from membrane phospholipids for the subsequent production of prostaglandins, thromboxanes and leukotrienes.

The present report deals with recent findings on cholinergic stimulation of phospholipid labeling in a nerve ending fraction from guinea pig brain, an effect which has been under investigation in this (49) and other laboratories (59) for a number of years. It has been stated that stimulated labeling effects are seen only in intact cells (43). While the nerve ending preparation requires brain homogenization, the particles maintain many of the properties of intact cells and retain their vectorial (inside-outside) boundary conditions. Thus they should in the present context be considered as resealed anucleate neurons. Unsealed membrane fragments do not support a stimulated phospholipid labeling effect, even in the presence of added $[\gamma-^{32}P]ATP$ (50). Since $^{32}P_i$ added to nerve ending particles must be taken up into the cytosol and be converted to $[\gamma-^{32}P]ATP$ prior to lipid labeling, most, or all of the labeled PhA and PhI is assumed to be on inner membrane surface in contact with this intracellular pool. Cell membrane receptors are located on the external membrane leaflet and it therefore follows that the stimulation of lipid labeling from added $^{32}P_i$ is a transmembrane phenomenon. The nerve ending preparation provides a useful model for the investigation of this phenomenon, as well as for the study of the biochemistry of CNS muscarinic action.

PHARMACOLOGY

Addition of as little as 10^{-6} M ACh or carbamylcholine to nerve ending preparations results in a stimulation of PhI and PhA labeling, although maximal stimulation (40-100%) requires an agonist concentration of 10^{-4} to 10^{-3} M. The relatively high concentrations of agonists required might appear to argue against a possible relationship between stimulated phospholipid labeling and events associated with synaptic transmission. However, it should be remembered that the biochemical correlates of receptor activation typically show this apparent insensitivity, in contrast to the attendant physiological responses for which minimal receptor occupancy is required (44). Of the cholinergic agents tested, only muscarinic agonists such as muscarine and methacholine are effective, while nicotinic agonists such as nicotine or 1,1-dimethyl-4-phenyl piperazinium iodide are without effect. There is also a separate class of known muscarinic agonists which appear to act only as "partial" agonists at muscarinic receptors in the nerve ending preparation. This group, which includes pilocarpine, bethanechol, arecoline and oxotremorine, typically induces only a small stimulation of PhA and PhI labeling, and can, in fact, block the larger stimulatory effect of ACh in a manner analogous to that of an antago-

nist (23). The muscarinic nature of the cholinergic response is confirmed by studies with antagonists. The
inclusion of 10^{-5} M atropine or 10^{-8} M quinuclidinylbenzi-
late (QNB) completely prevents stimulated phospholipid labeling, while in contrast, nicotinic antagonists such as
d-tubocurarine or hexamethonium are ineffective at concentrations as high as 10^{-4} M (23). In summary, all available
evidence suggests the sole involvement of muscarinic cholinergic receptors in stimulated phospholipid labeling. As
yet, there is little evidence to implicate nicotinic receptors in lipid labeling of either the nerve ending preparation, or indeed, of any other cell preparation (43). Even
in the bovine chromaffin cell, a cell type which possesses
both nicotinic and muscarinic cholinergic receptors, only
the muscarinic receptors have been found to be coupled to
phospholipid turnover (24).

THE LOCUS OF LABELING

The textbook "synaptosome" is generally depicted as
mitochondria, synaptic vesicles and a limited amount of
smooth endoplasmic reticulum enclosed by a plasma membrane.
Under favorable conditions, electron microscopy of the
pelleted fraction reveals the complete synaptic complex
with attached fragments of a postsynaptic specialized membrane of the neighboring efferent cell body, dendrite or
axon. During nerve ending particle isolation under conditions used in our studies with guinea pig brain, the
postsynaptic membrane is generally lost (51). For this
reason as well as the fact that [^{32}P]ATP formed inside the
nerve ending particle is not accessible to the postsynaptic fragment, it would seem reasonable to conclude that
the stimulated labeling effect is presynaptic. Presynaptic muscarinic autoreceptors have been described and are
proposed to regulate ACh production or release (54). However, denervation studies in two neural preparations, the
sympathetic ganglion (31,40,41) and pineal gland (53) have
clearly indicated that stimulated phospholipid labeling
in these instances is localized at a postsynaptic site.
To determine more precisely the structure(s) in the nerve
ending preparation responsible for stimulated phospholipid
labeling, we used nerve ending preparations obtained from
the guinea pig hippocampus. The hippocampus represents a
specialized region of the cerebral cortex which has the
great advantage for present purposes that all of its cholinergic input is derived from the septal nuclei and ar-
rives via a single well-defined tract, the fimbria. One
can readily lesion the fimbria, with a resultant degenera-
tion of the cholinergic input within a few days. This
leaves intact the intrinsic neurons of the hippocampus,
including those with denuded postsynaptic specializations
in the region of their lost cholinergic presynaptic terminals. Conversely, we can stereotaxically inject the guinea
pig hippocampus with an excitatory neurotoxin (ibotenic

acid), which will selectively destroy the intrinsic cell
bodies of the hippocampus, while leaving the presynaptic
terminals intact (52). The extent of the surgical or
neurotoxin lesion can be established quantitatively by
means of appropriate biochemical markers. The enzyme choline acetyltransferase indicates the presence of presynaptic cholinergic terminals, while [^{3}H]QNB binding serves
as a marker for muscarinic receptors. We have demonstrated
(22) that the septal denervation produces a profound decrease in choline acetyltransferase, but no loss in [^{3}H]-
QNB binding, indicating a preponderance of postsynaptic
muscarinic receptors (see Fig. 1). ACh-stimulated labeling
of PhA and PhI from ^{32}P$_i$ is not significantly impaired in
nerve endings derived from this preparation, a result which
argues against a presynaptic locus for the effect. As anticipated, destruction of hippocampal neurons by injection
of the excitatory neurotoxin ibotenic acid produces a
marked drop in [^{3}H]QNB binding, but does not decrease
levels of choline acetyltransferase. In nerve ending preparations from ibotenate-lesioned hippocampus, there is a
dramatic loss in stimulation of phospholipid labeling by
added carbamylcholine consistent with the degree of loss
of [^{3}H]QNB binding (25), yet there is no impairment in
basal labeling, i.e., the ability to incorporate ^{32}P$_i$
into phospholipids in the absence of added agonist. These
experiments then indicate that the muscarinic receptors
that mediate the observed stimulation of phospholipid labeling in nerve ending preparations are derived from postsynaptic (cholinoceptive) structures. How then can this
conclusion be reconciled with our textbook nerve ending
preparation whose cytoplasm is not in direct contact with
postsynaptic membrane?

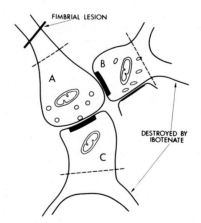

FIG. 1. Which hippocampal structures are the source of
nerve ending particles that mediate the muscarinic stimulation of lipid labeling? Particles are presumed to fragment
and reseal upon homogenization at sites indicated by broken
lines. ▬ = Muscarinic receptors.

Possible explanations are offered in the drawing in Figure 1, in which the cholinergic nerve ending A is severed. The observed stimulated labeling might be mediated by resealed dendrite-derived particles, or "dendrosomes" present in the hippocampal nerve ending preparation (Fig. 1, neuron C). Like their presynaptic equivalents, pinched-off postsynaptic endings contain cytosolic enzymes and mitochondria and can therefore support oxidative and substrate level conversion of $^{32}P_i$ to $[\gamma-^{32}P]ATP$. It is alternatively possible that the stimulated labeling is mediated by pinched-off presynaptic nerve endings which also contain some postsynaptic membrane surface (Fig. 1, neuron B) from the presynaptic input of a third neuron. In either event, presynaptic cholinergic nerve endings (A) are clearly not implicated in stimulated labeling. Ibotenate does not destroy glial cells, so that these experiments serve additionally to confirm that the observed muscarinic actions are attributable to neuronally-derived particles in the preparation. We conclude that the physiological significance of the stimulated muscarinic labeling is related to events that directly mediate or modulate the activity of cholinoceptive neurons.

A ROLE FOR CALCIUM

In non-CNS tissues such as the parotid gland, adrenal medulla, ileum, platelet or neutrophil, the activation of specific plasma membrane receptors results in both stimulated phospholipid labeling and a physiological response characteristic of the cell type (45). The latter, which may be as diverse as enzyme secretion, catecholamine or prostanoid release or muscle contraction, results from either a transient increase in the permeability of the plasma membrane to Ca^{2+} or from an intracellular mobilization of the cation. While there is general agreement that alterations in Ca^{2+} fluxes and in phospholipid labeling are intimately related events (46), there is presently a considerable difference of opinion as to whether changes in phospholipid turnover mediate Ca^{2+} fluxes (Fig. 2A), or whether stimulated phospholipid labeling results from the increased intracellular concentration of Ca^{2+} (Fig. 2B).

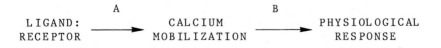

FIG. 2. Does the stimulated lipid labeling occur before (A) or after (B) calcium ion mobilization?

In the case of muscarinic-agonist stimulation of phospholipid labeling in nerve ending preparations, we initially found that the addition of Ca^{2+} was not obligatory for the labeling response (49). Subsequent studies, however, indicated that stimulated PhA and PhI labeling could be largely prevented by the inclusion of EGTA at concentrations (50-500 μM) that had no effect on the basal labeling of these two lipids (21). Moreover, the EGTA inhibition could be overcome by the addition of calcium. These apparently contradictory results may now be explained by the fact that micromolar concentrations of Ca^{2+} suffice to sustain stimulated phospholipid labeling, and that endogenous calcium concentrations fulfill this requirement (29). Further evidence for an involvement of calcium was obtained from studies in which addition of the ionophores A23187 or ionomycin to nerve ending preparations resulted in a selective stimulation of PhA and PhI labeling comparable in magnitude to that seen with ACh, and which was blocked by the additional presence of EGTA, but not by atropine (21). These observations support the hypothesis that in nerve ending fractions, the phospholipid labeling effect is a consequence rather than a predecessor of Ca^{2+} mobilization. A similar conclusion has been drawn for stimulated phosphoinositide turnover in neutrophils (16), mast cells (15), pancreas (20), chromaffin cells (24) and iris smooth muscle (1,2). That stimulated labeling is the result of calcium mobilization, however, is clearly not consonant with observations made on the blowfly salivary gland (11,19) or mammalian parotid gland (35), where results point to the operation of mechanism A, i.e., phospholipid turnover mediates Ca^{2+} mobilization (46). It is not yet known whether the relationship of Ca^{2+} mobilization and phospholipid labeling is fundamentally different in these tissues.

An interesting, if perplexing, complication of the ionophore studies in nerve ending preparations is the finding that ACh or carbamylcholine added together with A23187 results in a potentiation of the stimulation of lipid labeling, mediated through the muscarinic receptor (23). The result, a 2 to 3-fold stimulation of PhA and PhI labeling is about twice that anticipated from an additive effect. The enhancement has proven useful experimentally, for example in demonstrating the difference between partial and complete muscarinic agonists and in documenting a complementary receptor-mediated decrease in the radioactivity found in polyphosphoinositides under conditions in which PhA and PhI labeling is stimulated. The potentiation suggests an interaction of the muscarinic receptor and Ca^{2+} mobilization, possibly via Ca^{2+} gates in the plasma membrane. The ionophore and EGTA studies suggest that in our nerve ending preparation, ACh-receptor binding results in an elevation of cytosolic free Ca^{2+}, either by increased influx, or via release of Ca^{2+} from membrane-bound or intracellular stores. Changes in cytoplasmic Ca^{2+} concentrations could readily effect lipid labeling in a number of ways. It is known, for example, that phospholipases C and A_2, as well as the phosphomonoesterases that break down the polyphosphoinositides to PhI are all calcium-activated (18,36). In contrast, the lipid biosynthetic enzymes are generally unaffected or are inhibited by the presence of Ca^{2+} (3,27), thus making it improbable that the observed Ca^{2+} sensitivity of stimulated PhA and PhI labeling simply reflects a more efficient relabeling of these lipids. How the various calcium-dependent phosphomonoesterase and phosphodiesterase enzymes are capable of influencing the $^{32}P_i$-stimulated labeling is best considered in relation to the labeling cycle discussed in the following section. In addition, a number of lipids whose formation could directly or indirectly stem from PhA and PhI interconversion are claimed to have calcium ionophore activity, including PhA (48), lysophosphatidylinositol diphosphate (30), arachidonate (7) and the prostaglandins (58). Small increases in cytosolic Ca^{2+} could thus lead to cyclic cascades that maximize the cell response.

THE BIOCHEMICAL MECHANISM(S) OF STIMULATED PHOSPHOLIPID LABELING

The stimulated labeling of PhA and PhI from $^{32}P_i$ is thought to reflect an increased availability of diglyceride which could arise from either de novo synthesis or from the breakdown of preformed lipids. In the case of the nerve ending preparation, there is no evidence to suggest that increases in de novo synthesis are responsible, since the incorporation of [^{3}H]glycerol or [^{3}H]glucose into phospholipids is not increased by the addition of ACh or A23187, added singly or in combination (23). In addition, the stimulation of PhA and PhI labeling cannot be explained by an increased specific activity of intracellular ATP (23, 50). The stimulated labeling seen in nerve ending preparations is believed to occur via the steps shown in Figure 3.

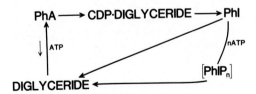

FIG. 3. Enzymatic interconversions in the phospholipid labeling cycle. The direct conversion of PhI to diglyceride is postulated for many tissues. Evidence at present suggests that in the case of the nervous system, diglyceride is furnished via the polyphosphoinositides (PhIP$_n$; n = 1 or 2).

Radioactivity from $^{32}P_i$ enters the labeling cycle via phosphorylation of diglyceride by $[^{32}P]ATP$, catalyzed by diglyceride kinase. Labeled PhA is then converted to labeled PhI via CDP-diglyceride. In nerve ending preparations stimulated by ACh or A23187, the incorporation of $[^3H]$inositol into PhI increased less than that of $^{32}P_i$ (23). This suggests that either added inositol does not exchange with the pool of inositol involved in stimulated PhI synthesis, or alternatively, that much of the observed basal label incorporated can be accounted for by CDP-diglyceride independent inositol-PhI exchange (55). A phospholipase C activity which degrades PhI to reform diglyceride completes the cycle. In several non-neural tissues it has been proposed that activation of this ubiquitous Ca^{2+}-dependent enzyme is responsible for the subsequent stimulation of PhA and PhI labeling (45). While phospholipase C activity is present in brain (34), there is little evidence to implicate this enzyme in stimulated lipid labeling in the nerve ending preparation. The possibility is largely discounted on the basis of experiments in which neither ACh nor A23187 promoted a significant loss of label from PhI previously labeled with either $^{32}P_i$, $[^3H]$glycerol or $[^3H]$inositol (23). PhA breakdown has been proposed as a possible source of diglyceride (50), although it now appears more likely that the polyphosphoinositides (phosphatidylinositol phosphate and diphosphate; PhIP, $PhIP_2$) serve this purpose. In the iris smooth muscle there is substantial evidence that ACh accelerates the breakdown of $PhIP_2$ (1,2), and recently Griffin and Hawthorne (28) provided evidence that a guinea pig nerve ending preparation stimulated with A23187 results in the breakdown of both PhIP and $PhIP_2$. In all instances in which we have found PhA and PhI labeling to be stimulated, e.g., ACh, carbamylcholine, muscarine and methacholine, there is a small but measurable decrease in the labeling of both PhIP and $PhIP_2$ (23). Furthermore, the potentiated increase in labeling of PhA and PhI in the copresence of ionophore and muscarinic agents is accompanied by a potentiated <u>decrease</u> in PhIP and $PhIP_2$ labeling. While muscarinic antagonists do not block the effect of the ionophore, they do block the cholinergic component of both stimulated PhA and PhI labeling and the decreased PhIP and $PhIP_2$ labeling, reducing the effects produced to that seen upon addition of ionophore alone. These results indicate that the turnover of the polyphosphoinositides in nerve ending preparations is linked specifically to the activation of muscarinic receptors (23). When nerve ending preparations are prelabeled with $^{32}P_i$ until the polyphosphoinositides have achieved isotopic equilibrium, the subsequent addition of either ACh or A23187 results in an accelerated loss of label, which becomes potentiated when both agents are present. EGTA prevents this loss of label. Since the polyphosphoinositides are labeled primarily in the phosphomonoester positions by the combined action of specific kinases and phosphomonoesterases, their level of radioactivity generally equilibrates with the $[^{32}P]$ATP pool after 15-30 min of incubation, a time at which PhA and PhI labeling is still increasing. The radioactivity in the polyphosphoinositides is thus a measure of their amount, and the observed drop in their radioactivity in the presence of ionophore or ACh undoubtedly reflects a decrease in their content. This is presumably the result of the phospholipase C activity which degrades polyphosphoinositides. Enzymatic activity which breaks down PhIP and PhIP$_2$ with the production of inositol diphosphate and inositol triphosphate, respectively, has been reported in brain, although it is not clear whether or not the same enzyme is active with PhI as substrate (36). At present, then, polyphosphoinositides appear to be candidates for the source of the diglyceride that initiates the ^{32}P lipid labeling effect in nerve endings. A role for polyphosphoinositide breakdown has also recently been postulated for tissues such as the parotid gland and hepatocyte (38) in which PhI breakdown was previously considered to be the key initial event. While these results have led to more agreement than this field ordinarily enjoys, the popularity of the notion, it must be cautioned, does not constitute proof.

THE RELATIONSHIP OF STEAROYL ARACHIDONOYL (ST/AR) LIPIDS TO STIMULATED $^{32}P_i$ LABELING OF PHOSPHOLIPIDS

Diacylglycerol phospholipids generally have a saturated fatty acid in the 1-position of sn-glycerol and an unsaturated fatty acid in the 2-position. It has long been known that all of the inositol phosphoglycerides (PhI, PhIP, and PhIP$_2$) are particularly enriched in the 1-stearoyl (18:0), 2-arachidonoyl (20:4, ω6) species, referred to here as ST/AR. When ^{32}P-labeled PhI from ACh-stimulated nerve preparations is subjected to argentation thin-layer chromatography, much of the radioactivity resides in the tetraenoic fraction, in which the predominant lipid is ST/AR PhI (50). Diglycerides and polyphosphoinositides purified from crude lipid extracts of brain (37) are also found to be enriched in the ST/AR species, as is CDP-diglyceride (56,57), and to some extent, PhA (57) as well. If the isolated lipids represent steady state levels of metabolic intermediates in the biosynthesis of all of the phospholipids, the preponderance of the ST/AR species would not have been predicted, since the major glycerophospholipids phosphatidylcholine and phosphatidylethanolamine contain relatively small amounts of the ST/AR moiety. Furthermore, PhA and CDP-diglyceride are also precursors of the phosphatidylglycerols, and the latter are not enriched in the ST/AR species. The results suggest then that the isolated ST/AR lipids are not the steady state biosynthetic intermediates, but rather are derived from a separate compartment of phospholipid. The $^{32}P_i$ labeling effect, as indicated in Figure 3, can be considered a closed cycle in which ST/AR diglyceride exchanges its head group from P_i to cytidine 5'-mono-phosphate, and thence to the inositol phosphates. We have discussed elsewhere the possibility that membrane ST/AR diglyceride binding sites would mediate availability of head groups to membrane-bound and/or cytosolic enzymes that catalyze these interconversions (5). PhA may be biosynthesized either via sequential acylation of glycerol phosphate or from acyl dihydroxyacetone phosphate following reduction to lyso PhA (4). By either route, selective acylation with arachidonoyl CoA does not occur. The question then arises as to where in the ST/AR cycle arachidonate is introduced. At present, the balance of evidence from biosynthetic studies favors the formation of non-ST/AR PhI, followed by deacylation to lyso PhI and reacylation with arachidonoyl CoA (6). The possibility that the ST/AR cycle of $^{32}P_i$ labeling is related to arachidonate metabolism has been raised by recent studies in the thrombin-stimulated platelet, which exhibits stimulated labeling of PhA and PhI, as well as the release of arachidonate (38). However, the source of this arachidonic acid has yet to be unequivocally identified. PhI (13), diglyceride (10), PhA (12), or other phospholipids (14,42) remain possibilities. The relevance of these findings to events in the stimulated nerve ending is presently unknown. It is yet to be established whether the 1-stearoyl-2-arachidonoyl moiety of the lipids is conserved during the labeling cycle, and in addition, the metabolic site of introduction of arachidonate needs to be established. In the latter context, it is of interest to note that both PhI-specific phospholipase A_2 (26) and CDP-diglyceride:inositol phosphatidyltransferase (47) have recently been shown to be relatively inactive against their respective ST/AR phospholipid substrates. Arachidonate release from brain has been observed in seizures (8), and the role of the prostanoid lipids in brain ischemia and traumatic edema (8) suggest important physiological consequences for the release of this fatty acid.

COMPARISON OF THE NERVE ENDING FRACTION WITH OTHER SYSTEMS EVINCING A $^{32}P_i$ LABELING EFFECT

In the proposed $^{32}P_i$-labeling cycle, phosphoinositide breakdown in the plasma membrane gives rise to diglyceride which is rapidly converted to PhA via soluble or membrane-bound diglyceride kinase. PhI is then resynthesized from PhA at the endoplasmic reticulum. In a secretory tissue such as pancreas, however, the measurable reduction of PhI content in response to the addition of a secretagogue is far in excess of the amount present in the plasma membrane. One possible explanation for this is that the plasma membrane PhI is continuously replenished from internal stores, such as the endoplasmic reticulum, via phospholipid-exchange proteins. The newly arrived PhI would then be susceptible to breakdown at the plasma membrane and the cycle would resume. Alternatively, some of the changes in phospholipid content may also reflect release of intracellular granules as part of the resultant secretory process.

In the nerve ending preparation, events at the plasma membrane appear to dominate the observed labeling effect, with little involvement of the endoplasmic reticulum. This is consistent with the observation that stimulated labeling of PhA in nerve ending preparations is typically two or three times as large as that of PhI. This pattern is also observed in the avian salt gland, a tissue with a very restricted amount of endoplasmic reticulum relative to plasma membrane (33). In contrast, tissues with an elaborate endoplasmic reticulum (pancreas, hepatocyte and parotid gland) display a greater stimulation of PhI labeling than of PhA in response to an agonist. Thus, in the nerve ending preparation, conditions may be more favorable for measuring those aspects of phospholipid metabolism that are correlated with the initial biochemical consequences of receptor-ligand interaction at the plasma membrane, independent of subsequent events involving other intracellular membranes.

SUMMARY

The stimulated labeling of phospholipids observed following addition of $^{32}P_i$ to nerve ending preparations from guinea pig brain constitutes a model system of CNS muscarinic receptor activation. The effect is cholinoceptive, i.e., occurs on a postsynaptic specialization of the neuronal plasma membrane. Ca^{2+} plays an integral role, and evidence is presented to indicate that the stimulated labeling is a consequence of receptor-mediated Ca^{2+} mobilization. The labeling is explained by a closed cycle in which the diglyceride kinase step is rate-limiting, due to restricted availability of diglyceride substrate. In this preparation, polyphosphoinositide breakdown may prove to be a major source of diglyceride.

REFERENCES

1. Abdel-Latif, A.A., Akhtar, R.A., and Hawthorne, J.N. (1977): Biochem. J., 162:61-73.
2. Akhtar, R.A., and Abdel-Latif, A. (1978): J. Pharmacol. Exp. Ther., 204:655-668.
3. Agranoff, B.W., Bradley, R.M., and Brady, R.O. (1958): J. Biol. Chem., 233:1077-1083.
4. Agranoff, B.W., and Hajra, A.K. (1971): Proc. Natl. Acad. Sci., 68:411-415.
5. Agranoff, B.W., and Bleasdale, J. E. (1978): In: Cyclitols and Phosphoinositides, ed. by W.W. Wells and F. Eisenberg, pp. 105-119. Academic Press, New York.
6. Baker, R.R., and Thompson, W. (1972): Biochim. Biophys. Acta, 270:489-503.
7. Barritt, G.J. (1981): Cell Calcium, 2:53-63.

8.   Bazan, N.G., and Rodriguez De Turco, E.B. (1980): Adv. Neurol., 28:197-205.
9.   Bell, R.L., and Majerus, P.W. (1979): J. Biol. Chem., 255:1790-1792.
10. Bell, R.L., Kennedy, D.A., Stanford, N., and Majerus, P.W. (1979): Proc. Natl. Acad. Sci., 76:3238-3241.
11. Berridge, M.J., and Fain, J.N. (1979): Biochem. J., 178:59-69.
12. Billah, M.M., Lapetina, E.G., and Cuatrecasas, P. (1981): J. Biol. Chem., 256:5399-5403.
13. Broekman, M.J., Ward, J.W., and Marcus, A.J. (1980): J. Clin. Invest., 66:275-283.
14. Broekman, M.J., Ward, J.W., and Marcus, A.J. (1981): J. Biol. Chem., 256:8271-8274.
15. Cockroft, S., and Gomperts, B.D. (1980): Biochem. J., 188:789-798.
16. Cockroft, S., Bennett, J.P., and Gomperts, B.D. (1980): FEBS Lett., 110:115-118.
17. Cockroft, S., Bennett, J.P., and Gomperts, B.D. (1980): Nature, 288:275-277.
18. Dawson, R.M.C., and Thompson, W. (1964) Biochem. J., 91:244-250.
19. Fain, J.N., and Berridge, M.J. (1979): Biochem. J., 178:45-58.
20. Farese, R.V., Larson, R.E., and Sabir, M.A. (1980): Biochim. Biophys. Acta, 633:479-484.
21. Fisher, S.K., and Agranoff, B.W. (1980): J. Neurochem., 34:1231-1240.
22. Fisher, S.K., Boast, C.A., and Agranoff, B.W. (1980): Brain Res., 189:284-288.
23. Fisher, S.K., and Agranoff, B.W. (1981): J. Neurochem., 37:968-977.
24. Fisher, S.K., Holz, R.W., and Agranoff, B.W. (1981): J. Neurochem., 37:491-497.
25. Fisher, S.K., Frey, K.A., and Agranoff, B.W. (1981): J. Neuroscience, in press.
26. Gray, N.C.C., and Strickland, K.P. (1982): This book.
27. Gibson, A., and Brammer, M.J. (1981): J. Neurochem., 868-874.
28. Griffin, H.D., and Hawthorne, J.N. (1978): Biochem. J., 176:541-552.
29. Griffin, H.D., Hawthorne, J.N., Sykes, M., and Orlacchio, A. (1979): Biochem. Pharmacol., 28:1143-1147.
30. Hayashi, F., Sokabe, M., Takagi, M., Hayashi, K., and Kishimoto, U. (1978): Biochim. Biophys. Acta, 510:305-315.
31. Hokin, L.E. (1966): J. Neurochem., 13:179-184.
32. Hokin, M.R., and Hokin, L.E. (1953): J. Biol. Chem., 203:967-977.
33. Hokin, M.R., and Hokin, L.E. (1967): J. Gen. Physiol., 50:793-811.
34. Irvine, R.F., Hemington, N., and Dawson, R.M.C. (1979): Eur. J. Biochem., 99:525-530.

35. Jones, L.M., and Michell, R.H. (1975): Biochem. J., 148:479-485.
36. Keough, K.M.W., and Thompson, W. (1972): Biochim. Biophys. Acta, 270:324-336.
37. Keough, K.M.W., MacDonald G., and Thompson, W. (1972): Biochim. Biophys. Acta, 270:337-347.
38. Kirk, C.J., Creba, J.A., Downes, C.P., and Michell, R.H. (1981): Biochem. Soc. Trans., 9:377-379.
39. Lapetina, E.G., and Cuatrecasas, P. (1979): Biochim. Biophys. Acta, 573:394-402.
40. Larrabee, M.G. (1968): J. Neurochem., 15:803-808.
41. Larrabee, M.G., and Leicht, W.S. (1965): J. Neurochem., 12:1-13.
42. McKean, M.L., Smith, J.B., and Silver, M.J. (1981): J. Biol. Chem., 256:1522-1524.
43. Michell, R.H. (1975): Biochim. Biophys. Acta, 415:81-147.
44. Michell, R.H., Jafferji, S.S., and Jones, L.M. (1976): FEBS Lett., 69:1-5.
45. Michell, R.H. (1979): Trends Biochem. Sci., 4:128-131.
46. Michell, R.H., and Kirk, C.J. (1981): Trends Pharmacol. Sci., 2:86-89.
47. Murthy, P.P.N., and Agranoff, B.W. (1982): This book.
48. Putney, J.W., Weiss, S.J., Van de Walle, C.M., and Haddas, R.A. (1980): Nature, 284:345-346.
49. Schacht, J., and Agranoff, B.W. (1972): J. Biol. Chem., 247:771-777.
50. Schacht, J., and Agranoff, B.W. (1973): J. Biol. Chem., 249:1551-1557.
51. Schacht, J., Neale, E.A., and Agranoff, B.W. (1974): J. Neurochem., 23:211-218.
52. Schwarcz, R., Hokfelt, T., Fuxe, K., Jonsson, G., Goldstein, M., and Terenius, L. (1979): Exp. Brain Res., 37:199-216.
53. Smith, T.L., Eichberg, J., and Hauser, G. (1979): Life Sci., 24:2179-2184.
54. Szerb, J.C., Hadhazy, P., and Dudar, J.D. (1977): Brain Res., 128:285-291.
55. Takenawa, T., Saito, M., Nagai, Y., and Egawa, K. (1977): Arch. Biochem. Biophys., 182:244-250.
56. Thompson, W., and MacDonald, G. (1975): J. Biol. Chem., 250:6779-6785.
57. Thompson, W., and MacDonald, G. (1976): Eur. J. Biochem., 65:107-111.
58. Weissman, G., Anderson, P., Serhan, C., Samuelsson, E., and Good, E. (1980): Proc. Natl. Acad. Sci., 77:1506-1510.
59. Yagihara, Y., and Hawthorne, J.N. (1972): J. Neurochem., 19:355-367.

Phospholipids in the Nervous System, Vol. 1: Metabolism, edited by L. Horrocks, et al. Raven Press, New York © 1982.

Perturbed Lipid Metabolism in the Brain: Not So Much a Summing-Up, More a Provocation

R. H. Michell

Department of Biochemistry, University of Birmingham, Birmingham B15 2TT, United Kingdom

I generally approach summing-up sessions at meetings with apprehension and expectation of boredom, so the idea of being the purveyor of that anticlimax made me feel like the victim in Pierre de Meyts's cartoon. This provided the introduction to his summing up at the 4th Hormones and Cell Regulation meeting at Bischenberg in 1979 (reproduced with the permission of the author and Elsevier/North Holland Biomedical Press).

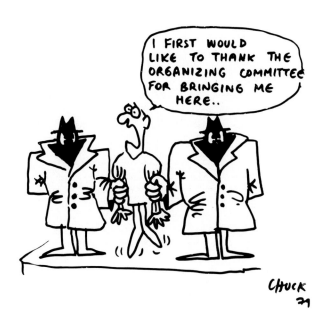

In self-defence I decided not to sum up but to comment critically on a personal selection of the material presented by our main speakers and in the poster sessions. Of the comments I made at the meeting, I have committed to paper only those related to the dramatic changes in glycerolipid metabolism that occur in stimulated tissues. In the nervous system the modes of experimental stimulation that produce such effects include defined chemical ligands (e.g. neurotransmitters) and much more general 'insults' (e.g. ischemia, anoxia, bicuculline-induced epileptiform seizures).

My comments will tend to fall into four groups: on the locus of stimulated inositol lipid metabolism in the brain; on the nature and mechanism of the changes in glycerolipid metabolism that are seen in insulted brains; on the meaning of the 'phosphatidylinositol response'; and on some weaknesses, arising both from limitations of experimental design and from inadequate prior formulation of working hypotheses, that characterize many of the reported studies.

I will open with two general criticisms. First, I wonder for how much longer 'classical' neurochemists can continue to make, either implicitly or explicitly, the obviously invalid assumption that changes in lipid metabolism in a neural region such as the cerebral cortex can usefully be interpreted as changes in a single metabolic pool. Grace Sun did point out the metabolic heterogeneity of phosphatidylinositol (PtdIns) and phosphatidylcholine in brain, but only to the extent of admitting the presence of two metabolically distinguishable pools of each lipid. But the brain is not a homogeneous cellular mass: surely there must be as many metabolic pools as there are cell-types? I suppose that the essence of this criticism, stated in broader terms, is that relatively little of the lipid neurochemistry to which we listened seemed to have been influenced much by the subtleties of modern neurobiology, either in terms of ideas or of experimental approaches. Surely we must make far more use of techniques such as selective lesioning or the culture of defined cellular populations; they seem likely to provide definitive experimental approaches to at least some of the problems that are not accessible within the complexity of the intact and unperturbed organ.

My second basic criticism is similar. Many of the studies that we learned of, especially in the 'insulted' brains, were of perturbed inositol lipid metabolism. Sometimes they were direct, and sometimes in the guise of changes in tissue turnover of diacylglycerol or arachidonate. Mechanistic information on the processes involved in modifying inositol lipid metabolism in the nervous sytem is still scanty as compared with the equivalent, but still limited, information on receptor-controlled phosphoinositide metabolism in peripheral tissues. Several of these presentations neither made any explicit comparison between the neural effects and the effects seen in simpler non-neural tissues nor attempted any hypothetical reconstruction of the observed changes. Surely such parochialism and caution are counter-productive. The apparent differences between cell-cell communication in the CNS and in peripheral tissues seem to be becoming less and less real as time passes, so it seems odd that lipid neurochemists are not making the maximum use of information from relatively simple peripheral tissue models in order to help generate an understanding of the events evoked by neurotransmitters in the CNS.

THE 'PHOSPHATIDYLINOSITOL RESPONSE' OF BRAIN: PRESYNAPTIC OR POST-
SYNAPTIC?

Brain was one of the first tissues in which Hokin and Hokin observed
neurotransmitter-stimulated labelling of PtdIns (17). However, it is probably not unfair to suggest that it has been a relatively unhelpful tissue
insofar as deciphering the mechanism and function of this response is concerned, probably because of its complexity. Pickard and Hawthorne (28)
and Grace Sun (this book) have shown that it possesses PtdIns pools of
very different metabolic characteristics, but it is not clear where in the
tissue these occur or where in the tissue stimulated PtdIns metabolism occurs. Are the metabolic compartments glial or neuronal and, if neuronal,
are they presynaptic or postsynaptic?
In 1966 Lowell Hokin showed autoradiographically that acetylcholine-
stimulated PtdIns labelling in sympathetic ganglia occurs in individual
acetylcholine-sensitive neurones (15). Moreover, PtdIns labelling response to acetylcholine or to high K^+ persists in ganglia that have been
deprived of their afferent innervation (16,27). Gene Anderson and his
colleagues, having technically improved the radioautographic approach,
have now shown that the small overall increase in PtdIns metabolism that
occurs during illumination of Xenopus retinas is entirely accounted for by
a large and unique change in the turnover of the PtdIns in the outer
plexiform layer, a response that is probably attributable to horizontal
cells. Each of these observations points to a postsynaptic neuronal locus
for neurotransmitter-stimulated PtdIns metabolism.
On the other hand, Lunt and Pickard (21), when they stimulated brain
that had been labelled in vitro for 20 h with $^{32}P_i$, interpreted their
data as indicating a selective presynaptic loss of label from the PtdIns
of synaptic vesicles (but inspection of the data in their paper suggests
that the recoveries of labelled lipids in the subcellular fractions were
uncomfortably low, making any interpretation somewhat ambiguous). In
later experiments, Pickard and Hawthorne (28) found that there was selective labelling of a 'synaptosome'-associated PtdIns pool in rat brain 2 h
after injection of $^{32}P_i$, and that electrical stimulation of an isolated 'synaptosomal' fraction caused breakdown of the ^{32}P-PtdIns of its
'synaptic vesicles'. It has also been known for many years that isolated
synaptosome-enriched fractions can, on stimulation with acetylcholine,
show a stimulated metabolism of PtdIns and phosphatidate (see 14). Most
recently the usual inference has been that this response occurs in
pinched-off presynaptic nerve terminals and that it might have a specific
presynaptic function that is somehow related to neurotransmitter release.
Pickard and Hawthorne (28) went so far as to suggest that diacylglycerol
released from PtdIns on stimulation of synaptosomes might be responsible
for the fusion of synaptic vesicles with the presynaptic plasma membrane.
But the 'synaptosome' data present two substantial problems. First,
when the highly active PtdIns of Pickard and Hawthorne's 'synaptosomes'
broke down upon electrical stimulation there was no concomitant loss of
unlabelled PtdIns from the fraction (28). The simplest explanation of
this is that the highly labeled and sensitive pool of PtdIns was not a
component of the presynaptic terminals that quantitatively dominated their
'synaptosomal' fraction, but was in some minor, but metabolically very
active, 'contaminant' of the fraction. Secondly, stimulation of brain
slices causes up to a threefold increase in the turnover of PtdIns
(admittedly when assayed by a $^{32}P_i$ incorporation, a flawed measure)
(see 22). But this response decreases substantially when the tissue is

fragmented into pieces smaller than 0.2-0.3 mm across: the maximum stimulation of PtdIns metabolism in isolated 'synaptosomal' fractions is only
a small fraction of this original response [see 14,22].   If a major fraction of the tissue's total response occurred in presynaptic terminals,
then the expectation should be that it would be fully preserved, or even
accentuated, in a relatively homogeneous preparation of nerve endings.
Instead its magnitude declines greatly during the progression from intact
tissue to isolated nerve endings.

This apparent paradox seems to be at least partly resolved by the experiments of Fisher et al. [this book and ref. 12] who showed, by using
ibotenate-induced lesions to kill hippocampal neurones, that the pool of
inositol lipids that displays acetylcholine-sensitive metabolism in 'synaptosomal' fractions isolated from the hippocampus occurs in postsynaptic
elements that are in the minority in the mixed 'synaptosome' fractions:
these postsynaptic elements are probably 'dendrosomes' (pinched off de-
ndritic elements).

If this interpretation were to prove applicable to all experiments on
stimulated inositol lipid metabolism in 'synaptosomal' fractions, then the
following conclusions would follow naturally from the postsynaptic neuronal site of the PtdIns response.   [1] The small pool of PtdIns in 'synaptosomal' fractions that is metabolically active and is rapidly and
selectively broken down is in postsynaptic neuronal fragments rather than
in nerve-endings.   [2] As corollary to this, the metabolically inert 'synaptosomal' PtdIns pool that constitutes the bulk of the PtdIns in such
fractions and does not respond to stimulation of these fractions is the
PtdIns of the presynaptic terminal.   [3] There is therefore no basis for
hypotheses that attempt to implicate PtdIns breakdown in specific presynaptic functions such as neurotransmitter release.   [4] The PtdIns response of a 'synaptosomal' fraction to cholinergic stimuli is a response
mediated by typical postsynaptic muscarinic receptors, so that problems
encountered in trying to interpret its function in relation to the 'odd'
functional behaviour of presynaptic muscarinic autoreceptors can be for-
gotten.   [5] The reason that the PtdIns response is lost as neural tissue
is chopped into smaller fragments is because the integrity of large, responsive neurones is destroyed, even though much smaller, but non-respon-
sive, nerve terminals survive.

To summarise, present evidence seems compatible with the view that the
PtdIns response of neural tissue is largely in postsynaptic neurones and
maybe also in glia (35).   The metabolism of nerve terminals is modest and
unresponsive to stimulation, and at present there is no experimental
information to suggest that it merits any special study.

PERTURBED PHOSPHOLIPID METABOLISM IN 'INSULTED' BRAIN

We heard a lot about what happens to lipid metabolism when the brain
is subjected to various degrees of insult, ranging from a complete
cessation of blood flow (after decapitation or carotid ligation) to
bicuculline-induced epileptiform seizures.   Presumably the latter, in
which the inhibitory action of brain GABA is cancelled out, represents the
excitatory neural equivalent of a 'howl-round' in an overloaded acoustic
circuit: this is stimulating both for the listener and for the participating electronics (neurones).   In all of these studies it was agreed that
the major easily assessed lipid change in such situations of massive brain
insult is a mobilisation of unesterified stearic and arachidonic acids.

So where did these fatty acids come from? The obvious candidates, given their characteristic stearic/arachidonic fatty acid pattern, are the inositol lipids, in which case one might expect the release to be initiated by phospholipase C action on PtdIns or polyphosphoinositides. If this were to happen the released fatty acids should initially be seen as liberated diacylglycerol: this is what Bazan and his colleagues observed. Going further, it was apparent from the data of Horrocks et al. that the first glycerophospholipid to decrease in concentration after insult was PtdIns (within 30 sec) and that this was followed only later by phosphatidylethanolamine and then phosphatidylcholine. In order to attempt some interpetation of this temporal sequence we must first make the assumption, as yet unproven, that all of these metabolically perturbed lipid pools are indeed in one set of equivalent cellular sites and that they display precursor-product relationships with one another. If we are lucky they might even be the metabolically active and responsive neuronal lipid pools that have been discussed in terms of their changes in phosphate metabolism in the previous section. At least this seems until proved false, likely to be the most useful working hypothesis.

Even then, further hypothesising can only continue fruitfully by relating the problem to existing data on non-neural tissues, where it is clear that many hormones and neurotransmitters do stimulate the breakdown of PtdIns to diacylglycerol. Moreover, it is also generally agreed that receptor-stimulated PtdIns breakdown is a response that frequently, and probably always, occurs at the same time as a receptor-controlled increase in cytosol $[Ca^{2+}]$ in stimulated cells (23,24). This was the reasoning that led me recently to suggest (22) that neurotransmitter-stimulated PtdIns metabolism, assessed as ^{3}H-inositol incorporation, might be used as a general, though indirect, biochemical correlate by which to radioautographically map the distribution amongst neurones of particular transmitter receptors whose activation leads to a rise in cytosol $[Ca^{2+}]$. Here one would predict that the light-stimulated PtdIns turnover in the horizontal cells of illuminated retinas [4] probably accompanies the action of some, as yet unidentified, neurotransmitter that uses Ca^{2+} as its intracellular messenger.

If the reader would like to see the entire sequence of events in inositol lipid metabolism that seems likely to be emerging from the studies in whole brain described in a different context, but in great detail, my advice is simply to read some of the platelet literature (e.g. refs. 5,7,8,20,23,31,32,34). Fig. 1 represents an attempt to summarise the many processes with which stimulated inositol lipid breakdown has, at least tentatively, been linked in peripheral tissues: surely some of these ideas should inform the design of future experiments on brain?

Amongst the receptors that produce stimulation of inositol lipid breakdown in peripheral tissues are several that are responsive to small amine neurotransmitters (muscarinic cholinergic, α_1-adrenergic, 5-HT$_1$, H$_1$-histamine) and several that respond to small peptides that are putative neurotransmitters (pancreozymin, substance P, angiotensin, vasopressin, bombesin, thyrotropin) (6,22,24). There is either unambiguous evidence or a clear indication that each of the former group of receptors also controls PtdIns metabolism in brain (see 14,22); few similar experiments on the CNS have yet been attempted with the peptides (see 22).

Given the pattern of events seen in 'insulted' brain, I think that it would be reasonable to propose, as a working hypothesis, that the occurrence of PtdIns breakdown, diacylglycerol accumulation and arachidonate liberation in the cell bodies and dendrites of the neurones of 'insulted'

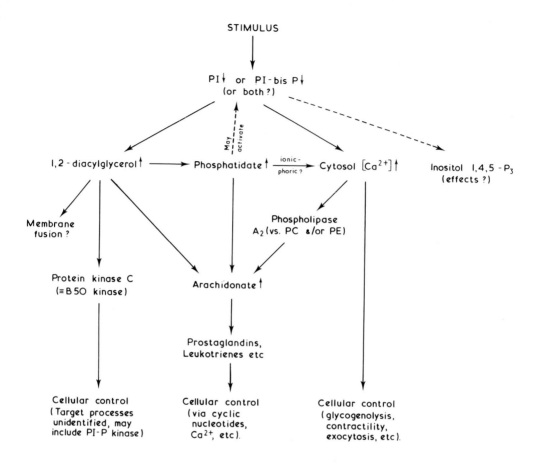

Fig. 1. A hypothetical scheme that summarises many of the functions that have been tentatively ascribed to receptor-stimulated inositol lipid breakdown. An alternative view, that inositol lipid breakdown follows rather than precedes calcium mobilization, is summarised by Cockcroft (9). The information summarised here arises from work with a variety of cell-types, especially the platelet (5,7,20,23,24,31,32,34). Interrelationships are also likely between these changes and: [a] the changes in phospholipid methylation that characterise some stimulated cells (see the paper by Crews in this volume); [b] changes in cellular cycle nucleotide concentrations (e.g. ref. 8). These additional complications were omitted from this scheme for the sake of simplicity.

brain are all caused by a massive and uncontrolled relase of excitatory
neurotransmitters. Moreover, it seems likely that many (though not all)
of these transmitters share a mode of action on their target neurones in
which breakdown of inositol lipids and the mobilization of Ca^{2+} in the
cytosol are the key factors. We do not yet know which of the many endogenously released transmitters act in this way in neural tissue, but the
published data both from peripheral tissues and from brain and ganglia
offer strong hints as to which may be good candidates.

How could this type of hypothesis best be tested? Surely not very
easily in tissue models as uncontrolled as those that exist inside the
skull of a decapitated or carotid-ligated rat! The obvious alternative
would appear to be relatively thick (> 0.3 mm) tissue slices, but these
are relatively small and they may not preserve an intact enough neural
'wiring pattern' for an excitatory 'howl-round' to be set up and sustained
during insults such as anoxia. Studies which start by selecting and adding effective individual neurotransmitters will be valuable, but they by-
pass the important question as to which transmitters are implicated in
situ. One possibility might be to resurrect, for the purposes of lipid
biochemistry, the electrically stimulated brain slice preparation in which
Pumphrey showed enhanced metabolism of PtdIns many years ago (29).
Although such slices are deprived of their normal input from external
afferent pathways, their response to electrical stimulation may well be
mediated by the endogenous release of transmitters and it may therefore be
somwhat like what happens in the insulted brain in situ. One wonders
whether bicuculline would release inhibitory control in such slices.
There might then be dramatic changes in lipid metabolism even during a
very mild level of electrical stimulation that would, in the absence of
bicuculline, produce little effect on lipid metabolism. If this were to
happen, could one then use pharmacological antagonists to identify participating endogenous neurotransmitters? Nemoto and his colleagues told
us that barbiturates ameliorate the effects of anoxia. They also inhibit
acetylcholine-stimulated PtdIns turnover in synaptosomes (26). One
wonders what they would do to the responses of electrically stimulated
slices.

WHAT IS THE MECHANISM AND FUNCTION OF STIMULATED INOSITOL LIPID METABOLISM?

First I shall state a couple of points that appear generally not to be
controversial. First, receptor-stimulated inositol lipid metabolism appears to be a universal accompaniment of the mobilisation of cytosol
Ca^{2+} by receptors (6,9,23,24). Even this is now cast in some doubt by
the adrenal medulla experiments of Hawthorne, Agranoff and their colleagues. Secondly, the initiating reaction in this type of response seems
always to be the breakdown of an inositol lipid to diacylglycerol.

When we proceed to points over which there is disagreement, the first
problem is to decide which lipid is initially broken down on stimulation.
Most evidence points to controlled PtdIns breakdown (24), but Abdel-Latif
argues for an important effect of α-adrenergic and muscarinic stimuli upon
breakdown of PtdIns(4,5)P_2 in iris smooth muscle. The significance of
this effect is difficult to assess, since it is not detectable until 10
min after stimulation (i.e. long after the muscle has contracted), needs
the tissue to be metabolically poisoned before it can be seen, and depends
upon the presence of extracellular Ca^{2+} (2). However, it does seem that
the rise in cytosol Ca^{2+} that occurs in receptor-stimulated healthy

tissue can't evoke it. This is reminiscent of the human erythrocyte, where Ca^{2+} can stimulate phosphodiesterase-catalyzed $PtdIns(4,5)P_2$ breakdown, but only after elevation of cytosol $[Ca^{2+}]$ to a level far higher than would ever occur in a healthy cell [11].

However, our own recent work on isolated liver cells has shown a very rapid breakdown of $PtdIns(4,5)P_2$ upon stimulation with Ca^{2+}-mobilising ligands such as vasopressin (15,18,23). This response, like PtdIns breakdown in the same cells, shows the expected characteristics for a coupling reaction involved in receptor-controlled Ca^{2+} mobilisation. Our current working hypothesis is that the stimulated breakdown, or rather disappearance, of PtdIns that we and others have been studying for several years may itself be a secondary event, merely a measure of the stimulated consumption of PtdIns by the kinases that replenish the stimulated cell's store of $PtdIns(4,5)P_2$. If this is correct, then the worries that arise from the inability of either our own group (19) or Hawthorne and Azila (this book) to see any clear subcellular localization of stimulated PtdIns 'breakdown' may be groundless. What we now need to know is where in the cell $PtdIns(4,5)P_2$ breaks down, and not whence came the PtdIns for its resynthesis. This information is not yet available for any cell.

The other important fuel for recent challenges to the view that PtdIns or $PtdIns(4,5)P_2$ breakdown might be a coupling reaction in Ca^{2+} mobilization by receptors (e.g. 9) has been a collection of observations that have suggested inositol lipid breakdown is caused by, rather than a cause of, a rise in cytosol $[Ca^{2+}]$. There is now no doubt that PtdIns can sometimes be broken down as a consequence of the mobilization of Ca^{2+} by receptors (see 9,23 for reviews), but that does not answer the more difficult question as to whether the available data demonstrates in any tissue that all inositol lipid breakdown is Ca^{2+}-mediated (i.e. none is receptor-mediated). My own judgement is that the only system in which, on the available evidence, this appears probable is the leucocyte stimulated with fmet-leu-phe (8,20,23).

Others who have independently drawn the conclusion that Ca^{2+} controls inositol lipid breakdown have usually done so on the basis of experiments on the Ca^{2+} requirement either of receptor-stimulated inositol lipid labelling in intact cells or of inositol lipid-degrading enzymes in broken cell preparations. For reasons discussed elsewhere (8,23), I think that attempts to interpret cell function on the basis of these experiments are so inherently ambiguous that they cannot be regarded as useful evidence in the answering of so important a question. PtdIns labelling is far too indirect a measure of cellular response (see below), and the requirement of an enzyme in isolation for a trace of Ca^{2+} cannot be interpreted as strong evidence that it is controlled by Ca^{2+} when in an intact cell.

On balance, therefore, I think the occurrence in neural tissue of a PtdIns response to any individual receptor-directed stimulus, whether measured as PtdIns or $PtdIns(4,5)P_2$ (or, less satisfactorily, as PtdIns or phosphatidate labelling) can still be regarded an an indirect indication that the relevant receptor uses Ca^{2+} as its intracellular messenger in neural tissue, probably in neurones. At least for the H_1-histamine receptor of cerebral cortex, this view is strongly supported by the demonstration of a Ca^{2+}-mediated glycogenolytic response to H_1-histamine receptor activation (33).

METHODOLOGICAL PROBLEMS

Two major problems of experimental approach still greatly reduce the value of much of the information published in this field.

The first is the continued use by many workers of lipid labelling as their major or only measure of stimulated inositol phospholipid metabolism (see 23,25): much of the information provided by such studies is un-interpretable. Labelling studies can be of particular use when it is possible either to pulse-label a lipid or to label it until it reaches isotopic equilibrium with an isotopically equilibrated cellular precursor pool (e.g. ATP). Under such carefully defined circumstances a loss of label from pulse-labelled lipid can validly be used to study lipid breakdown (e.g. 19) and changes in equilibrium labelling of a lipid reflect changes in its steady-state concentration (e.g. 18). Most labelling studies, however, have simply followed isotope incorporation via a multi-step synthetic route to a complex lipid, e.g. PtdIns. Attempts to use such non-equilibrium experiments to analyze quantitatively the mechanisms or kinetics of some preceding event such as PtdIns breakdown are invalid, since every step in the intervening pathways might be independently susceptible to a variety of environmental variations (e.g. Ca^{2+} concentration). There is a temptation, in the absence of extensive data on lipid breakdown, to continue optimistically to overinterpret those labelling experiments whose results accord with one's prejudices and unceremoniously to dismiss those that do not. In the longer term it would be better to disregard them all. I do not wish to deny the continued usefulness of simple labelling studies for carefully defined and limited purposes (e.g. for studying relative potencies of agonists or antagonists under otherwise constant conditions (e.g. 13), but simply to oppose their uncritical use for attempting to answer mechanistic questions.

The second major methodological problem relates to the choice of appropriate assay conditions under which to study, in broken-cell systems, those enzymes that are candidates for a role in stimulated lipid metabolism. We often seem to lose sight of the simple requirement that our experiments should tell us how an enzyme is likely to behave under the conditions that it normally encounters within healthy cells. This can be well illustrated by reference to the Ca^{2+}-dependent phosphodiesterases that degrade PtdIns and $PtdIns(4,5)P_2$. The best characterized PtdIns phosphodiesterase is a cytosol enzyme found in many, if not all, eukaryote cells. When offered pure PtdIns it attacks it avidly, but when offered a mixed lipid phase that is similar to a natural membrane then it acts only slowly (see the paper by Dawson and his colleagues). It is unfortunate that until recently almost all published studies of this enzyme utilized pure substrate, making their relevance to its normal behaviour very doubtful. The Ca^{2+} requirement of this enzyme renders superficially attractive the notion that cytosol $[Ca^{2+}]$ might control it, especially since it can be activated by very low concentrations of buffered Ca^{2+} (3). On the other hand, it is equally possible that it simply requires a trace of Ca^{2+}, but is controlled by some other route (23,24). Many studies still study its Ca^{2+} requirement in the absence of an added Ca^{2+} buffer, forgetting that PtdIns is itself an effective Ca^{2+} buffer and thus rendering impossible the interpretation of their results. In addition, the ability of other ions (Mg^{2+}, Na^+, etc.) to inhibit this enzyme (probably by competition with Ca^{2+}?) has meant that these inhibitory ions are usually omitted from incubations. But they are normally around in the cell, so that it is the activity of the phosphodiesterase in their presence that is of relevance to the intracellular situation. Moreover, amphiphilic ions are often included in assays of these enzymes because of their ability (as detergents) to modify the activities of lipid metabolising enzymes. They may interact with the enzymes, they may disperse and/or modify the charge characteristics of lipid substrates, and they may change the concentrations of free ions (e.g. Ca^{2+}) in solution (due to displacement from binding to lipid). Any of these effects may change expressed enzyme activities. For example, do Irvine and Dawson's studies of the effects of phosphatidate and fatty acids on PtdIns phosphodiesterase represent anything more than the effects of any anionic amphiphile on this activity under 'artificial' assay conditions?

The importance of using incubation conditions like those in the cell impressed itself upon us particularly strongly during a recent study by Pete Downes of the Ca^{2+}-dependent polyphosphoinositide phosphodiesterase of the human erythrocyte membrane (28). At low ionic strength, in the absence of Mg^{2+}, this enzyme was appreciably activated by ~1 μM Ca^{2+}, i.e. a concentration only one or two orders of magnitude above the ambient Ca^{2+} concentration of the healthy erythrocyte (~10^{-8} M). This seemed odd, since the survival of the polyphosphoinositides throughout the lifespan of healthy erythrocytes suggested that the phosphodiesterase was never switched on during their 120 days in the circulation. This paradox was resolved when we found that the inclusion of approximately physiological concentrations of Na^+ and Mg^{2+} in our assay medium decreased the apparent Ca^{2+} affinity of the polyphosphoinositide phosphodiesterase more than 100-fold: it then became clear that it would never be activated by Ca^{2+} under conditions compatible with erythrocyte survival. I hope we manage to remember this lesson in our future work.

CONCLUDING REMARKS

I would like to thank the participants in this meeting for helping me to focus these, I hope useful, thoughts. My criticisms are not of the meeting: they also apply to much of the other work in this field. These criticisms are stated here (maybe sometimes overstated?) in a deliberately pointed and provocative style. This is in the hope that they will evoke from the reader either a reasoned, and equally spirited, defense of his approach or else a change in that approach.

ACKNOWLEDGEMENTS

I am grateful to my colleagues Chris Kirk, Lynne Jones, Pete Downes, Judith Creba, and Phillip Hawkins for the discussions that led to many of these comments, and the MRC and the Wellcome Trust for financial support.

REFERENCES

1. Abdel-Latif, A.A., Yau, S.-J. and Smith, J.P. (1974): J. Neurochem., 22:383-393.
2. Abdel-Latif, A.A., Akhtar, R.A. and Smith, J.P. (1979): In: Cyclitols and Phosphoinositides, edited by W.W. Wells and F. Eisenberg, pp. 121-143, Academic Press, New York.
3. Allan, D. and Michell, R.H. (1974): Biochem. J., 142:599-604.
4. Anderson, R.E. and Hollyfield, J. (1981): Biochim. Biophys. Acta., 665:619-622.

5. Bell, R.L., Kennerly, D.A., Stanford, N. and Majerus, P.A. (1979): J. Biol. Chem., 76:3238-3241.
6. Berridge, M.J. (1980): Trends in Pharmacol. Sci., 1:419-424.
7. Broekman, M.J., Ward, J.W. and Marcus, A.J. (1980): J. Clin. Invest., 66:275-283.
8. Chau, L.-Y. and TAi, H.-H. (1981): Biochem. Biophys. Res. Commun., 100:1688-1695.
9. Cockcroft, S. (1981): Trends in Pharmacol. Sci., in press.
10. Cockcroft, S., Bennett, J.P. and Gomperts, B.D. (1981): Biochem. J., in press.
11. Downes, C.P. and Michell, R.H. (1981): Biochem. J., in press.
12. Fisher, S.K., Frey, K.A. and Agranoff, B.W. J. Neurosci., in press.
13. Hanley, M.R., Lee, C.M., Jones, L.M. and Michell, R.H. (1980): Mol. Pharmacol., 18:78-83.
14. Hawthorne, J.N. and Pickard, M.R. (1979): J. Neurochem., 32:5-14.
15. Hokin, L.E. (1965): Proc. Natl. Acad. Sci. U.S.A., 53:1369-1376.
16. Hokin, L.E. (1966): J. Neurochem., 13:179-184.
17. Hokin, L.E. (1979): In: Structure and Function of Nervous Tissue, edited by G. Bourne, Vol. 3, pp. 161-184, Academic Press, New York.
18. Kirk, C.J., Creba, J.A., Downes, C.P. and Michell, R.H. (1981): Biochem. Soc. Trans., 9:377-379.
19. Kirk, C.J., Michell, R.H. and Hems, D.A. (1981): Biochem. J., 194:155-165.
20. Lapetina, E.G., Billah, M.M. and Cuatrecasas, P. (1981): Nature, 292:367-369.
21. Lunt, G.G. and Pickard, M.R. (1975): J. Neurochem., 24:1203-1208.
22. Michell, R.H. (1979): Neurosciences Research Program meeting, to be published.
23. Michell, R.H., Kirk, C.J., Jones, L.M., Downes, C.P. and Creba, J.A. (1981): Phil. Trans. Roy. Soc. Lond. Ser. B., in press.
24. Michell, R.H. and Kirk, C.J. (1981): Trends in Pharmacol. Sci., 2:86-90.
25. Michell, R.H. and Kirk, C.J. (1981): Biochem. J., 198:247-248.
26. Miller, J.C. and Leung, I. (1979): Biochem. J., 178:9-13.
27. Nagata, Y., Mikoshiba, K. and Tsukada, Y. (1973): Brain Res., 56:259-269.
28. Pickard, M.R. and Hawthorne, J.N. (1978): J. Neurochem., 30:16-23.
29. Pumphrey, A.M. (1969): Biochem. J., 112:61-70.
30. Reddy, P.V. and Sastry, P.S. (1979): Brain Res., 168:287-298.
31. Rittenhouse-Simmons, S. and Deykin, D. (1981): In: Platelets in Biology and Pathology, edited by J.L. Gordon, Vol. 2, pp. 349-372, Elsevier/North Holland, Amsterdam.
32. Rittenhouse-Simmons, S. (1981): J. Biol. Chem., 256:4153-4155.
33. Schwartz, J.-C., Pollard, H. and Quach, T.T. (1980): J. Neurochem., 35:26-33.
34. Takai, Y., Kaibuchi, K., Matsubara, T. and Nishizuka, Y. (1981): Biochem. Biophys. Res. Commun., 101:61-67.
35. Woelk, H., Kanig, K. and Peiler-Ichikawa, K. (1974): J. Neurochem., 23:1057-1063.

Alterations of Phospholipid Methylation and Viscosity in Brain Membranes of Old Rats

S. Teolato, A. C. Bonetti, G. Calderini, *A. Gaiti, **F. Crews, and G. Toffano

*Department of Biochemistry, Fidia Research Laboratories, Abano Terme, Italy; *Department of Biochemistry, University of Perugia, Perugia, Italy; **Department of Pharmacology, University of Florida, College of Medicine, Gainesville, Florida 32610*

Enzymatic conversion of phosphatidylethanolamine into phosphatidylcholine appears to be related to the capability of an external signal to translate information into the cells (Hirata, F. and Axelrod, J.: Science, 209:1082-1090, 1980). This phospholipid methylation is catalyzed by two methyltrnasferases which were recently detected also in synaptosomal plasma membranes prepared from rat brain (Crews, F., Hirata, F. and Axelrod, J.: J. Neurochem., 34:1491-1498, 1980). Since alterations of normal physiological functions observed during aging might be associated with biochemical changes of cell membranes, we have studied the methyltransferase activities in rat brain at different ages. With increasing age membrane phospholipid methylation is stimulated. This effect is due to an increase of methyltransferase I activity, the rate limiting step of phosphatidylethanolamine transformation, while methyltransferase II activity remains unchanged. The highest increase is detected in the cerebellum while a lower but significant activation is present in other brain areas such as the striatum, cerebral cortex and limbic system. On the contrary, the enzymatic activity decreases in the brain stem.
In addition, membrane viscosity is altered during aging. As the enzymatic phospholipid methylation could be involved in maintaining the membrane viscosity, the possible relationship between these two biochemical changes is under investigation.

Serine Decarboxylation as a Source of Phosphoglyceride Ethanolamine in Myelinating Organ Cultures of Cerebellum

Keith Bradbury

Department of Pathology, University of Leeds, Leeds LS2 9JT, United Kingdom

Myelinating cultures of newborn rat cerebellum (1) were maintained in vitro for 28 days. On labelling cultures with $[3-^{14}C]$-L-serine the rise in labelling of phosphatidylserine (PS) over 24h was progressive but more rapid at earlier times. In contrast acid stable and acid labile ethanolamine phosphoglycerides (EPG) exhibited a pronounced labelling lag up to 3h followed by rapid accretion up to 24h suggesting that PS label might be entering EPG metabolism. A comparison of $[3-^{14}C]$-L-serine and $[1-^{14}C]$-DL-serine labelling of culture EPG showed a labelling ratio of 50:1. This would be expected if serine were being decarboxylated to ethanolamine with the loss C_1. Mild hydrolysis of culture lipids at 21 days in vitro showed that base labelling was: PS 86%, acid labile EPG 91%, acid stable EPG 95%, of the molecular label indicating that secondary metabolism of label into phospholipid glycerol and FA was small. Pulse labelling for 1h with $[3-^{14}C]$-L-serine gave initial sp. act. (d.p.m./nmol lipid phosphorus) of 16×10^2 for PS and 2×10^2 for acid stable EPG. After a 12h cold chase the respective values were 11×10^2 and 8×10^2. This rise in acid stable EPG labelling in the absence of an extracellular pool of labelled serine and in the presence of a very small water soluble intracellular pool of label strongly indicates that serine in PS was being decarboxylated to form the ethanolamine of EPG. While the role of serine decarboxylation in brain in vivo remains uncertain, the present study indicates that a truly organoid culture can ultilize the pathway in common with less differentiated dissociated cells previously reported (2).

(1) Bradbury, K. & C.E. Lumsden (1979) J. Neurochem. 32, 145-154.
(2) Yavin, E. & B.P. Zeigler (1977) J. biol. Chem. 252, 260-267.

Distribution and Packing of Phosphatidylethanolamine and Phosphatidylcholine in Microsomal Membranes

M. Mersel, A. Benenson, P. Mandel, and L. Freysz

Centre de Neurochimie du CNRS, 67084 Strasbourg Cedex, France

The distribution of phosphatidylethanolamine (PE) and phosphatidylcholine (PC) and the packing of their acyl moieties (AM) in microsomal membranes of chicken brains were investigated using different approaches:

(a) Labeling or removal of the hydrophilic moiety of the phospholipids by TNBS or phospholipase C from C. welchii (PhC).

(b) Labeling of the hydrophobic moieties (AM) by $^{125}I_3$ in saturating conditions (4 molecules I_3/molecule phospholipid).

(c) Labeling of the hydrophobic moieties (AM) of surface phospholipids by lactoperoxidase (LPO) catalysed radioiodination in non-saturating conditions (7 atoms $^{125}I^-$/100 molecules of phospholipids).

The determination of external phospholipids (PE_{ex} and PC_{ex}) and of total phospholipids (PE_{tot}/PE_{tot}) by TNBS and PhC showed an asymmetric distribution of the phospholipids between the two membrane leaflets: PC_{ex}/PE_{ex} = 2.95; PC_{tot}/PE_{tot} = 1.05 (cf. this book, Freysz et al. Labeling of membrane with $^{125}I_3$ in saturating conditions showed results which were in agreement with those obtained by PhC and TNBS, i.e. the distribution of label between PC and PE (*PC/*PE) was 3.00 and 0.71 when the membranes were incubated for 10 minutes and 12 hours respectively. However when AM were labeled for 10 minutes at 20°C by LPO catalyzed radioiodination almost all the radioactivity was found to be associated with PE (*PC/*PE = 0.083). When the temperature was raised to 37°C the rate of labeling increased more in PC_{ex} than in PE_{ex} (*PC/*PE = 0.20). These data suggest that:

(a) Probing of AM with I_3 in saturating conditions allows the investigation of the intramembrane distribution of PE and PC.

(b) AM composing surface PE are more accessible to the LPO (I^-) catalyzed radioiodination than those composing surface PC.

(c) LPO catalysed radioiodination permits to follow the differential order of packing of the AM in surface PE and PC under various physical conditions.

Sidedness of Phosphatidylethanolamine Synthesis in Rat Brain Microsomes

R. Roberti, L. Corazzi, L. Binaglia, G. Arienti, and G. Porcellati

Institute of Biological Chemistry, The Medical School, University of Perugia, Perugia, Italy

Phosphatidylethanolamine (PE) can be synthesized in brain through two pathways: net synthesis and base-exchange. The sideness of these reactions has been examined in rat brain microsomes both <u>in vivo</u> and <u>in vitro</u>. Brain microsomes were incubated with $[1-^3H]$ ethanolamine of high specific activity in the base-exchange conditions and then treated with non-penetrating concentrations of 2,4,6-trinitrobenzenesulfonic acid (TNBS). Most (90% or more) of labelled PE was accessible to the probe, indicating a localization of the base-exchange reaction at the cytoplasmic side of the membranes.

Likewise, about 95% of the labelled PE formed from CDP-$[1,2-^{14}C]$ ethanolamine and membrane-bound diacylglycerol was available for the reaction with TNBS, in the same non-penetrating conditions.

In the <u>in vivo</u> experiments rats were injected intracerebrally with $[1-^3H]$ ethanolamine and sacrificed after different times from the injection of the isotope. Microsomes were prepared in the cold and incubated with TNBS at non-penetrating concentrations in order to determine the transverse distribution of the labelled lipid. These experiments showed that labelled PE was not restricted to the cytoplasmic face of microsomes. Moreover the ratio between the specific activity of trinitrophenyl-PE and that of PE decreased with time.

These results indicate that the mechanisms of PE formation in brain are active on the cytoplasmic side of the endoplasmic reticulum. On the other hand, the results coming from the <u>in vivo</u> experiments suggest that the transfer of the newly formed phospholipid to the luminal side is effective.

Supported by the grant N° 80.00543.04 from CNR, Rome.

Modification of Membrane Lipid Composition of Glioma Cells in Tissue Culture and Its Effect on β-Adrenergic Receptor Function

R. C. McKenzie and P. J. Brophy

Department of Biochemistry, University of Stirling, Stirling FK9 4LA, Scotland

Rat glioma cells were grown in a medium supplemented with
N,N'-dimethylethanolamine.   Phosphatidyl-N,N'-dimethylethanolamine
accumulated in the cell membranes at the expense of
phosphatidylcholine.   After 48 hours of culture the phosphatidyl-
-N,N'-dimethylethanolamine content had increased to 32% of total
phospholipid.   The effects of altering membrane lipid composition
on membrane fluidity, phospholipid methylation, and β-adrenergic
receptor-adenylate cyclase coupling will be discussed.

Stimulation of Sphingomyelin Degradation in Synaptosomal Plasma Membranes by Melittin and by Increased Membrane Fluidity

R. Pellkofer and K. Sandhoff

*Institut für Organische Chemie und Biochemie der Universität Bonn 1, D-5300 Bonn 1,
Federal Republic of Germany*

The general anaesthetic halothane increases membrane
fluidity as determined by fluorescence depolarization
of diphenylhexatriene. Simultaneously it stimulates up
to 40-fold the sphingomyelin degradation, by membrane-
bound neutral sphingomyelinase in calf brain synaptosomal
plasma membranes. On the other hand addition of melittin,
an amphiphilic peptide from bee venom, at concentrations
ranging from 25 to 100μM, increases fluidity in these
membranes only slightly but results in a 25-fold stimulation of sphingomyelin hydrolysis. Higher concentrations
of melittin (up to 1mM) results in a decreased membrane
fluidity and sphingomyelin degradation as compared to
the concentrations mentioned above. Experiments on the
binding of melittin to different phospholipids will be
presented.

Rapid HPLC Determination of Specific Radioactivities of Free Fatty Acids

M. I. Aveldaño de Caldironi, M. Vanrollins, and L. A. Horrocks

Department of Physiological Chemistry, The Ohio State University, Columbus, Ohio 43210

A method for the rapid, accurate determination of specific radioactivities of free fatty acids is described. The procedure involves HPLC resolution on Zorbax-ODS reverse phase columns using mixtures of acetonitrile and aqueous H_3PO_4 (0.04 M, pH 2). Detection at 192 nm enables determination of polyenoic fatty acids in the nanomole range, and radioactivity from ^3H- or ^{14}C-labeled compounds can be accurately measured using standard liquid scintillation techniques. Free fatty acids obtained after saponification of brain lipid fractions were resolved using 60% (v/v) acetonitrile in aqueous H_3PO_4. Major components appeared in the order 22:6, 20:4, 18:2, 20:3, 22:4, 16:0, 18:1, 18:0. The elution of 18:0 and other strongly retained fatty acids was speeded up by increasing the acetonitrile concentration to 90%. Distributions of radioactivity from intraventricularly injected ^3H-20:4(n-6) and $1-^{14}C$-22:4 (n-6), as well as individual specific activities, were measured. At 60 min after injection, the ^3H distribution in fatty acids from glycerophospholipids was 93% in 20:4 (n-6), 2.7% in 22:4 (n-6), and 3.8% in an unidentified fatty acid. The procedure gave resolution of underivatized free fatty acids at room temperature comparable to that obtained by GLC (180-205°C) after their conversion into methyl esters. Positional isomers of polyenoic fatty acids, difficult to resolve by GLC, were neatly separated under these conditions. For example, the (n-3), (n-6), and (n-7) isomers of 20:4 were baseline separated and well apart from the (n-3), (n-6), and (n-9) isomers of 20:3. A major drawback of the HPLC approach as opposed to GLC is the low sensitivity of the detection at 192 nm for saturated fatty acids. However, this can be overcome by increasing sample size or by using labeled standards to establish their position on chromatograms. Eluted free fatty acids can be extracted into hexane and subjected to further study, such as GC-MS identification or analysis of intramolecular radiocarbon distributions (Schmidt decarboxylation procedures). The method can also be used for the preparative isolation of free fatty acids from biological or synthetic origins.

Comparison of the Metabolism of Arachidonate, 20:4 (n-6), and Adrenate, 22:4 (n-6)

H. W. Harder, L. A. Horrocks, M. Vanrollins, and
M. I. Aveldaño de Caldironi

Department of Physiological Chemistry, The Ohio State University, Columbus, Ohio 43210

We have begun metabolic studies to help define the role, if any, of adrenate as a precursor of prostaglandins and lipoxygenase products in brain. The homology of adrenate with arachidonate, its known retroconversion to arachidonate in liver (Sprecher, 1967), and its relatively high concentration in brain support the possibility of such a role of adrenate.

$[1-^{14}C]$Adrenate provided by H. Sprecher was mixed with $[^3H]$ arachidonate and complexed with BSA giving concentrations of 0.013 μmol adrenate/μl and and 0.030 nmol arachidonate/μl. A volume of 4.0 μl of this solution was injected into the right lateral ventricles of C3H mice at a rate of 2 μl/min through chronically implanted cannulae. A stereotactic apparatus was used to implant the cannulae 1.5 mm lateral to bregma to a depth of 2.5 mm and dye added to the solution verified its entry into the ventricular system. The mice were killed by liquid nitrogen 60 min after injection, their frozen brains were removed, and their brain lipids were extracted. Recovery of the injected isotopes in the lipids was about 25% for both ^3H and ^{14}C. Saponification and HPLC analysis of a portion of the phospholipid fatty acids showed for ^3H, 93% in 20:4, 3% in 22:4, and 4% in an unidentified fatty acid. For ^{14}C, about 80% was in 22:4 and the remainder was in 16:0. The percentage distribution of ^3H and ^{14}C within the phospholipids, free fatty acids, and less polar lipids was as follows:

	^3H	^{14}C
Choline glycerophospholipids	42.0±1.1	30.7±1.0
Ethanolamine glycerophospholipids	13.9±0.6	14.5±0.6
Inositol glycerophospholipids	20.3±0.7	7.4±0.3
Serine glycerophospholipids	3.3±0.2	3.1±0.3
Phosphatidic acid	1.0±0.2	1.0±0.1
Less polar lipids	17.0±1.2	39.9±0.7
Free fatty acids	2.5±0.2	3.4±0.5

For both ^3H and ^{14}C about 4% was in diacylglycerol, about 1% was in monoacylglycerol, and less than 1% was in cholesterol. However, about 30% of the ^{14}C was in triacylglycerol as compared to only 11% of the ^3H. The distribution for ^3H corresponds closely to that found by Yau and Sun (1974) for arachidonate injected alone suggesting that arachidonate was metabolized independently of adrenate in our study.

Accumulation of Free Fatty Acids in Ischemia, Hypoxia, Hypoglycemia, and Status Epilepticus: Total Amounts and Distribution

E. Westerberg, C.-D. Agardh, S. Rehncrona, T. Wieloch, and B. K. Siesjö

Laboratory of Experimental Brain Research, University Hospital, S-221 85 Lund, Sweden

Conditions, like ischemia and epileptic seizures lead to a marked increase in the free fatty acid (FFA) content of brain tissues, with arachidonic acid showing the largest relative increase. Using an identical basic model (rats ventilated on 70% N_2O) we have recently measured FFA composition and tissue energy state in cerebral cortex during hypoglycemia, bicuculline-induced status epilepticus, ischemia, and arterial hypoxia. The pathophysiological conditions differ between the models since only hypoxia and ischemia lead to cellular hypoxia while hypoglycemia and status epilepticus allow a continued oxygen supply. In ischemia and hypoglycemia recovery events were studied as well. In these conditions and in hypoxia, accumulation of FFA was found to correlate with deterioration of tissue energy state, but in status epilepticus the phosphorylation state of the adenine nucleotide pool was only marginally affected. It seems possible that the adverse conditions studied could be associated with activation of different phospholipases, and that different membrane structures may be affected. In order to shed light on this possibility we have compared changes in FFA concentrations at various times following the induction of ischemia, hypoglycemia, and status epilepticus and considered changes observed in hypoxia as well. Particular attention was paid to alterations in concentrations of polyenoic FFAs, particularly arachidonic acid.

FFA (μmol/g)	Complete ischemia 5'	30'	Hypoglycemia 5'	30'	St.epilepticus 1'	30'
TOTAL	0.65 +0.07	1.85 +0.05	0.75 +0.07	0.75 +0.08	0.37 +0.04	0.41 +0.04
20:4	0.19 +0.02	0.44 +0.01	0.15 +0.02	0.08 +0.01	0.08 +0.01	0.05 +0.01

(Mean +S.E.M.)

The results demonstrate (1) that in the acute phases of all three conditions there are increased levels of FFAs (2) that arachidonic acid shows the largest relative increase, and (3) that when the hypoglycemia and status epilepticus (but not ischemia) are prolonged, the arachidonic acid concentration progressively decreases. It is suggested that oxidation of polyenoic fatty acid occurs in conditions with maintained oxygen supply. We propose that oxidative conversion of arachidonic acid is a common pathway leading to cell damage during hypoglycemia and epileptic seizures and in the recirculation period following ischemia.

Attenuation of Brain Free Fatty Acid Liberation During Global Brain Ischemia to Screen Potentially Effective Drugs for Treatment of Postischemic and Hypoxic Encephalopathy

E. M. Nemoto, G. K. Shiu, J. P. Nemmer, and A. L. Bleyaert

Department of Anesthesiology and Critical Care Medicine, The Anesthesia and Critical Care Medicine Research Laboratories, University of Pittsburgh, Pittsburgh, Pennsylvania 15261

We previously showed in rats, that whole brain total free fatty acids (FFA) increased linearly with time after normothermic decapitation ischemia and especially arachidonic and stearic acids, was significantly attenuated by barbiturate anesthesia which effectively reduces neurologic dysfunction after cerebral ischemic or hypoxic insults. The direct correlation between the severity of brain damage and brain FFA liberation with duration of global ischemia suggests that brain FFA liberation <u>during</u> global ischemia is involved in the pathogenesis of brain injury. Thus, its attenuation by drugs may indicate their efficacy in ameliorating ischemic brain injury. We studied the effects of ketamine, lofentanil, R41-468 a serotonin S_2 receptor blocker, Y-9179 an immidazole derivative, halothane, etomidate, innovar, pentobarbital and thiopental on brain FFAs after 10 min normothermic decapitation ischemia in rats. Total FFAs were significantly attenuated by all drugs except ketamine and R41-468. The most effective drugs were Innovar, phenytoin, pentobarbital and thiopental which were the only drugs that attenuated arachidonic acid release. Our results suggest that they would also be most effective in treating postischemic encephalopathy while the others are decidedly less effective and ketamine, ineffective. In general, our findings corroborate the results obtained in long-term recovery studies in animals.

Rapid Changes in Endogenous Pools Containing Arachidonic Acid in Cerebrum and Cerebellum During Experimental Epilepsy

N. G. Bazán and E. B. Rodríguez de Turco

INIBIBB, UNS-CONICET, 8000 Bahía Blanca, Argentina

Although there is a widespread distribution of arachidonate containing lipids and there is a high content of this acyl group in the CNS only a small proportion is released during early ischemia or convulsions and recovered as free arachidonic acid and as arachidonoyldiglycerides. The pool size and composition of FFA rapidly increases in cerebrum during bicuculline-induced status epilepticus. Stearic and arachidonic acid are the major FFA to increase as a function of time after seizures begin. Palmitic, oleic and docosahexaenoic acids do not increase any further after the first tonic clonic fit (3-4 min). In cerebellum much smaller changes take place in all FFA. A sharp decrease of stearoyl-arachidonoyl-glycerol is observed in cerebrum from 3-4 min to 5-7 min. Pretreatment with α-methyl-p-tyrosine does not change basal levels of FFA in the CNS and does not alter the bicuculline-stimulated production of these lipids in cerebrum either. However, a significant proportion of the bicuculline effect is observed in cerebellum on free stearic, oleic and arachidonic acid. On the other hand, this drug in hibits by 70% the production of stearoyl-arachidonoyl-glycerol due to bicuculline in cerebellum and cerebrum. A stimulated release of FFA also takes place upon pretreatment with p-chlorophenylalanine. Although more than one degradative reaction is involved in the described effects, a very specific phospholipid pool of membranes predominates: the one containing arachidonoyl-stearoyl. It is of interest to point out that marked differences between cerebrum and cerebellum were shown in so far as their capability to rapidly change arachidonic acid containing lipids. In cerebellum an indirect adrenergic mechanism is suggested to control the deacylation of membrane lipids based upon the results obtained by α-methyl-p-tyrosine pretreatment on the seizure-induced lipid changes. There seems to be a maximal capacity to produce FFA in the CNS. The seizure-induced changes may involve mechanisms different from those of late post decapitation ischemia. Moreover, enhancement of excitatory systems (electroconvulsive shock or pentylenetetrazol) or blockade of inhibitory systems (bicuculline) trigger the release of FFA, mainly arachidonic acid and of arachidonoyl-diglycerols. The use of this experimental model will help to understand the role of arachidonic acid and of arachidonate containing membrane lipids in the initiation, maintenance and propagation of the seizure discharges. The overshooting of the mechanism that releases free arachidonic acid during repeated convulsions such as in status epilepticus might be limited by drugs. If this can be done the harmful and often morbid consequences of status epilepticus due to irreversible brain damage could be circunvented.

Diffusion of Intracerebrally Injected ^{14}C-Arachidonic Acid or ^{14}C-Palmitic Acid in the Mouse Brain: Effects of Ischemia and Electroconvulsive Shock

E. B. Rodríguez de Turco, M. F. Pediconi, and N. G. Bazán

INIBIBB, UNS-CONICET, 8000 Bahía Blanca, Argentina

Further studies of the action of a single electroconvulsive shock and of postdecapitation ischemia on the brain phospholipid metabolism were carried out after intracerebral injections of ^{14}C-20:4 or ^{14}C-16:0 (both complexed with free fatty acid-free bovine serum albumin). A rapid diffusion of ^{14}C-20:4 took place throughout the cerebral hemispheres, brain stem and cerebellum. Ischemia or electroshock inhibited diffusion. Acylation of both fatty acids in individual phospholipids and in neutral glycerides was differentially affected by the above mentioned treatments. After one min of injection and ischemia unchanged acylation of ^{14}C-16:0 was found whereas almost maximal inhibition of ^{14}C-20:4 in all lipids, except for phosphatidyl ethanolamine, was observed. A time-course study showed that an uneven inhibition took place in phospholipids. Electroconvulsive shock also affected mainly ^{14}C-20:4 acylation, triacylglycerol being the most affected after 5 min. Phosphatidylinositol and diacylglycerol were strongly inhibited after 1 min and then partial recovery took place. Although phosphatidylethanolamine and phosphatidylserine were also·deeply inhibited at 1 min, a tendency to an enhanced acylation was observed at 10 min. Dimethylimipramine plus pargyline pretreatment increased the inhibitory effect of electroconvulsive shock on ^{14}C-20:4 labeling of all lipids, mainly on phosphatidic acid, diglycerides and triglycerides. It is concluded that the effect of ischemia and of electroconvulsive shock can be differentiated in so far as their actions on lipid metabolism. Arachidonate of membrane lipids was more altered than palmitate metabolism and drug-induced modifications suggested the involvement of an adrenergic mechanism in these changes.

Lipid Modifications in the Brain Cellular Membranes of an Hibernating Mammal, the European Hamster, During Its Circannual Rhythm

J. Robert, D. Montaudon, L. Dubourg, and *B. Canguilhem

*Laboratoire de Biochimie médicale A, Université de Bordeaux II, Bordeaux; *Institut de Physiologie, Faculté de Médecine de Strasbourg, Strasbourg, France*

Hibernating mammals have a body temperature of about 6 C during the periods of deep hibernation which occur in Winter. One of the basic questions about hibernation concerns the existence of a membrane adaptation, which allows the membrane to function at low temperatures. Numerous studies on temperature acclimation in bacteria, plants or poikilothermic vertebrates have shown that a membrane lipid adaptation occurred when the environmental temperature was lowered. An increase in fatty acyl unsaturation is considered to be responsible for the maintenance of the fluid liquid-crystalline state of the membranes in these species.

We have studied the lipid composition of the brain cellular membranes of European hamsters (*Cricetus cricetus*) sacrificed at various times in the year : in Winter (during both torpid and active states), in Spring, Summer and Autumn. We have studied the proportion of cholesterol, the phospholipid distribution, the acyl group composition of phosphoglycerides and the ganglioside distribution in whole brain hemispheres. We have also studied some of these parameters in subcellular fractions of brain. The variations encountered were extremely small and most of them were at the limit of significance. No differece at all was observed between active and torpid animals sacrificed in Winter. A small increase of the cholesterol level was observed in Winter compared to other seasons. Ethanolamine plasmalogens tended to be higher in Summer than in Winter, while the other phospholipids did not change significantly during the year. Very small differences in acyl group compositions were observed, the main ones being an increase of linoleic acid in Winter and an increase of docosahexaenoic acid in Summer. In Spring and Summer, a slight increase of stearic acid and a slight decrease of palmitoleic and oleic acids were also observed. The changes concerned in fact less than 5 % of the total phosphoglycerides acyl chains. Synaptosomes were the subcellular fraction in which the changes described above in total brain actually occurred. Gangliosides were the lipids subjected to the most significant changes, as already observed by Hilbig & Rahmann in Golden hamsters. A decrease of GM1 and an increase of GD1b, GD2 and GQ1 were observed in Winter animals.

We can therefore conclude that the lipid adaptation of cellular membranes is extremely low in hibernating mammals as compared to that described in non-mammalian species submitted to important environmental temperature changes. Other mechanisms must therefore be postulated to explain the maintenance of membrane functions at low temperatures in these animals.

(Supported by a grant from INSERM : CRL n° 81.3020)

Turnover Rates of Molecular Species of Ethanolamine Ether Phospholipids of Rat Brain *In Vivo*

Y. Masuzawa, K. Waku, and *Y. Ishima

Faculty of Pharmaceutical Sciences, Teikyo University, Sagamiko, Tsukuigun, Kanagawa; Laboratory of Neurophysiology, Tomobe Hospital Medical Centre, Tomobe, Nishiibaragigun, Ibaragi, Japan

[1-^{3}H]Glycerol was intracerebrally injected into the brain of 18-days old rat and the lipids were extracted after selected periods. 1-Acyl-, 1-O-alkyl- and 1-O-alkenyl-2-acyl-3-acetylglycerol were prepared from the ethanolamine phosphoglycerides and fractionated by $AgNO_3$-impregnated TLC into six molecular species. Bands 1-6 obtained in this way can be designated as saturated, monoene, diene, tetraene, tetraene+pentaene and hexaene. Band 4 and 6 are predominant among those derived from ether phospholipids. The specific radioactivities of the fractionated species were determined. In the three kinds of ethanolamine phosphoglycerides, monoene and hexaene species turned over rapidly, while tetraene species turned over rather slowly. Since it was established that plasmalogen was biosynthesized from alkyl ether phospholipid in mammals, the turnover time, turnover rate and turnover rate constant of each molecular species of plasmalogen were calculated from the kinetic data of 1-O-alkyl- and 1-O-alkenyl-2-acyl-3-acetylglycerol derived from the corresponding ethanolamine phospholipids.

molecular species	turnover time(min)	turnover rate (μmole/gtissue/min)	turnover rate const. min^{-1}
(01)	252	0.0040	0.021
(11)	212	0.0017	0.017
(04)	362	0.0095	0.037
(14)+(05)	276	0.0030	0.038
(06)	310	0.0140	0.064

The above data shows that a highest turnover rate was observed in 06 species and high content of 22:6 in plasmalogen may be due to this turnover rate.

Axonal Transport of Phospholipids, Including the Mitochondria-Specific Diphosphatidylglycerol, in Rat Sciatic Nerve

A. D. Toews, W. D. Blaker, and P. Morell

Biological Sciences Research Center and Department of Biochemistry and Nutrition, University of North Carolina at Chapel Hill, Chapel Hill, North Carolina 27514

The axonal transport of choline-, ethanolamine-, serine- and inositol-phosphoglycerides, as well as the mitochondria-specific diphosphatidyl glycerol (cardiolipin), was examined in adult rat sciatic nerve following injection of 200 μCi [2-^{3}H]glycerol into the L-5 dorsal root ganglion. [2-^{3}H]glycerol was rapidly incorporated into phospholipids with maximal labeling in the ganglion occurring by 2 hours; radioactivity in dorsal root ganglion then decayed with an apparent half-life of 3 days during the next 2 weeks. The bulk of the labeled phospholipids were transported at a rapid rate of 280 mm/day after a synthesis and/or processing lag of 12 minutes. Choline and ethanolamine phosphoglycerides were the major transported species, accounting for approximately 80% of the total transported lipid radioactivity. Labeled phospholipids in the crest of transported radioactivity were enriched in choline phosphoglycerides relative to ethanolamine phosphoglycerides, indicating that choline phosphoglycerides were committed to transport sooner and/or were transported at a more rapid rate than ethanolamine phosphoglycerides. Maximal accumulation of labeled phospholipids in the first 70 mm of sciatic nerve distal to the dorsal root ganglion occurred at 2 days after injection. Phospholipid radioactivity in this portion of the nerve declined with an apparent half-life of approximately 3 days between 1 and 2 weeks after injection.

Diphosphatidylglycerol, which accounted for approximately 3-5% of the total transported lipid radioactivity and is probably indicative of the axonal transport of mitochondria, was transported at a rate of 120 mm/day, somewhat slower than the bulk of the phospholipids. Maximal accumulation of diphosphatidylglycerol in the nerve did not occur until 7 days after injection; however, radioactivity in this lipid also decayed with an apparent half-life of approximately 3 days between 1 and 2 weeks after injection.

The kinetics of transport for phospholipids in the rat sciatic nerve (PNS) are generally similar to those we have previously reported for the rat visual system (CNS). Diphosphatidylglycerol transport kinetics are consistent with a model we have previously proposed (Blaker, W.D., et al., J. Cell Biol., in press, 1981) in which the apparent "transport" of mitochondria is actually the result of random bidirectional saltatory movements of individual mitochondria which equilibrate them among the cell body, axon and nerve ending pools.

Supported in part by USPHS grants NS-11615, NS-16371 and HD-03110.

Reversibility of the Propranolol-Induced Change in Retinal Phospholipid Biosynthesis

N. M. Giusto, M. G. Ilincheta de Boschero, and N. G. Bazán

Instituto de Investigaciones Bioquímicas, UNS-CONICET, Gorriti 43, Bahía Blanca, Argentina

Glycerolipid biosynthesis is rapidly modified in the retina by dl-propranolol, d-propranolol, haloperidol, phentolamine and bromo-ergocryptine. Although different pharmacological actions are elicited, similar changes are observed on lipid metabolism.

This study was carried out with bovine retinas and $(2-^3H)$ glycerol was used as a precursor. De novo synthesis of phosphatidic acid, phosphatidylserine and phosphatidylinositol are enhanced by propranolol. However, rapid reversal of the effect is obtained by transferring the retina to a drug-free medium. By the same procedure the inhibitory effect on the synthesis of phosphatidylcholine and triglycerides is overcome.

The content of phosphatidic acid is enhanced two-fold by short-term incubation with propranolol and is further increased by 20 min incubation with the drug. However, subsequent incubation of the retina in drug-free media also reverts the effect.

Subcellular fractionation studies show that although most of the described changes are microsomal, also other fractions show the effect suggesting a rapid spreading of the changes.

The biosynthesis of phosphatidylserine and of CDP-DG were also studied by separately incubating retinas with $(2-^3H)$ glycerol, (^3H) serine or (^3H) cytidine and a modified procedure was used to identify the isolated lipids and to assess the labeling of CDP-DG. Propranolol stimulates six-fold the synthesis of phosphatidylserine from labeled glycerol or serine. In addition, labeling of CDP-DG by cytidine or glycerol is increased in drug treated retinas 10-fold.

The reversibility of the effect helps to understand the drug-induced shifts of several sites of membrane lipid synthesis and to suggest the existance of controlling points that may be modulated by endogenous metabolites. Moreover, it adds further support to an alternate pathway for phosphatidylserine in neuronal tissues.

Properties and Regulation of Monoacylglycerol Lipase in the Cerebral Cortex

Joanna Strosznajder, *Harjit Singh, and *Lloyd A. Horrocks

*Experimental and Clinical Medical Research Centre, Polish Academy of Sciences, 00-784 Warsaw, Poland; *Department of Physiological Chemistry, The Ohio State University, Columbus, Ohio 43210*

Diacylglycerols in brain may be hydrolyzed by a diacylglycerol lipase to give fatty acids and monoacylglycerols. The latter is further hydrolyzed by a monoacylglycerol lipase. We have solubilized both enzymes from acetone-dried powders and have developed spectrophotometric assays based on the thioester substrate analogs synthesized by Cox and Horrocks (J. Lipid Res. 22:496-505, 1981). The substrate for monoacylglycerol lipase, 1-S-decanoyl-1-mercapto- 2,3-propanediol, was suspended as a 1.5 mM semi-stable microcrystalline dispersion by sonication with 2.5 mM of lysophosphatidyl choline. Background thiol substrate isomerization was monitored and subtracted from the observed rates to yield enzyme activity. All assays were linear with respect to time and with protein concentration up to 300 µg/ml. Monoacylglycerol lipase activity was heat labile, rapidly losing activity at temperatures over 40°C. At pH 7.4, similar activities were found in bovine and rat brain but the activities were 1.8-2.7 fold greater in bovine white matter than in gray matter. The K_m for 1-S-decanoyl-1-mercapto-2,3-propanediol is 52 µM and the V_{max} is 190 nmol/mg tissue protein/h. Both Ca^{2+} and Mg^{2+} have no effect on the activity but 250-500 µM Zn^{2+} causes a 50% inhibition. Free fatty acids at concentrations between 50 µM and 1 mM inhibit the activity by 22-90%. Stimulation of activity was found with noradrenaline between 10 and 100 µM but not at 1 mM and with 5-hydroxytryptamine between 10 µM and 1 mM concentrations. No significant effects were found with acetylcholine or cAMP. Increased activities were found after exposure of rats to hypoxic hypoxia with 5% O_2 and after 30 sec of post-decapitation ischemia. The activity had returned to normal after 5 min of ischemia. These increased activities of monoacylglycerol lipase may contribute to the increased concentrations of free fatty acids during hypoxia and ischemia.

Catabolism of Plasmalogen in Rat Brain

H. Debuch and J. Gunawan

Institute of Physiological Chemistry, University of Cologne, Federal Republic of Germany

We found an enzyme in 21-day-old rat brain, which liberates the aldehyde from 1-[^{14}C]alk-1'-enyl-sn-glycero-phosphoethanolamine (lysoplasmalogen) as substrate. Comparing the different cell fractions, the enzyme was enriched in the light microsomes. It has a pH optimum between 7.1 and 7.3. The enzymatic activity is lower in younger as well as in older animals. Mg^{++} and Ca^{++} ions inhibit the reaction to some extent, whereas Na deoxycholate is a strong inhibitor.

We found the same enzyme activity in rat liver microsomes (3), however, the specific activity was 700 fold higher. Another enzyme of brain microsomes hydrolyses ethanolamine-lysoplasmalogen to alkenylglycerol (2). This enzyme action reaches about the same activity as that of aldehyde liberation. In presence of Mg^{++} however, the former is stimulated 4 times.

Plasmalogenase, detected by Ansell and Spanner (1), has been described by several authors (for review see 4). We used 1-[^{14}C]alk-1'-enyl-2-acyl GPE as well as unlabelled plasmalogen as substrates, however we did not succeed in finding [^{14}C] labelled aldehyde after incubation neither with acetone dried powder nor with any of the cell fractions from rat brain of different ages.

REFERENCES

1. Ansell, G.B. and Spanner, S. (1968): Biochem. J., 108: 207-209.

2. Gunawan, J., Vierbuchen, M., an Debuch, H. (1979): Hoppe-Seyler's Z. Physiol. Chem., 360:971-978.

3. Gunawan, J. and Debuch, H. (1981): Hoppe-Seyler's Z. Physiol. Chem., 362:445-452.

4. Horrocks, L.A., Spanner, S., Mozzi, R., Fu, S. C., D'Amato, R.A., and Krakowka, S. (1978): In: Myelination and Demyelination, edited by J. Palo, pp. 423-438. Plenum Publishing Corporation.

Different Glia Cell Cultures Models for Studies on Phospholipid Metabolism

B. Witter, J. Gunawan, and H. Debuch

Institute of Physiological Chemistry, University of Cologne, Federal Republic of Germany

Two different primary cultures were prepared:
i) brains of newborn rats were dissociated and cultivated according to the method of Booher and Sensenbrenner (1) in the presence of 20% fetal calf serum. A "mixed" - populated culture of astrocytes and oligodendrocytes was achieved by addition of brain extract from newborn rats to the medium after 5 days in culture (Sensenbrenner et al. (2)). Neurons were not detectable.
ii) A 5-fold dilution of initial inoculation and addition of brain extract after 9 days in culture produced a nearly "pure" astrocyte culture. Harvest on the 16th or 18th day, respectively.

Both types of cultures were incubated with the substrate 1-[^{3}H]alkyl-GPE for different times: after 3 h incubation not only the total uptake of the substrate but also the acylation to 1-alkyl-2-acyl-GPE proceeds to a greater extent in the "mixed" populated cultures than in the astrocyte cultures. However, during the course of incubation time up to 20 h the acylation in both cultures approached nearly the same values, whereas another enzyme reaction such as "base-exchange" into the PC-analogue showed a remarkable retardation in the astrocyte culture. Some choline plasmalogen formation was also observed in both cultures.

REFERENCES

1. Booher, J. and Sensenbrenner, M. (1972): Neurobiology, 2:97-105.

2. Sensenbrenner, M., Springer, N., Booher, J., and Mandel, P. (1972): Neurobiology, 2:49-60.

Phospholipase Activities in Primary Neuronal Cultures

A. D. Edgar, L. Freysz, and G. Vincendon

Centre de Neurochimie du CNRS, 67084 Strasbourg Cedex, France

Phospholipase activities were examined in primary neuronal cultures prepared from 15 day old rat embryos, and the results compared with the phospholipase activities previously reported for primary glial cultures. Primary neuronal cultures contain phospholipase A_1, A_2 and C activities with phosphatidylcholine (PC) and phosphatidylethanolamine (PE). The pH profiles of these enzymes were slightly different from those present in glial cells. In both cell types the different phospholipases A_1 and A_2 did not exhibit an absolute Ca^{2+} dependency. In neurons the specific activities of the phospholipases A_2 and C with PC or PE were similar and much lower than the specific activities of the phospholipase A_1. Nicergoline, propanolol and phentolamine (adrenergic antogonists) inhibited the neuronal phospholipase A_1, A_2 and C activities at different rates, while atropine (cholinergic antagonist) had no effect. Since neurons contain also very active diglyceride lipase and lysophospholipase these results may suggest that phospholipases A_1 and C could be modulators of the polyunsaturated fatty acid release.

Production of Unesterified Choline by Homogenates of Rat Brain

Steven H. Zeisel

Department of Nutrition and Food Science, Laboratory of Neuroendocrine Regulation, Massachusetts Institute of Technology, Cambridge, Massachusetts 02139

There is a net efflux of unesterified (free) choline from the brain in vivo, probably as a result of hydrolysis of phosphatidylcholine (lecithin). In vitro, preparations of rat brain also produce large amounts of free choline. We attempted to elucidate the factors which influence the formation of choline.

Homogenates of rat brain were incubated in 0.2M Hepes buffer (pH 7.4) containing 0.05M magnesium chloride at 37°C. Lecithin concentrations in the incubation mixture decreased from 300 to 200 nmol/mg protein during a 2 hr incubation. At the same time free choline rose from 2 to 10 nmol/mg protein. If the brains were microwaved prior to incubation (fixing all proteins), no lecithin was degraded and no choline was formed. Brain specimens from rats killed by microwave irradiation had higher lecithin concentrations (450 nmol/mg protein) and lower choline concentrations (0.8 nmol/mg protein) than specimens from decapitated rats (300 and 2 nmol/mg protein, respectively). ^{14}C-(methyl)-lecithin was metabolized during incubations to form ^{14}C-choline as well as ^{14}C-phosphorylcholine and ^{14}C-glycerophosphorylcholine. These compounds do not seem to be obligatory intermediates in the formation of choline, as choline appears prior to phosphorylcholine.

Maximal production of choline by brain homogenates occurs at pH 7.4-8.5, at 37°C, and at buffer osmolarities of 200-300 mOsms. The addition of magnesium greatly stimulates choline production. (Calcium and manganese are less potent.) Nickel and zinc are inhibitors of these reactions, as is EDTA. Addition of EGTA has no effect. Variations in atmospheric oxygen or the addition of dinitrophenol also had no effects on choline formation. ATP inhibited the production of choline. This inhibition could be reversed by adding equimolar amounts of magnesium. ADP, AMP and CTP did not alter choline formation. The effects of the above treatments could not be explained by their actions on the formation of lecithin or phosphorylcholine.

The subcellular distribution of the choline production activity was also studied. It was found in all membrane containing fractions (P2, myelin, mitochondria, synaptosomes and microsomes) with maximal activity in the microsomal fraction. No activity was found in soluble fractions.

When ^{14}C-(methyl)-lecithin was injected into the dorsal hippocampus of living rats, significant amounts of ^{14}C-phosphorylcholine and ^{14}C-choline were formed within 3 hours.

These data are consistant with the hypothesis that, within brain, lecithin is metabolized to form free choline. Though many enzyme activities are probably involved, choline production has characteristics (magnesium stimulated, zinc inhibited, pH optimum of 7.5) similar to those described for lysophospholipase D activity. In vivo, lecithin is metabolized to form free choline; however, recycling of choline during lecithin synthesis limits the accumulation of free choline. In vitro, the degradation of lecithin predominates (possibly due to lower ATP concentrations) and large amounts of choline accumulate. A lecithin cycle, in which the phospholipid is continuously degraded and reformed could facilitate moment-to-moment regulation of membrane composition.

(Dr. Zeisel is a John A. and George L. Hartford Fellow of the John A. Hartford Foundation.)

Choline Synthesis in Neurons and Glial Cells

R. Massarelli, F. Dainou, J. C. Louis, H. Dreyfus, R. Mozzi,
G. Porcellati, and L. Freysz

*Centre de Neurochimie du CNRS, U44 de l'INSERM, 67084 Strasbourg Cedex, France;
Institute of Biological Chemistry, University of Perugia, 06100 Perugia, Italy*

In recent years the supply of choline to nerve cells has been considered as a possible step in the regulation of acetylcholine synthesis. Many studies have led to the conclusion that choline may be transported into nerve cells via two mechanisms of uptake which differ in their affinity for the substrate. However recent observations have shown that the regulation of the metabolism of acetylcholine is not strictly correlated to its uptake. The presence of methyltransferases in nervous tissue, described recently by various groups, prompted us to investigate the possible synthesis of choline in neurons and glial cells.

Pure primary neuronal and glial cultures from chick embryo cerebral hemispheres were incubated with various concentrations of radioactive ethanolamine and the distribution of radioactivity in different phospholipids and acid soluble compounds was analyzed as a function of time.

In the acid soluble fraction of both cell types, the highest radioactivity was observed in phosphorylethanolamine and phosphorylcholine followed by CDPethanolamine and CDPcholine. The radioactivity of these four compounds increased as a function of the incubation time and was higher in neurons than in glial cells. Only very low amounts of radioactivity could be detected in free ethanolamine and choline. In the lipid fraction the highest incorporation of radioactivity was found in phosphatidylethanolamine and the corresponding plasmalogens. Notable radioactivity was also found in monomethylphosphatidylethanolamine and phosphatidylcholine. The incorporation of the radioactivity into these two compounds increased with time. In opposite, the radioactivity in the dimethylphosphatidylethanolamine was very low and reached a plateau after 1 hour of incubation in neurons. The radioactivity in the various phospholipids was higher in neurons than in glial cells. Moreover in both cells the incorporation of ethanolamine into phosphorylcholine was much higher than into the phosphatidylcholine.

These data indicate that both neurons and glial cells contain methyltransferases which are able to methylate ethanolamine derivatives. The occurence of radioactive monomethyl- and dimethyl-phosphatidyl-ethanolamine suggests that in both cell types phosphatidylethanolamine can be methylated to phosphatidylcholine. However the much higher radioactivity present in phosphorylcholine than in phosphatidylcholine may also suggest that these cells contain an enzymatic system capable of methylating phosphorylethanolamine.

Biosynthesis of Choline from Phosphatidylethanolamine in Synaptosomes: The Role of Serine as a Precursor of Phosphatidylethanolamine

J. K. Blusztajn and R. J. Wurtman

Department of Nutrition and Food Science, Laboratory of Neuroendocrine Regulation, Massachusetts Institute of Technology, Cambridge, Massachusetts 02139

We have previously shown (<u>Nature</u> 290, 417, 1981) that brain synaptosomes synthesize phosphatidylcholine by sequential methylation of phosphatidylethanolamine, catalyzed by an enzyme(s), phosphatidylethanolamine N-methyltransferase which utilizes S-adenosylmethionine as a methyl donor. The phosphatidylcholine formed in 30 minutes constitutes 1.9 ppm of total synaptosomal phosphatidylcholine. Free choline, quickly liberated from the phosphatidylcholine, constitutes 88 ppm of synaptosomal free choline. Thus the enrichment of the choline pool is 50 fold higher than the enrichment of the phosphatidylcholine pool.

We now report that incubation of synaptosomes in the presence of [U^{14}C]-serine resulted in its incorporation to phosphatidylserine (PS) which was subsequently decarboxylated to ethanolamine phospholipids (E-PL). PS formation was activated by calcium, nickel, sodium, potassium and was inhibited by zinc. [The effect of nickel on the formation of PS apparently is mediated by an increase in the affinity for serine of the enzyme(s) that catalyzes the formation of PS.] ^{14}C-E-PL present after a 15 min. incubation with ^{14}C-serine exceeded that of ^{14}C-PS. Nickel affected E-PL and PS formation in a similar fashion.

We conclude that serine may be a precursor in the neuronal synthesis of choline <u>in situ</u>.

Phospholipid Turnover and Cyclic Nucleotide for Bidirectional Regulation of Protein Phosphorylation in Synaptic Transmission

Y. Takai, R. Minakuchi, U. Kikkawa, K. Sano, K. Kaibuchi, B. Yu,
T. Matsubara, and Y. Nishizuka

Department of Biochemistry, Kobe University School of Medicine, Kobe 650; Department of Cell Biology, National Institute for Basic Biology, Okazaki 444, Japan

Both excitatory and inhibitory processes in neuron are initiated by interaction of various transmitters with cell surface receptors, and the molecular basis for such cellular communication has attracted great attention. We have recently isolated a new protein kinase from rat brain as a nearly homogeneous form. This enzyme (C-kinase) is most abundant in brain tissue, particularly in synaptic membranes. The activation of C-kinase is not related to cyclic nucleotide, but apparently coupled to phosphatidylinositol (PI) turnover (Hokin & Hokin, 1955), which is provoked by various signals such as muscarinic cholinergic and α-adrenergic stimulators, many neuropeptides as well as by depolarization (Michell, 1975; Hawthorne & White, 1975). This enzyme is activated by the simultaneous presence of phosphatidylserine (PS) and Ca^{2+}. A small quantity of unsaturated diacylglycerol (DG) greatly increases the affinity of enzyme for PS, and dramatically decreases Ka for Ca^{2+} to the 10^{-7} $\underline{M}$ range. Thus, it is conceivable that excitatory signals may induce PI hydrolysis to produce DG, which in turn serves as an initiator for the selective activation of C-kinase. Phosphatidylethanolamine enhances further, whereas phosphatidylcholine and sphingomyelin diminishes C-kinase activation. The enzyme activated in this way phosphorylates many proteins, particularly those associated with membranes. A series of studies with human platelets as a model system indicates that DG formation, C-kinase-specific phosphorylation and release reaction always proceed in parallel manners, and such transmembrane control of protein phosphorylation seems to operate in physiological processes. It is noted that cyclic AMP strongly inhibits the signal-induced formation of DG and thereby blocks C-kinase activation. It is possible, therefore, that inhibitory signals such as β-adrenergic and dopaminergic stimulators may counteract C-kinase activation at the level of DG formation presumably through the action of cyclic AMP-dependent protein kinase. (supported by Ministry of Edu., Sci. & Cult., Japan)

The Distribution of the γ-Aminobutyric Acid and Glycine Carrier in Cerebral Cortex

M. Giesing and U. Gerken

Laboratory for Nerve Tissue Culture, Institute for Physiological Chemistry, 5300 Bonn, Federal Republic of Germany

Experimental changes in the phospholipid composition of living cells stemming from rat cerebral cortex have been used to study the carrier systems for the inhibitory amino acid neurotransmitters GABA and glycine. The cellular density of the GABA carrier and the dissociation constant in viable cells previously enriched with phosphatidylcholine (PC) or -ethanolamine (PE), were dependent both on the polar head group and the fatty acid (FA) composition. The FA-composition of PC played a less significant role for the function of the glycine carrier. PE was even ineffective. The activity of the GABA carrier changed with temperature exhibiting two continuities in Arrhenius plots. The transport curves were shifted within the discontinuities as a function of the cellular lipid composition. Both observations were not made for glycine.-Enzymatic digestion of plasma membrane components resulted in a reduced Na^+-dependent binding of the two ligands. Trypsin treatment of living cells inactivated more rapidly the binding of glycine whereas phospholipase C affected more the GABA carrier.-It is concluded that the two carrier systems differ in the distribution in plasma membranes. The GABA carrier molecules seem to be completely integrated into the membrane thus facing the cytoplasmic and the external surface. The proteins may also undergoe a FA-specific partitioning between the fluid and ordered lipid domains of the membrane. In contrast to GABA the proteins that bind and transport glycine, are rather distributed on the external surface of the plasma membrane. The functioning of the carrier molecules is not affected by the fluid or ordered state of lipids.-It is tempting to speculate that these findings may explain at least in part why only GABA is a major inhibitory neurotransmitter in cerebral cortex.

Lipid Composition of Rat Brain Synaptosome, Myelin, and Mitochondrial Fractions After Chronic Ethanol Administration

C. Alling, *J. Engel, and *S. Liljequist

Departments of Psychiatry and Neurochemistry and Pharmacology, University of Göteborg, Göteborg, Sweden

The aim of the study was to measure whether or not lipid changes occurred in rat brain membranes as a consequense of long-term ethanol administration. Sprague-Dawley rats were presented an ethanol solution (8% w/v) as their only drinking fluid. The ethanol concentration was gradually increased to 16% (w/v). The 9 ethanol treated and 9 control rats were killed at 150 days of age and analysed individually. Forebrains were homogenized and myelin, synaptosomes and mitochondria were obtained by centrifugation in a sucrose gradient. The fractions were analysed for their concentrations of major lipids, phospholipid composition, fatty acid composition of major phosphoglycerides. The ratios between the concentrations of cholesterol, phospholipids and total proteins were the same between the groups in all fractions. In the synaptosomes ethanolaminephosphoglycerides had a smaller proportion of arachidonic acid (p<0.01) and cholinphosphoglycerides had a larger proportion of oleic acid (p<0.01), in ethanol treated rats compared to control rats. These two fatty acids had abnormal values also in blood serum and changes in brain correlated significantly with those in serum. These findings indicate, that brain membranes pertubated by ethanol, acquire aberrations also found in the environmental biochemistry. Myelin and mitochondria were less affected, indicating that phospholipids in synaptosomes are less spared than those of the other two fractions.

Supported by the Swedish Medical Research Council (projects nos. 2157, 4247, 5249), and the Swedish Council for Planning and Coordination of Research.

Prostaglandins Turnover in Torpedo Electric Organ: Presynaptic Muscarinic Modulation

I. Pinchasi, M. Schwartzman, A. Raz, and D. M. Michaelson

Department of Biochemistry, Tel Aviv University, Ramat Aviv, Israel

Acetylcholine (ACh) release from Torpedo electric organ is regulated by presynaptic muscarinic receptors; the muscarinic agonist, oxotremorine (oxo), inhibits ACh release, and atropine (atro) reverses this effect. Recent findings suggest that muscarinic inhibition is due to the uncoupling of intra-terminal Ca^{2+} and ACh release, and not to the inhibition of K^+-depolarization-induced Ca^{2+} entry into the terminals.

Since prostaglandins (PG's) were found to inhibit neurotransmission in various systems, we investigated their possible involvement in muscarinic regulation of ACh release. K^+-depolarization of Torpedo synaptosomes in the presence of Ca^{2+} and oxo resulted in a concentration-dependent increase in the level of bioassayable PG's. This effect was blocked by both atro and the PG's synthesis blocker, indomethacin.

Incubation of electric organ tissue slices with ^{14}C-arachidonic acid (AA) resulted in 30% conversion into PGE_2 and about 10% conversion into various PG-hydroxy derivatives. About 2% of the added AA were incorporated into phospholipids. Upon homogenization of the tissue there was a 10-fold decrease in the ability to convert ^{14}C-AA into PGE_2. Sub-cellular fractionation revealed that the highest specific activity resides in the pure synaptosomal fraction. In preliminary experiments oxo led to a marked increase both in the extent of incorporation of ^{14}C-AA into phospholipids and in its conversion to PGE_2.

The above experiments demonstrate that the Torpedo electric organ possesses a very active PG's synthesis apparatus and that muscarinic activation is accompanied by changes in PG's synthesis and turnover, suggesting a role for the latter in the regulation of ACh release.

Effect of Prostaglandins on the Ca^{++}-Stimulated ATPase Activity of Rat Myometrium Plasma Membranes (MPM)

G. Deliconstantinos, D. Aravantinos, N. Louros, and S. G. A. Alivisatos

Department of Physiology, University of Athens Medical School, Athens 609, Greece

Prostaglandins, if incubated in aqueous solutions ($\sim 10^{-6}$M) with MPM from near delivery pregnant rats bind, similar to steroid hormones, onto the membranes[1]. The mechanism of this binding is not yet elucidated but binding evokes enzymatic changes of the membranous proteins, including the Ca^{++}-stimulated ATPase. There are striking differences between the amount of binding and the evoked effects. Most drastic, in this respect, appears the PGE_2 whose action is approximately twice as that of progesterone[2] (decrease of the Ca^{++}-stimulated ATPase down to 10% of its original value, (i.e., 90% inhibition). Maximum inhibition, after a sigmoid course, in our experiments, was observed using 1 x 10^{-5}M PGE_2 in the presence of 10 mM Ca^{++}. Upward of this Ca^{++}-concentration, the effect remains unchanged. Similar, but less noted evoked effects are observed by arachidonic acid and mutual exclusion, commensured to the aqueous concentration, are observed, as with the steroid hormones[2]. Considering that maintenance of Ca^{++} into the myometrial cells is a *sine qua non* condition for the function of this system and that prostaglandins PGF_{2a} and E_2 are related to reproductive physiology, our findings suggest that the described enzymatic changes are involved in stimulating uterine contractions[3].

[1] G. Deliconstantinos, N. Louros and S.G.A. Alivisatos, Biochem. Soc. Transactions of FEBS 9 (2), Wed-S23-12 (1981)

[2] S.G.A. Alivisatos, G. Deliconstantinos and G. Theodosiadis, Biochim. Biophys. Acta 643, 650-658 (1981)

[3] N.C. Louros, International Surgery 61, 73 (1976)

Anticonvulsant Activity of Phosphatidylserine Liposomes Containing GABA

S. Mazzari, A. Zanotti, R. Borsato, *P. Orlando, and G. Toffano

*Department of Biochemistry, Fidia Research Laboratories, Abano Terme; *Radiochemical Center, Università Cattolica, Rome, Italy*

Liposomes have been proposed as drug carriers in different biological systems. When this delivery system is used, carried drug distribution is determined by that of liposomes (Gregoriadis, G.: New England J. Med., 295:704-710 and 765-770, 1976). Phosphatidylserine (PS) liposomes have been shown to influence cerebral metabolism in animal and man (Toffano, G. and Bruni, A.: Pharm. Res. Commun., 12:829-845, 1980); in addition PS liposomes containing GABA antagonized penicillin induced epileptic activity in rats (Loeb et al.: IRCS Med. Sci., 6:488, 1978). These findings suggest the potential use of PS liposomes as a drug delivery system in the CNS for substances that do not cross the blood brain barrier as the GABA itself. To investigate this possibility we have studied the effect of PS liposome entrapped GABA on the convulsions induced by isoniazide, a drug known to inhibit the GABA synthesis. PS and GABA were sonicated together and injected intravenously into mice pretreated with isoniazide (160 mg/kg, s.c.). PS liposomes containing GABA were capable to reduce the number of convulsant animals (from 93 to 42%), delay the appearance of clonic convulsions (from 56,5 to 92,2 min) and decrease the mortality rate (from 83 to 21%). In contrast PS liposomes by themselves (100 mg/kg i.v.) delayed only the appearance of clonic convulsions (from 56,5 to 75,3 min), while GABA alone (100 or 200 mg/kg i.v.) was ineffective in the same experimental condition. Phosphatidylcholine liposomes containing GABA were not capable to reproduce the same effect, suggesting a different distribution with respect to PS liposomes.

Present results indicate that carried GABA is capable to antagonize the central effect of isoniazide and provide indirect evidence that part of PS liposomes can cross, as intact structure, the brain blood barrier.

Interaction of Cultured Neuroblastoma Cells with Sonicated Phosphatidylserine

A. Vecchini, *P. Orlando, L. Binaglia, *P. Massari, *C. Giordano, and G. Porcellati

*Institute of Biological Chemistry, The Medical School, University of Perugia; *Radioisotope Laboratory, Università Cattolica del Sacro Cuore, Rome, Italy

The Interaction of cultured N2A Neuroblastoma cells with sonicated phosphatidylserine (PS) has been studied. 1-acyl-2-[9,10-^{3}H-oleoyl]-sn-glycerol-3-phosphoryl-[U-^{14}C] serine was sonicated in PBS (10 nmols/ml; ^{3}H: 1.04 µCi/ml; ^{14}C: 220 nCi/ml). Neuroblastoma cells were incubated with 5 ml of this suspension in Falcon flasks for times ranging from 5 min to 1 hour. At stated times, the lipid suspension was removed. The cells were exhaustively washed with cold PBS and incubated at 4°C with 20 ml of 4 mM trinitrobenzenesulfonic acid (TNBS) in physiological solution (pH 8.5). After 2 hours of incubation, TNBS was removed and the cells were exhaustively washed with buffered physiological solution (pH 7.0). The cells were recovered and the lipid extracted. Lipid classes were separated by two-dimensional TLC and radioactivity measured by scintillation.

All lipid classes were labelled, already after 5 min incubation, and labelling was clearly time-dependent. Trinitrophenyl-PS (TNPh-PS), formed by reaction of the PS molecules exposed to the extracellular milieu with the non penetrating probe, exhibited a specific activity higher than that of unreacted PS.

^{3}H/^{14}C ratio of TNPh-PS was the same of the sonicated lipid, while the same ratio was smaller in the unreacted PS. Moreover, ^{3}H-labelling was constantly higher in the unreacted PS than in other lipid classes.

On this basis, PS is supposed to be only in part deacylated and reacylated, the most part entering intact into the cells.

CDP-Diglycerides: Stereospecific Synthesis and Enzyme Studies

P. P. N. Murthy and B. W. Agranoff

Neuroscience Laboratory, University of Michigan, Ann Arbor, Michigan 48109

We have synthesized a number of CDP-diglycerides and employed them to study the specificity of two enzymes of their metabolism:

$$\text{CDP-diglyceride} \xrightarrow{\text{CDP-diglyceride hydrolase}} \text{phosphatidic acid} + \text{CMP} \qquad (I)$$

$$\text{CDP-diglyceride} + \text{inositol} \xrightarrow{\text{CDP-diglyceride inositol phosphatidyl transferase}} \text{phosphatidyl inositol} + \text{CMP} \qquad (II)$$

CDP-diglyceride formation is generally considered to be a rate-limiting step in phosphoinositide formation in eukaryotes. Other fates of CDP-diglyceride include conversion to phosphatidylglycerols or degradation via (I). The latter activity, originally described in bacteria, was recently demonstrated in mammalian tissues, including brain (Rittenhouse et al., J. Neurochem. 36:991-999, 1981). For the present studies, dipalmitoyl or distearoyl-sn-glycero-3-phosphorylcholines were obtained commercially and converted to the 1-acyl lyso derivatives by treatment with snake venom phospholipase A_2. The lysophosphatidylcholines were reacylated with various fatty acid anhydrides using dimethylaminopyridine as catalyst. The resulting lecithins were converted to phosphatidates by treatment with cabbage phospholipase D, which were then reacted with CMP-morpholidate to give CDP-diglycerides. The purified CDP-diglycerides, some of which have been synthesized for the first time, include (as the 1,2-diacyl-sn-glycero-3-pyrophosphoryl-5'-cytidine derivative): distearoyl, dipalmitoyl, stearoyl arachidonoyl, stearoyl oleoyl, diarachidonoyl, and arachidonoyl stearoyl. For the latter two CDP-diglycerides, diarachidonoyl lecithin was first synthesized from sn-glycero-3-phosphorylcholine. Purity of each product was confirmed by TLC and physical measurements, including high resolution NMR. Preliminary results indicate that enzyme (II) exhibits much higher fatty acid specificity than enzyme (I). Results are discussed in relation to the hypothesis that the inositides are precursors of the labile arachidonate precursor pool. (Supported by NIH Grant #NS 15413.)

357

Properties of Human Lysosomal Sphingomyelinase with Emphasis on the Substrate Specificity

C. S. Jones, D. J. Davidson, P. Shankaran, and J. W. Callahan

Research Institute, The Hospital for Sick Children, and the Departments of Pediatrics and Biochemistry, University of Toronto, Toronto, Canada

Sphingomyelinase, purified to apparent homogeneity, contains a single major polypeptide chain of 89,000 daltons and two minor components (47,500 and 30,700 daltons respectively). Urea-electrofocusing gels have shown microheterogeneity of the major component which has an acidic isoelectric point (pI range of 4.6-5.0). The composition includes hydrophobic, acidic and basic amino acid contents of 26.8, 22.9 and 11.7 per cent respectively. The enzyme hydrolyzes two synthetic phosphodiesters bis(MU)-phosphate and bis(NP)phosphate in addition to sphingomyelin and hexadecanoyl (NP) phosphocholine. MU phosphocholine is hydrolyzed but at a very slow rate. Hydrolysis of bis(MU)phosphate displays a sigmoidal substrate dependency with inhibition at concentrations above 2.5 mM. Total activity was also influenced by Triton X-100 at all concentrations tested (0.075-1.75 mg/ml). Chromatography on Sephadex G-25 and dialysis experiments indicate that bis(MU)phosphate does not enter a micelle with the detergent. Hexadecanoyl (NP) phosphocholine hydrolysis also shows a dependency on Triton X-100. At substrate concentrations below 4mM, detergent inhibits the enzyme reaction whereas at higher concentrations of the hexadecanoyl-derivative (above 4mM), Triton X-100 stimulates the reaction. Sphingomyelin analogs such as ceramide phosphoinositol and ceramide phosphoinositol-mannose are totally hydrolyzed by the enzyme. We conclude that bis(MU) phosphate is hydrolyzed following interaction of enzyme and Triton X-100. The latter alters the enzyme probably by inducing a conformational change which allows binding and hydrolysis of bis(MU)phosphate at the catalytic site. The hexadecanoyl (NP) phosphocholine on the other hand micellized by itself and is an excellent substrate for sphingomyelinase at very low detergent concentrations. The data suggest that hydrolysis of substrates by sphingomyelinase may occur through cooperative interactions.

Phospholipid Metabolism in Acetylcholine-Stimulated Synaptosomes from Ox Caudate Nucleus

K. A. Foster and J. N. Hawthorne

Department of Biochemistry, University of Nottingham Medical School, Queen's Medical Centre, Nottingham NG7 2UH, United Kingdom

Previous studies have reported changes in the metabolism, studied using ^{32}P labelling, of phosphatidylinositol and phosphatidic acid in synaptosomes stimulated by either acetylcholine (1,2) or depolarization (3,4). These studies used synaptosomes prepared from whole guinea pig cortices. Such a preparation would contain a heterogeneous population of synaptosomes, and this precludes a precise characterization of the relationship between such phospholipid effects and synaptic transmission. Phospholipid effects seen in synaptosome preparations are likely to be a presynaptic event (3), and so a preparation in which cholinergic receptors are known to play a presynaptic role would provide a more defined system for a study of the biological significance of any phospholipid effects seen during acetylcholine stimulation of the synaptosomes. Synaptosomes from the caudate nucleus have been shown to possess cholinergic receptors (both muscarinic and nicotinic) which modulate the release of dopamine from the synaptosomes (5).

Synaptosomes have been prepared and characterized from the caudate nucleus of ox brain, removed freshly post-mortem. Using such a synaptosome preparation the effect of acetylcholine stimulation on phospholipid metabolism within the synaptosomes is being studied. Studies have initially been conducted using ^{32}P labelling of lipids to detect any changes caused by acetylcholine. Preliminary results indicate an increased labelling of synaptosomal phosphatidic acid during acetylcholine stimulation.

1) Schacht, J. & Agranoff, B.W. (1972) J. Biol. Chem. 247, 771-777
2) Yagihara, Y. & Hawthorne, J.N. (1972) J. Neurochem. 19, 355-367
3) Hawthorne, J.N. & Bleasdale, J.E. (1975) Mol. Cell. Biochem. 8, 83-87
4) Bleasdale, J.E. & Hawthorne, J.N. (1975) J. Neurochem. 24, 373-379
5) De Belleroche, J. & Bradford, H.F. (1978) Brain Res. 142, 53-68

Effects of Calcium and Cinchocaine on Phosphoinositide Metabolism in Isolated Vagus and Phrenic Nerves of Rats

G. L. White, P. Broom, and A. Weir

School of Pharmacy, Portsmouth Polytechnic, Portsmouth, United Kingdom

Vagus and phrenic nerves were excised from albino rats (Wistar Strain) and incubated in 1.5 ml of Earle's medium containing (^{3}H) inositol. Usually a 3h incubation at 37°C was used while gasing with moist O_2-CO_2 (95:5, v/v). Phospholipids were extracted with chloroform-methanol-conc. HCl (800:400:3, by vol.), washed and chromatographed on oxalate-impregnated silicic acid plates. Spots were stained, scraped and counted in water-Aquasol in a scintillation counter. Phosphatidylinositol was more highly labelled than the higher inosities in both vagus and phrenic nerves. Using rat vagus nerve, when calcium was omitted from the medium the labelling of phosphatidylinositol was highly significantly increased. The divalent ionophore A23187 also appeared to increase the radioactivity in this particular phospholipid. Cinchocaine (a local anaesthetic) caused a significant increase in labelling of phosphatidylinositol in rat vagus nerve but this appeared to be dependent upon the dose used. Thus several compounds have been shown to have a marked effect upon phosphatidylinositol metabolism and this may well be related to the intracellular and extracellular calcium concentrations.

The Blood–Brain Barrier is Impermeable to Inositol, Indicating Synthesis in Brain

C. Font, A. Gjedde, A. J. Hansen, and E. Siemkowicz

*Medical Physiology Department A, The Panum Institute, Copenhagen University,
Copenhagen, Denmark 2200*

The cyclohexitol myo-inositol is a precursor of phosphatidylinositol and hence for the phosphoinositides in brain. It is present in brain tissue in concentrations 100 times higher than those of plasma, indicating either active transport into brain, or an impermeable blood-brain barrier and local synthesis. In order to distinguish between these possibilities and thus to determine the mode and rate of inositol transport into rat brain, we injected male Wistar rats with mixtures of labelled inositol and mannitol and followed the rate of uptake by brain for times not exceeding five minutes. The results are shown in the figure. As previously described (GJEDDE 1981), the initial slope of the uptake curve represents the blood-brain barrier permeability, and the ordinate intercept the plasma volume of brain. The blood-brain barrier permeability of inositol averaged 0.27 ± 0.02 ($\bar{x}\pm$ S.E., $n=7$) ml $100g^{-1}min^{-1}$ or $4\cdot10^{-7}$ cm s^{-1} at a cerebral capillary surface area of 100 cm^2g^{-1}. The permeability of mannitol was 0.08 ± 0.01 ml $100g^{-1}min^{-1}$ or $1\cdot10^{-7}$ cm s^{-1}. The values are compatible with the measured passive permeability of cell membranes to hydrophilic molecules the size of inositol and mannitol. Both inositol and mannitol are subject to chemical change in plasma. Therefore, the permeabilities increase somewhat with longer exposure times of the isotopes. At a brain concentration of 5 mM, inositol must leak out of brain at a rate of 1.4 μmol $100g^{-1}min^{-1}$. Neither glucose nor galactose affected the inositol permeability. It is concluded that the high concentration in brain is caused by local synthesis.

Reference:
GJEDDE, A. J. Neurochem. 36:1463–1471, 1981

Supported by the Medical Research Council (Denmark).

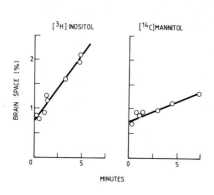

Studies on Bovine Brain Phosphatidylinositol Transfer Protein Using Fluorescent Phospholipid Analogues

P. J. Somerharju, P. Van Paridon, and K. W. A. Wirtz

Biochemical Laboratory, Rijksuniversiteit Utrecht, Utrecht 2506, The Netherlands

Bovine brain contains a protein which catalyses transfer of phosphatidylinositol and phosphatidylcholine between membranes. When these lipids are present in the same membrane the protein preferentially complexes phosphatidylinositol (Demel,R.A., Kalsbeek,R., Wirtz, K.W. A. and van Deenen,L.L.M. (1977) Biochim. Biophys. Acta 466,10-22). In order to obtain additional information on the mode of action of this protein we have developed a method which allows one to follow continuously protein catalyzed phospholipid transfer. This method is based on the use of fluorescent phosphatidylinositol and -choline derivatives (synthesis and purification of these lipids will be descibed). In vesicles prepared of these lipids the fluorescence is effectively quenched due to interactions between the fluorescent groups. When an excess of unlabeled vesicles and a transfer protein is added, a time and protein concentration dependent increase of fluorescence is observed. This increase results from insertion of the labeled phospholipids into the unlabeled (i.e. nonquenching) acceptor membranes. This fluorimetric assay is especially suitable for kinetic studies and was applied to study further the substrate specifity of the phosphatidylinositol transfer protein. First we studied the headgroup specifity by comparing transfer of phosphatidylinositol and various headgroup analogues obtained by periodate oxidation of phosphatidylinositol. It was observed that that the rate of transfer was markedly decreased upon oxidative degradation of the inositol moiety suggesting that the protein has a specific recognition site for the inositol group.The fluorimetric assay was also used to measure protein-mediated transfer of diester, diether and dialkyl phosphatidylcholines. Similar rates of transfer were observed for all these derivatives indicating that the glycerol-hydrocarbon bonding region plays less important role in the protein-lipid interactions.

A Postsynaptic Locus for the Stimulation of Phospholipid Labeling by Muscarinic Agonists in Synaptosomes Derived from Hippocampus

S. K. Fisher, K. A. Frey, and B. W. Agranoff

Neuroscience Laboratory, University of Michigan, Ann Arbor, Michigan 48109

Metabolic consequences, including enhanced phospholipid turnover, in response to the addition of various cell surface ligands to tissue preparations, is generally considered to reflect the activator of postsynaptic receptors. An apparent exception to this is the muscarinic-agonist stimulation of phosphatidic acid (PhA) and phosphatidylinositol (PhI) labeling in brain synaptosome preparations, which has been considered to reflect the activation of presynaptic receptors. A previous study from this laboratory (Brain Res. <u>189</u>, 284-288, 1980) has cast doubt on this assumption, since we observed that destruction of the sole cholinergic afferent input to the hippocampus reduced neither the number of muscarinic receptors present in the hippocampal synaptosome fraction, nor did it alter the muscarinic agonist-stimulation of PhA and PhI labeling from $^{32}P_i$. This result suggested that the muscarinic receptors linked to phospholipid turnover in hippocampal synaptosomes are present on cholinoceptive rather than cholinergic structures. To further investigate this possibility, we have used the neurotoxin, ibotenic acid, to selectively destroy intrinsic neurons in the hippocampus. Male guinea pigs received 3 x 10 ug ibotenic acid injections in one side of the hippocampus. Twelve days later, completeness of the procedure was evaluated histologically. Following unilateral ibotenic acid lesion, the specific activity of glutamate decarboxylase in synaptosomes derived from the lesioned side was reduced by 30 $\pm$ 7%, and [^{3}H]quinuclidinyl benzilate binding was reduced by 42 $\pm$ 6% ($p<0.005$). While there was a loss in yield of synaptosomes (23 $\pm$ 4%), activity of basal phospholipid labeling from $^{32}P_i$ computed per mg protein from lesioned hippocampus was not reduced. There was, however, a marked reduction in carbachol-stimulated labeling of PhA (91 $\pm$ 9% in the control vs. 52 $\pm$ 7% in the lesion, $p<0.005$) and in that of PhI (31 $\pm$ 5% in the control vs. 19 $\pm$ 4% in the lesion, $p<0.02$). These results, taken together with those previously obtained from fornix lesions, confirm that muscarinic receptors in hippocampus coupled to PhA and PhI turnover are located predominantly on postsynaptic cholinoceptive structures. Thus, in this respect, the locus for enhanced phospholipid turnover in synaptosome preparations is in accord with that observed in other tissues. (Supported by NIH Grant #NS 15413. S.K.F. was supported by NIMH Training Grant #MH 15794-01.)

363

Cholinergic Agonist-Induced Changes in Phospholipid Turnover Are Independent of Catecholamine Secretion in Bovine Adrenal Chromaffin Cells

S. K. Fisher, *R. W. Holz, and B. W. Agranoff

*Neuroscience Laboratory, University of Michigan, Ann Arbor, Michigan 48109; *Department of Pharmacology, Medical School, University of Michigan, Ann Arbor, Michigan 48109*

A possible link between enhanced phospholipid turnover, calcium influx and catecholamine secretion in response to cholinergic agonists has been examined in bovine adrenal chromaffin cell preparations maintained in monolayer culture. The addition of carbachol (3×10^{-4} M) to cells preincubated for 30 min in a physiological salt solution containing $^{32}P_i$ and [^{3}H]glycerol resulted in a selective stimulation of incorporation of both precursors into phosphatidic acid (70-160%) and phosphatidylinositol (97-120%). Stimulated labeling was detectable 1-2 min after the addition of carbachol. Muscarinic cholinergic agonists consistently resulted in a stimulation of phosphatidic acid and phosphatidylinositol labeling, while the addition of nicotinic agonists resulted in little or no change in phospholipid labeling. Stimulated phosphatidic acid and phosphatidylinositol labeling could be blocked by inclusion of atropine (10^{-6} M) but not by d-tubocurarine (4×10^{-5} M). In contrast to stimulated phospholipid labeling, however, only nicotinic cholinergic agonists were effective in stimulating catecholamine release, and this could be inhibited by d-tubocurarine, but not by atropine. Nicotinic agonists also facilitated $^{45}Ca^{2+}$ influx into chromaffin cells (42-84% stimulation), whereas muscarinic agonists had no measurable effect on calcium influx. Catecholamine release and stimulated phospholipid labeling also displayed different requirements for extracellular calcium. Thus, carbachol-stimulated catecholamine release was absolutely dependent on the presence of added calcium whereas no such requirement existed for stimulated phospholipid labeling. Nevertheless, a role for calcium in muscarinic agonist-stimulated labeling can be inferred from the observation that inclusion of EGTA (5×10^{-4} M) reduced stimulated phosphatidic acid and phosphatidylinositol labeling by <85%. These results suggest that catecholamine secretion and phospholipid turnover are mediated through pharmacologically distinct cholinergic receptor populations. In bovine chromaffin cell preparations, stimulated phospholipid turnover appears then to be neither a prerequisite for secretion nor a consequence of it. (Supported by NIH Grant #NS 15413 to B.W.A. and NSF Grant #BNS 78 24494 to R.W.H. S.K.F. was supported by NIMH Training Grant #MH 15794-01.)

Studies on the *In Vivo* Metabolism of Polyphosphoinositides in Rat Brain and in Intact Cultured Cells

P. R. Bär, L. H. Schrama, W. H. Gispen, and J. Jolles

Division of Molecular Neurobiology, Rudolf Magnus Institute for Pharmacology and Laboratory of Physiological Chemistry, Institute of Molecular Biology, State University of Utrecht, The Netherlands

Rat brain phospholipids were labelled in vivo by an intracerebroventricular injection of ^{32}Pi. The method of sacrifice used (immersion into liquid nitrogen for 8 sec followed by rapid dissection of the cold but not frozen brain) enabled subcellular fractionation and subsequent in vitro assay of the prelabeled phospholipids, while no breakdown of the polyphosphoinositides occurred, once the material was at 0-4°C. In comparing different subcellular fractions, it appeared that purified mitochondria contain highly labelled PI (phosphatidylinositol) but no DPI (phosphatidylinositol 4-phosphate) and TPI (phosphatidylinositol 4,5-diphosphate). Purified synaptosomes, and especially myelin contain highly labeled TPI; myelin contains only a small amount of radiolabelled PI. The rate of in vivo incorporation into synaptosomes and myelin was similar. Upon incubation in vitro after prelabelling in vivo, both DPI and TPI rapidly lost the radiolabel. Half of the labile portion of the incorporated ^{32}p was removed within 2 min and this breakdown was Ca^{2+}-dependent.

Intact neuroblastoma x glioma hybrid cells (108 CC 15) and neuroblastoma cells (NIE 115) were incubated in suspension with ^{32}Pi or [γ-^{32}P] ATP. A very quick labeling of PI, DPI, TPI and PA (phosphatidic acid) resulted, already after 10-60 sec. After short incubation times, DPI and TPI were preferably labeled (50% of total incorporation after 2 min) whereas PI and PA incorporated 35% in the same time. When the incubation time was shorter than 10-30 min, only very little labelling of other phospholipids was observed (PC,PE,PS and cardiolipin). After longer incubations (30-240 min), DPI, TPI and PA reach a plateau but PI and the other phospholipids incorporate label linearly up to 4 hours. It is concluded that these cells are useful to study the polyphosphoinositide metabolism. Short incubation times should then be used.

ACTH and β-Endorphin Modulate Brain Polyphosphoinositide Metabolism

J. Jolles, P. R. Bär, and W. H. Gispen

Division of Molecular Neurobiology, Rudolf Magnus Institute for Pharmacology and Laboratory of Physiological Chemistry, Institute of Molecular Biology, University of Utrecht, The Netherlands

Effects of neuropeptides on the interconversion of the polyphospho-inositides was studied in vitro. A brain subcellular fraction containing both light membranes and cytosolic proteins was incubated under hypotonic conditions with $[\gamma\text{-}^{32}P]$ATP. Of the membrane phospholipids only DPI (phosphatidylinositol 4-phosphate), TPI (phosphatidylinositol 4,5-diphosphate) and PA (phosphatidic acid) became labelled. The reference peptide ACTH (1-24) stimulated the formation of TPI and inhibited the production of PA. For effects on TPI formation both the sequences ACTH (5-7) and ACTH (10-16) were needed. Effect on PA formation required the sequences ACTH (5-7) and ACTH (10-16). The basic aminoacids in ACTH (10-16) seemed to be of crucial importance for the peptide effects. A stimulatory effect on DPI instead of TPI was visible when ACTH was shortened from the N-terminus. β-endorphin inhibited PA formation and this effect was abolished by C-terminal shortening to γ-endorphin. Other endorphins, including the enkephalins, were ineffective. High concentrations of naloxone inhibited TPI and PA formation but did not counteract the effects of ACTH(1-24), indicating that the opiate antagonist does not antagonise ACTH. In a partially purified enzyme preparation incubated with DPI as exogenous lipid substrate, similar effects of ACTH1-24 and β-endorphin were found: Thus, ACTH and β-endorphin dose-dependently inhibited the formation of PA: ACTH stimulated the production of TPI whereas β-endorphin had only minor influence on this polyphosphoinositide. It is concluded that the structure activity relationship correlates with a similar relationship obtained on the phosphorylation of a protein, present in synaptic plasma membranes (B-50 protein, molecular weight 48.000). This finding adds support to the notion that a functional relationship may exist between protein phosphorylation and polyphosphoinositide metabolism (Jolles et al., Nature 286 (1978) 623).

A Phospholipase A_2 Purified from Bovine Brain Microsomes Which Shows Selectivity Towards Phosphatidylinositol (PI)

N. C. C. Gray and K. P. Strickland

*Department of Biochemistry, Health Sciences Centre, University of Western Ontario,
London, Ontario N6A 5C1, Canada*

A phospholipase A_2 with a pH optimum of 7.5 has been purified 1600 times from bovine brain microsomes (106,000g pellet obtained from 12,000g supernate). The enzyme was extracted and stabilized into medium containing Triton X-100, glycerol, asolecithin and β-mercaptoethanol. Purification, keeping the enzyme in the above medium where possible, was achieved by ammonium sulphate fractionation, column chromatography (Sephadex G-200 and DEAE-Sephacel) and polyacrylamide gel electrophoresis. The purified enzyme runs as a single band on a SDS-polyacrylamide gel and gives a molecular weight of 18,000 daltons. The enzyme is heat resistant (70°C) and stimulated by Ca^{2+} (2-5mM) and the detergents, Triton X-100 (0.025%) and octylglucoside (25mM). The kinetic parameters are: K_m = 0.52mM and V_{max} = 1440 nanomoles ^{14}C-oleic acid released/min/mg protein using PI labelled with ^{14}C-oleic acid in the 2-position. PI's, labelled in the 2-position with different fatty acids, gave the following order of release with the enzyme: $C_{16:0} > C_{18:0} > C_{18:1} > C_{20:4}$. The addition of these fatty acids (5μM and 10μM) caused an inhibition of fatty acid release in the reverse order to that just noted. There was little or no release from PI's labelled with fatty acid in the 1-position. These evaluations were made based on ^{14}C or ^{3}H counts and glc analysis of the fatty acids released. The enzyme showed the following order of activity towards phosphoglycerides containing ^{14}C-oleic acid in the 2-position: PI (set at 100%); phosphatidylcholine, 61.2%; phosphatidylserine, 51.9%; phosphatidic acid, 31.8% and phosphatidylethanolamine, 24.6%. The above phospholipase A_2 has the appropriate properties required of an enzyme to function in a deacylation-reacylation cycle for PI, in particular, and possibly for other phosphoglycerides. (supported by the MRC of Canada).

Comparison of Binding of Cholesterol and Steroid Hormones onto Dog Brain Synaptosomal Plasma Membranes (SPM)

S. G. A. Alivisatos, G. Deliconstantinos, G. Theodosiadis, and N. Louros

Department of Physiology, University of Athens Medical School, Athens 609, Greece

All steroids including testosterone, progesterone, oestrone, cortisol and some other compounds like dodecanol and octanol, bind onto SPM[1,2,3]. The binding follows in all cases a sigmoid path with changing concentrations of the ligand (incubation time with the membranes 3 to 4 hours). This binding of all above compounds evoke drastic functional changes of all integral membranous proteins including those of SPM, (e.g., the ouabain sensitive ATPase) and the mitochondria, if exposed to the steroid aqueous solutions. The binding of one of this compound can be mutually excluded by another, if the direction of the change (decrease or increase of a specific activity) is the same for the testing compounds and if any two compounds are used in concentration commensured with the number of binding sites for each of them (e.g., testosterone binds 30 times less than cholesterol) producing the same evoked effect in ouabain sensitive ATPase in the same time interval. These effects, and others in vivo (electrophysiological effects in dog's heart)[4] indicate, that these hormones, in addition to the effects at the nuclear level, show additional direct effects upon membranes, controlling for example the water content of the cells, their adenyl cyclase activity[5], etc. They also affect the fluidity of membranes, depending on the amount of bounding. The mechanism of this bounding, which occurs from the monomeric forms of the steroids in aqueous solution, is cooperative[3]. Glucosides of cholesterol, dodecanol and octanol, bind onto biological membranes in a similar manner as the non-glucosidated compounds and evoke the same qualitatively actions. The greater water-solubility of the glucosides permitted recently experiments in which the cholesterol/phospholipid ratio (C/P) from 0.82 in SPM, approaches unity. The mechanical and evoked effects of this overload of the membranes with cholesterol are now studied.

1. S.G.A. Alivisatos et al, B.B.R.C. 79, 677 (1977)
2. S.G.A. Alivisatos et al, B.B.A. 643, 642-649 (1981)
3. S.G.A. Alivisatos et al, B.B.A. 643, 650-658 (1981)
4. S.G.A. Alivisatos et al, Fed. Proc. 37, 536 (1978)
5. A. Papaphilis and G. Deliconstantinos, Biochem. Pharmacol. 29, 3325 (1980)

Cytotrophic and Cytotropic Properties of Phospholipids (PHL) and Globuline Induced (Gl. In) Phospholipids: Studies of Complex Phospholipids Marked by Globulins

G. C. Velley

Psychophysiological Laboratory, French University, 75006 Paris, France

Irradiation made of pregnant females induces disorders in phospholipids metabolism (C.N.S.). In new-born rats post-natal maturation is disturbed. Psychosomatic disorders were observed: (thermoregulation, immune response, puberty, learning,...ovary tumors and others troubles suggesting precocious ageing). In foeto injections of phospholipids or/and antigens-tissues (mitochondria (M), microcosms (m), ribosoms (r)) before or after irradiation restores partially functional injuries and Central Nervous System metabolism. Electroencephalography and immunobiological studies of these animals after in foeto injection (of M+m+r) reveals three facts: 1) The immune response is difered, elongated, and diminished in intensity. 2°) Before the antibody formation appear cytotropic and cytotrophic properties of globulines; we call them "induced globulins" 3°) These induced globulins give complexes with phospholipids. These complexes behave as "marked" phospholipids (PHL-Gl. In). These complexes were used to prepare "vesicles" able to transfer and direct these (M+m+r) towards injured regions restoring their function. Results are resumed on the chart below.

Behaviour of:	irradiation before	800/400 rad after	irradiated and treated
thermoregulation	+++	800 rad +-	800 rad +++
sleep (slow)	30-42 %	" 23-27 %	" 33-38 %
PPS sleep ("paradoxical")	10-12 %	" 0,5-2 %	" 9-11 %
Ulcer (induced by swimming)	3 to 6	400 rad 11-17	400 rad 5-8
Ovary tumor	8-11 %	" 30-47 %	" 11-17 %
age by tumor advention (m.)	9-11 months	" 6-8 m.	" 8-11 m.

Myotonic Muscular Dystrophy: Calcium-Dependent Phosphatidate Metabolism in the Erythrocyte Membrane

L. H. Yamaoka, J. M. Vance, and A. D. Roses

Department of Medicine and Department of Biochemistry, Division of Neurology, Duke University Medical Center, Durham, North Carolina 27710

Myotonic muscular dystrophy (MyD) is a systemic genetic disorder which may be the result of a defect in cellular membrane function. Grey, et al. (J. Clin. Invest. 65: 1478, 1980) have suggested that the erythrocytes of MyD patients have a decreased calcium-stimulated phosphatidic acid (PA) accumulation which, in turn, may reflect alterations in membrane properties which have been documented in MyD. This alteration in PA metabolism could be the result of a defect in the calcium-stimulated hydrolysis of the polyphosphoinositols (calcium-dependent phosphodiesterase) or in the subsequent formation of PA from its precursors (diglyceride kinase). In vitro assays were established for both enzymes in erythrocyte membranes (ghosts) prepared from MyDs and normal controls.

Calcium-dependent phosphodiesterase activity has been assayed with both endogenously labelled erythrocyte $[^{32}P]$-diphosphoinositol (DPI) and $[^{32}P]$-triphosphoinositol (TPI) and with the same phospholipids isolated from rat brain. In the presence of 0.5 mM calcium, radioactivity associated with erythrocyte $[^{32}P]$-DPI and $[^{32}P]$-TPI decreased by 50% and 70% respectively in comparison to membranes incubated in the absence of calcium. In contrast, when assayed with isolated rat brain DPI and TPI, maximum activity occurred at 0.3 µM free Ca^{2+} and activity was inhibited by >300 µM. It was not calmodulin sensitive. No differences in enzyme activity were found between MyDs and normal controls.

Diglyceride kinase activity was assayed by measuring the incorporation of $[^{32}P]$ from $[\gamma-^{32}P]$-ATP into either 1,2 diolein or 1,2 dipalmitin. The assay conditions were consistent with previous studies of the enzyme, being dependent on [ATP] and $[Mg^{2+}]$, although our ghost preparations were inhibited by EGTA (2.5 mM). Calcium restores the original level of activity but does not stimulate the kinase. No differences in activity were found between ghosts prepared from MyDs and normal controls.

Our results do not support an alteration in PA accumulation accounted for by differences in the membrane associated enzymes of PA metabolism.

Subject Index

Acetylcholine (ACh)
  in choline, 142, 143
  in PC, 155
  in phosphatidylcholine biosynthesis, 148
  in phosphoinositides, 254, 259–262
  phospholipid metabolism in, 359
  in Pi, 259, 261
  PS in, 168–171
  in torpedo electric organ, 353
Acyl-CoA, metabolism of, 118–119
l-Acyl-sn-glycero-3-phosphoryl-choline, 66, 67
Acylation of phospholipids, 63–73
Acylation-reacylation cycle, 8
Acylglycerol-3-phosphate, 51
Acyltransferases, in fatty acid uptake, 85
S-Adenosylmethionine (SAM)
  in interconversion, 3, 4, 6, 7
  in membrane fluidity, 24
  in PC, 157
Adrenate, arachidonate metabolism compared
    with, 334
β-Adrenergic-receptor-adenylate cyclase complex,
    22
Aging, lipid metabolism in, 106–107
l-Alkenyl-2-acyl-glycerophospholipids, 211
Alkenylglycerol, 8
γ-Aminobutyric acid (GABA)
  in cerebral cortex, distribution of, 351
  in epilepsy, 160
  in Huntington's chorea, 160
  in Parkinson's disease, 160
  in PC biosynthesis, 160–162
  in phosphatidylserine, 355
  in PS, 178
Arachidonate
  in acute hypoxia, 116–117, 120
  adrenate metabolism compared with, 334
  CDPamines in, 131
  ischemia and, 131
  in ischemic brain, 125
  in phosphatidylcholine, 114
  in phosphatidylinositol, 114
  in phospholipid labeling, 310
  release of, 80–81
  synaptosomal phospholipid uptake of, 114
Arachidonic acid
  3-DZA in, 26

  in epilepsy, 337
  in GPC, 75
  in GPI, 75
  in mouse brain, 338
Arachidonoyl-GPI, turnover of, 76
Arachidonoyl groups, turnover of, 75–86
Astroglia, plasmalogenase in, 212–213
Atropine
  FFA and, 84
  Na in, 255–258
  in PC formation, 151, 153
  in phosphoinosites, 262
  in Pi, 259, 261
Axonal smooth endoplasmic reticulum, 231
Axonal transport
  pathways for, 232
  of phospholipids to nerve endings, 231–235
  study of, 235
Axons
  distribution of labeled lipids formed in,
    224–225
  radioactive choline released from, 234
Axoplasm
  distribution of labeled lipids formed in,
    224–225
  ganglia compared with, 226
  synaptosomes compared with, 226

Base exchange enzymes
  phospholipase D and, 13–19
  topographic localization of, 19
Bicuculline
  in epileptiform seizures, 318
  FFA in, 80–82
  in GABA binding, 161, 162
  lysophospholipids in, 82–83
Brain cells, phospholipids of, 201
Brain cellular membranes, lipid modifications in,
    339
Brain cholinergic mechanisms, 165–171
Brain membranes
  asymmetry of, 37–46
  cholesterol in, 368
  fatty acids in, 111–121
Brain tissue, lipid turnover of, 105–109
Bromocriptine, in ACh, 169

371